P9-DBW-070

THOMSON DELMAR LEARNING'S
CASE STUDY SERIES

Medical-Surgical
Nursing

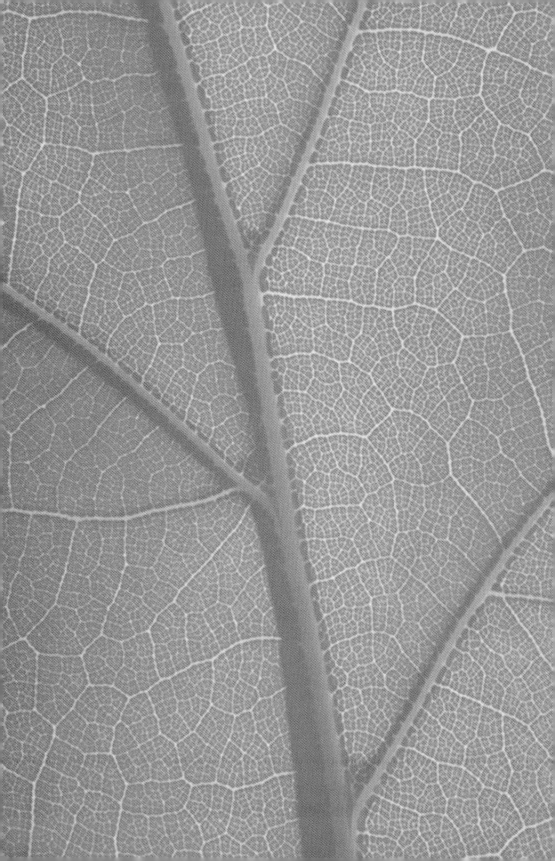

THOMSON DELMAR LEARNING'S
CASE STUDY SERIES

Medical-Surgical Nursing

Gina M. Ankner

RN, APRN, BC

THOMSON

DELMAR LEARNING

Australia   Canada   Mexico   Singapore   Spain   United Kingdom   United States

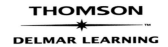

THOMSON
DELMAR LEARNING

Thomson Delmar Learning's Case Study Series: Medical-Surgical Nursing
by Gina M. Ankner, RN, APRN, BC

**Vice President,
Health Care Business Unit:**
William Brottmiller

Director of Learning Solutions:
Matthew Kane

Managing Editor:
Marah Bellegarde

Acquisitions Editor:
Tamara Caruso

Marketing Director:
Jennifer McAvery

Marketing Manager:
Michele McTighe

Technology Director:
Laurie Davis

Editorial Assistant:
Jennifer Waters

Production Director:
Carolyn Miller

Content Project Manager:
Anne Sherman

Art Director:
Jack Pendleton

COPYRIGHT © 2008 Thomson Delmar Learning, a part of the Thomson Corporation. Thomson, the Star logo, and Delmar Learning are trademarks used herein under license.

Printed in the United States
1 2 3 4 5 6 7 8 XXX 11 10 09 08 07

For more information, contact Thomson Delmar Learning, 5 Maxwell Drive, Clifton Park, NY 12065.
Or, find us on the World Wide Web at http://www.delmarlearning.com

ALL RIGHTS RESERVED. No part of this work covered by the copyright hereon may be reproduced or used in any form or by any means— graphic, electronic, or mechanical, including photocopying, recording, taping, Web distribution or informa- tion storage and retrieval systems— without the written permission of the publisher.

For permission to use material from this text or product, contact us by Tel (800) 730-2214
Fax (800) 730-2215

www.thomsonrights.com

Library of Congress Cataloging-in- Publication Data

Ankner, Gina M.
  Medical-surgical nursing / Gina M. Ankner.
    p. ; cm. —
  (Thomson Delmar Learning's case study series)
  Includes bibliographical references and index.
  ISBN 978-1-4180-4087-1 (alk. paper)
  1. Nursing—Case studies. I. Title. II. Series.
    [DNLM: 1. Nursing Care—Case Reports. 2. Nursing Care—Problems and Exercises. 3. Perioperative Nursing—Case Reports.
  4. Perioperative Nursing—Problems and Exercises. WY 18.2 A611m 2008]

RT81.6.A553 2008
610.73—dc22
                          2007036084

Notice to the Reader

Publisher does not warrant or guarantee any of the products described herein or perform any independent analysis in connection with any of the product information contained herein. Publisher does not assume, and expressly disclaims, any obligation to obtain and include information other than that provided to it by the manufacturer.

The reader is expressly warned to consider and adopt all safety precautions that might be indicated by the activities described herein and to avoid all potential hazards. By following the instructions contained herein, the reader willingly assumes all risks in connection with such instructions.

The publisher makes no representations or warranties of any kind, including but not limited to, the warranties of fitness for particular purpose or merchantability, nor are any such representations implied with respect to the material set forth herein, and the publisher takes no responsibility with respect to such material. The publisher shall not be liable for any special, consequential, or exemplary damages resulting, in whole or part, from the readers' use of, or reliance upon, this material.

Contents

Reviewers   vii

Preface   ix

Cases by Topic   xiv

Comprehensive Table of Variables   xv

Part 1   **The Digestive System** **1**

Case Study **1** *Mrs. Kenton*   3

Part 2   **The Urinary System** **13**

Case Study **1** *Mrs. Reese*   15

Case Study **2** *Mr. Rossi*   25

Part 3   **The Respiratory System** **37**

Case Study **1** *Mr. Yang*   39

Case Study **2** *Mrs. Harriet*   51

Part 4   **The Cardiovascular System & the Blood** **71**

Case Study **1** *Mr. Cowen*   73

Case Study **2** *Mr. McCann*   85

Part 5   **The Musculoskeletal System** **101**

Case Study **1** *Mrs. DiCenzo*   103

Case Study **2** *Mrs. Bagnell*   117

Case Study **3** *Mr. Rodriquez*   127

Part 6   **The Integumentary System** **139**

Case Study **1** *Mr. Shannon*   141

Case Study **2** *Ms. Champlin*   151

Part 7   **The Nervous/Neurological System** **165**

Case Study   **1**   *Derek*   167

Case Study   **2**   *Mrs. Kahn*   179

Part 8   **The Endocrine/Metabolic System** **195**

Case Study   **1**   *Mrs. Duarte*   197

Case Study   **2**   *Mr. Kiley*   209

Part 9   **The Reproductive System** **219**

Case Study   **1**   *Ms. Swan*   221

Case Study   **2**   *Mr. Benjamin*   235

Case Study   **3**   *Ms. Dalton*   249

Part 10   **The Hepatobiliary System** **259**

Case Study   **1**   *Mr. Escobar*   261

Index **275**

Reviewers

Patricia N. Allen, MSN, APRN-BC
Clinical Assistant Professor
Indiana University School of Nursing
Bloomington, Indiana

Bonita E. Broyles, RN, BSN, PhD
Associate Degree Nursing Faculty
Piedmont Community College
Roxboro, North Carolina

Joyce Campbell, MSN, APRN, BC, CCRN
Associate Professor
Chattanooga State Technical Community College
Chattanooga, Tennessee

Marianne Curia, MSN, RN
Assistant Professor
University of St. Francis
Joliet, Illinois

Karen K. Gerbasich, RN, MSN
Faculty Assistant Professor
Ivy Tech Community College
South Bend, Indiana

Amanda M. Reynolds, MSN
Associate Professor
Grambling State University
Grambling, Louisiana

Preface

Delmar Learning's Case Studies Series was created to encourage nurses to bridge the gap between content knowledge and clinical application. The products within the series represent the most innovative and comprehensive approach to nursing case studies ever developed. Each title has been authored by experienced nurse educators and clinicians who understand the complexity of nursing practice, as well as the challenges of teaching and learning. All the cases are based on real-life clinical scenarios and demand thought and "action" from the nurse. Each case brings the user into the clinical setting and invites her to utilize the nursing process while considering all the variables that influence the client's condition and the care to be provided. Each case also represents a unique set of variables, to offer a breadth of learning experiences and to capture the reality of nursing practice. To gauge the progression of a user's knowledge and critical thinking ability, the cases have been categorized by difficulty level. Every section begins with basic cases and proceeds to more advanced scenarios, thereby presenting opportunities for learning and practice for both students and professionals.

All the cases have been reviewed by experts to ensure that as many variables as possible are represented in a truly realistic manner and that each case reflects consistency with realities of modern nursing practice.

Praise for Delmar Learning's Case Study Series

"[This text's] strength is the large variety of case studies—it seemed to be all inclusive. Another strength is the extensiveness built into each case study. You can almost see this person as they enter the ED because of the descriptions that are given."

—MARY BETH KIEFNER, R.N., M.S., Nursing Program Director/Nursing Faculty, Illinois Central College

"The cases . . . reflect the complexity of nursing practice. They are an excellent way to refine critical-thinking skills."

—DARLA R. URA, MA, RN, APRN, BC,
Clinical Associate Professor, Adult and Elder
Health Department, School of Nursing,
Emory University

"The case studies are very comprehensive and allow the undergraduate student an opportunity to apply knowledge gained in the classroom to a potentially real clinical situation."

—TAMELLA LIVENGOOD, APRN, BC, MSN, FNP,
Nursing Faculty, Northwestern Michigan College

"These cases and how you have approached them definitely stimulate the students to use critical-thinking skills. I thought the questions asked really pushed the students to think deeply and thoroughly."

—JOANNE SOLCHANY, PhD, ARNP, RN, CS,
Assistant Professor, Family & Child Nursing,
University of Washington, Seattle

"The use of case studies is pedagogically sound and very appealing to students and instructors. I think that some instructors avoid them because of the challenge of case development. You have provided the material for them."

—NANCY L. OLDENBURG, RN, MS, CPNP,
Clinical Instructor, Northern Illinois University

"[The author] has done an excellent job of assisting students to engage in critical thinking. I am very impressed with the cases, questions, and content. I rarely ask that students buy more than one . . . book . . . but, in this instance, I can't wait until this book is published."

—DEBORAH J. PERSELL, MSN, RN, CPNP,
Assistant Professor, Arkansas State University

"This is a groundbreaking book. . . . This book should be a required text for all undergraduate and graduate nursing programs and should be well-received by faculty."

—JANE H. BARNSTEINER, PhD, RN, FAAN,
Professor of Pediatric Nursing, University of
Pennsylvania School of Nursing

How to Use This Book

Every case begins with a table of variables that is encountered in practice, and that must be understood by the nurse in order to provide appropriate care to the client. Categories of variables include age, gender, setting, culture, ethnicity, cultural considerations, preexisting conditions, coexisting conditions, communication considerations, disability considerations, socioeconomic considerations, spiritual considerations, pharmacological considerations, legal considerations, ethical considerations, alternative therapy, prioritization considerations, and delegation considerations. If a case involves a variable that is considered to have a significant impact on care, the specific variable is included in the table. This allows the user an "at a glance" view of the issues that will need to be considered to provide care to the client in the scenario. The table of variables is followed by a presentation of the case, including the history of the client, current condition, clinical setting, and professionals involved. A series of questions follows each case that require the user to consider how she would handle the issues presented within the scenario. Suggested answers and rationales are provided for remediation and discussion.

Organization

Cases are grouped according to body system. Within each part, cases are organized by difficulty level from easy, to moderate, to difficult. This classification is somewhat subjective, but it is based upon a developed standard. In general, the difficulty level has been determined by the number of variables that impact the case and the complexity of the client's condition. Colored tabs are used to allow the user to distinguish the difficulty levels more easily. A comprehensive table of variables is also provided for reference to allow the user to quickly select cases containing a particular variable of care.

While every effort has been made to group cases into the most applicable body system, the scope of many of the cases may include more than one body system. In such instances, the case will still only appear in the section for one of the body systems addressed. The cases are fictitious; however, they are based on actual problems and/or situations the nurse will encounter. Any resemblance to actual cases or individuals is coincidental.

Also Available:

Clinical Decision Making: Case Studies in Medical-Surgical Nursing by Gina M. Ankner 1-4018-4085-1 (978-1-4018-4085-1)

An additional 40 case studies based on real-life clinical scenarios that demand thought and action from the nurse.

Also visit www.delmarhealthcare.com for more information on other titles in the Thomson Delmar Learning Nursing Case Study series!

Acknowledgments

Foremost, I would like to thank Libby Howe and Andrea Clemente, my Product Managers, whose guidance, encouragement, and support throughout the duration of this project is beyond measure. I am grateful to the hardworking team of Libby, Andrea, Matt Kane, Director of Learning Solutions, and Tamara Caruso, Acquisitions Editor, for the opportunity to be involved in the Case Study Series. Many thanks to those individuals who willingly shared their personal stories so future nurses could learn from them. The input from students, friends, and family was invaluable, especially the generosity of Kimberly Dodd, MD, and Kathleen Elliott, APRN, BC, whose contributions and support exemplify friendship and professional collaboration. With great appreciation, I wish to acknowledge the reviewers for the constructive comments and suggestions that helped to enhance the educational value of each case.

About the Author

Gina M. Ankner, RN, APRN, BC, earned her bachelors and masters degrees in nursing from Boston College. She began her nursing career on a cardiac telemetry unit working as a collegiate nurse intern while earning her bachelors degree and as a registered nurse for several years. In 1995, she was a research coordinator in the department of maternal-fetal medicine at Women & Infants' Hospital of Rhode Island where she currently works per diem in women's primary care. In 1997 she joined the College of Nursing faculty at the University of Massachusetts Dartmouth.

She has presented in a variety of venues on topics related to college health and the use of date rape and recreational drugs. Most recently, Gina presented a series of workshops in Southeastern Massachusetts titled The Clinical Nurse Instructor Role: Charting a Course for Success. Sponsored by a Nursing Career Ladder Initiative (NUCLI) grant, the workshops provided an understanding of the role of a clinical instructor and strategies for success. She is the principal lecturer, a clinical instructor, and the course and lab coordinator for the fundamentals of nursing course. Her teaching responsibilities also include clinical instruction in medical-surgical nursing.

Note from the Author

My students are the inspiration for this book. With rare exception, each case study is based on a client that a student has cared for. Through the student's eyes, I share stories of men and women who have turned to their nurses for care and support during their illness. Perhaps when reading a scenario, you will think, "It would not happen like that." Please know that it did and that it will. The most enjoyable part of writing each case was the realization that another nursing student will learn from the experience of a peer. The intent was not only to provide the more common patient scenarios, but also to present actual cases that encourage critical thinking and prompt a student to ask "what if?"

The wonderful thing about a case study is that the possibilities for learning abound! These cases provide a foundation upon which endless knowledge can be built. So feel free to be creative—change a client's gender, age, or ethnicity, and pose new questions. Most importantly, enjoy the journey of becoming a better nurse.

The author welcomes comments via e-mail at MedSurgCases@ yahoo.com.

Cases by Topic

Case #	Case Topic
CSS 1-1	Achalasia
CSS 2-1	Acute Pyelonephritis
CSS 2-2	End Stage Renal Disease
CSS 3-1	Hemothorax
CSS 3-2	Pneumonia
CSS 4-1	Hypertension
CSS 4-2	Chronic Lymphocytic Leukemia
CSS 5-1	Rheumatoid Arthritis
CSS 5-2	Lyme Disease
CSS 5-3	Spinal Cord Injury
CSS 6-1	Cellulitis
CSS 6-2	Burn
CSS 7-1	Meningitis
CSS 7-2	Cerebrovascular Accident
CSS 8-1	Graves' Disease
CSS 8-2	Hypoglycemia
CSS 9-1	Genital Herpes
CSS 9-2	Benign Prostatic Hypertrophy
CSS 9-3	Human Papillomavirus
CSS 10-1	Hepatic Encephalopathy

Comprehensive Table of Variables

CASE STUDY	AGE	SETTING	ETHNICITY	CULTURE	PREEXISTING CONDITIONS	COEXISTING CONDITIONS	COMMUNICATION	DISABILITY	SOCIOECONOMIC STATUS	SPIRITUALITY	PHARMACOLOGIC	LEGAL	ETHICAL	ALTERNATIVE THERAPY	PRIORITIZATION	DELEGATION
Part One: The Digestive System																
1	30	Primary care	White American			X					X	X				
Part Two: The Urinary System																
1	27	Hospital	White American		X	X			X	X	X			X		
2	58	Home	White American		X	X			X		X					
Part Three: The Respiratory System																
1	90	Hospital	Hmong	Language barrier; appropriate greetings; eye contact; touch	X	X	X		X			X	X		X	X
2	68	Hospital	Black American		X				X		X				X	X
Part Four: The Cardiovascular System & the Blood																
1	50	Primary care	Black American		X				X						X	X
2	60	Hospital	White American		X	X			X		X					
Part Five: The Musculoskeletal System																
1	59	Primary care	Italian American					X			X			X	X	X
2	36	Hospital	White American						X		X				X	X
3	23	Home	Hispanic	Injury resulting from act of violence				X	X							X

Part / #	Age	Setting	Ethnicity	Additional variable	1	2	3	4	5	6	7	8	9	10
Part Six: The Integumentary System														
1	80	Hospital	Irish American		X				X		X			X
2	52	Hospital	White American		X			X			X		X	
Part Seven: The Nervous/Neurological System														
1	21	Hospital	White American				X	X	X		X	X		X
2	88	Hospital	Arab American	Health care provider gender preference	X	X	X		X	X	X	X		X
Part Eight: The Endocrine/Metabolic System														
1	40	Primary care	White American			X			X		X			
2	33	Hospital	Black American		X	X			X		X		X	
Part Nine: The Reproductive System														
1	19	Walk-in	Black American		X			X		X	X	X	X	X
2	70	Primary care	White American								X	X	X	
3	25	GYN primary care	White American		X	X	X		X		X		X	
Part Ten: The Hepatobiliary System														
1	47	Hospital	Black American		X	X		X	X		X			

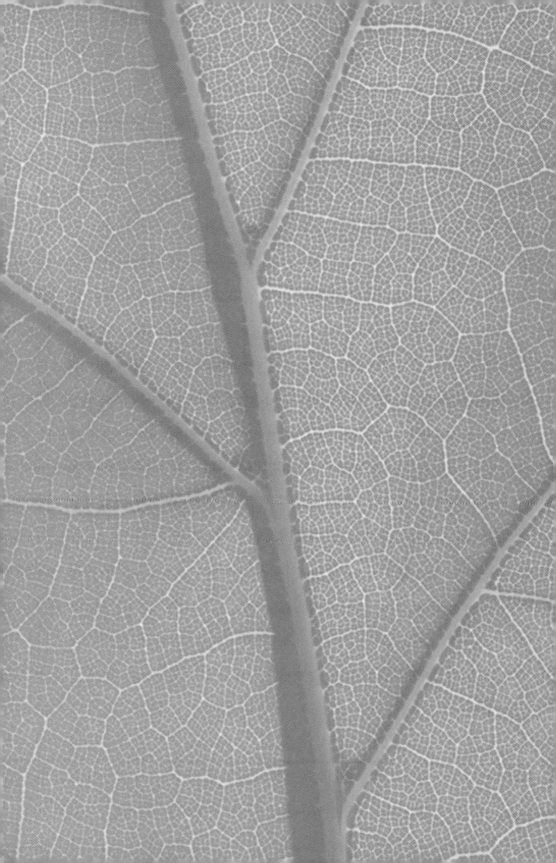

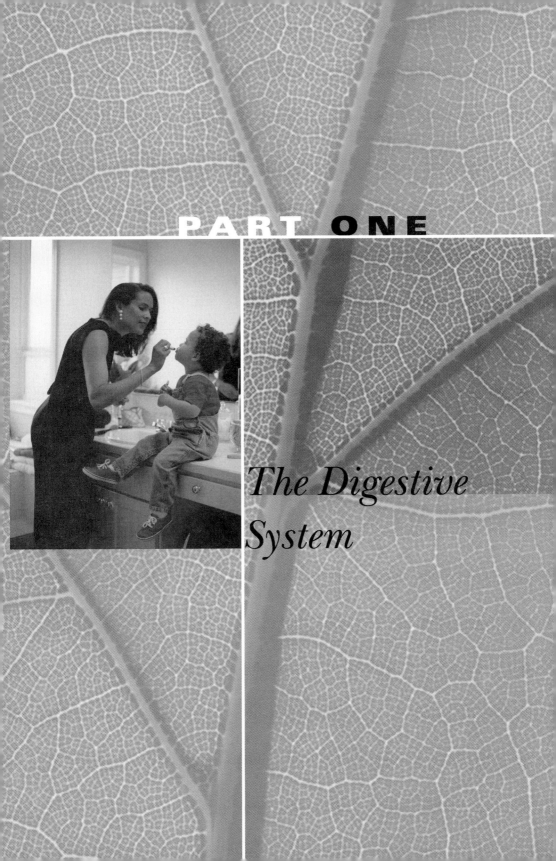

PART ONE

The Digestive
System

CASE STUDY 1

Mrs. Kenton

GENDER

Female

AGE

30

SETTING

- Primary Care

ETHNICITY

- White American

CULTURAL CONSIDERATIONS

PREEXISTING CONDITION

COEXISTING CONDITION

- Dysphagia, gastroesophageal reflux disease (GERD)

COMMUNICATION

DISABILITY

SOCIOECONOMIC

SPIRITUAL/RELIGIOUS

PHARMACOLOGIC

- Nifedipine (Procardia XL); verapamil (Calan); isosorbide dinitrate (Isordil); sublingual nitroglycerin (Nitrostat); botulinum toxin, type A (Botox); metoclopramide (Reglan)

LEGAL

- Informed consent

ETHICAL

ALTERNATIVE THERAPY

PRIORITIZATION

DELEGATION

THE DIGESTIVE SYSTEM

Level of Difficulty: Difficult

Overview: This case presents a woman diagnosed with achalasia. The potential implications of this motility disorder on a client's health maintenance and the treatment options to offer symptom relief are discussed. The differential diagnosis of scleroderma is considered, and diagnostic tests are explained. The indication for medication therapy prescribed postoperatively is reviewed. Nursing diagnoses appropriate for this client are prioritized.

DIFFICULT

3

Client Profile

Mrs. Kenton is a 30-year-old woman who is at her annual physical exam appointment with her primary health care provider (HCP). The HCP comments that Mrs. Kenton has lost weight since last year. She replies, "I'm not surprised. For the past four or five months, I have had a hard time swallowing certain foods and I get bad heartburn. I eat. But my diet has definitely changed. I can't eat certain foods. My husband says I eat like a bird, taking little bites at a time."

Case Study

Further assessment reveals that Mrs. Kenton has a difficult time swallowing what she refers to as "bulky or solid foods, like bread, pasta, and grapes." She states, "If I eat these foods, I have to take large sips of room temperature water and swallow very hard to push the food down my throat. Then the food just feels like it is sitting at the top of my stomach. It is very uncomfortable. I don't go anywhere without my bottled water. I am afraid I will choke." Mrs. Kenton denies that anyone else in her family has a similar problem and is unaware of anyone in her family who has been diagnosed with symptoms of scleroderma. The HCP refers her to a gastrointestinal specialist. The following diagnostic tests are prescribed: endoscopy, barium swallow, esophageal manometry, and serum antinuclear antibody (ANA) testing.

Results of the diagnostic tests conclude that Mrs. Kenton has moderately severe achalasia, and she is scheduled for a laproscopic esophagomyotomy with fundoplication.

Questions

1. The HCP considered the differential diagnosis of scleroderma. Discuss the pathophysiology of this disease. How are the clinical manifestations of scleroderma similar to the symptoms Mrs. Kenton described?

2. Provide Mrs. Kenton with a brief explanation of each of the diagnostic tests prescribed: endoscopy, barium swallow, esophageal manometry, and serum antinuclear antibody testing. Which tests require informed consent and for which procedures must Mrs. Kenton have nothing by mouth (NPO) for a minimum of eight hours beforehand?

3. Scleroderma has been ruled out and Mrs. Kenton is diagnosed with achalasia. Discuss the pathophysiology of this disorder, characteristic clinical manifestations, potential complications, and incidence.

4. What are five additional assessment findings that should be considered to gain a more thorough understanding of the severity of Mrs. Kenton's achalasia?

5. Identify three nursing diagnoses for the client with achalasia. List the diagnoses in priority order.

Questions (continued)

6. Mild cases of achalasia are treated with medication, diet therapy, and changes in position. Discuss these treatment recommendations.

7. Mrs. Kenton has been diagnosed with a moderately severe form of achalasia and will require surgical intervention. Discuss the traditional esophageal dilation procedure and the esophagomyotomy procedure. What are the risks and benefits of each procedure?

8. Mrs. Kenton has a laproscopic esophagomyotomy with fundoplication. At the follow-up appointment with her surgeon, she complains of nausea when she eats. "It is almost like my stomach got used to eating small meals. Now that I am trying to eat normally again, I feel too full and sick to my stomach." The surgeon would like Mrs. Kenton to take metoclopramide for a few weeks. Discuss how this medication works, suggested length of therapy, and common adverse effects, and provide the client with reminders about the most effective administration of the medication.

Questions and Suggested Answers

1. The HCP considered the differential diagnosis of scleroderma. Discuss the pathophysiology of this disease. How are the clinical manifestations of scleroderma similar to the symptoms Mrs. Kenton described? Progressive systemic sclerosis (PSS) is a generalized systemic disease more commonly referred to as systemic scleroderma. The term "scleroderma" means hardening of the skin, which is one of the clinical manifestations of PSS. Clients with only skin involvement have localized scleroderma. Skin thickening is visible on the trunk, face, neck, proximal, and distal extremities. Clients are described as having CREST syndrome: *C*alcinosis (calcium deposits), *R*aynaud's phenomenon, *E*sophageal dysmotility, *S*clerodactyly (scleroderma of the digits), and *T*elangiectasia (spiderlike hemangiomas). Clients with systemic sclerosis have a chronic connective tissue disease that is characterized by inflammation, fibrosis, and sclerosis of the skin and vital organs. Microvascular damage and fibrous degeneration of tissue and excess collagen cause fibrosis and malfunction of the involved organ(s). Major organ damage is likely to develop with diffuse scleroderma, specifically affecting the gastrointestinal tract, cardiovascular system, pulmonary system, and renal system. Respiratory involvement and hypertension are common and renal involvement is the leading cause of death (Ignatavicius & Matzko, 2006; Marek, 2007).

Women are affected with PSS three to four times more often than men. The onset of the disease is usually seen in individuals between 30- and 50 years old. Clinical characteristics of PSS that are similar to Mrs. Kenton's case include involvement of the gastrointestinal (GI) tract, particularly the esophagus. In the client with scleroderma, the esophagus loses its motility, resulting in dysphagia and gastroesophageal reflux disease (GERD). A small hiatal hernia may be present, and swallowing may be difficult. Peristalsis is impaired and reflux of the gastric contents can cause esophagitis and may lead to ulceration (Ignatavicius & Matzko, 2006). The commonalities between the client population affected by PSS, clinical manifestations, and Mrs. Kenton's reported symptoms warrant consideration of scleroderma as a differential diagnosis to be ruled out in this case.

2. Provide Mrs. Kenton with a brief explanation of each of the diagnostic tests prescribed: endoscopy, barium swallow, esophageal manometry, and serum antinuclear antibody testing. Which tests require informed consent and for which procedures must Mrs. Kenton have nothing by mouth (NPO) for a minimum of eight hours beforehand? An *endoscopy* introduces a flexible fiberoptic tube with a light and camera on the end (endoscope) into the client's esophagus. Clients with achalasia usually have resistance as the endoscope is passed from the esophagus into the stomach because of the high pressure in the lower esophageal sphincter. This test is helpful in diagnosing achalasia and is prescribed to evaluate the appearance of the esophageal mucosa, assess for dilation of the esophagus, note a lack of peristaltic waves and assess for changes associated with cancer or Candida. Findings, however, may be within normal limits early in the disease (Daniels, 2002; Sands, 2007; Visovsky, 2006).

A *barium swallow* is an X-ray study in which X-rays of the esophagus are taken after the client swallows barium, which fills the esophagus. The passage of the barium into the stomach is assessed. This is the most sensitive test for visualizing the esophagus and can reveal esophageal dilation and narrowing at the terminal esophagus (sometimes referred to as a "rat tail" or "bird's beak" narrowing), which is a hallmark finding of the lower esophageal sphincter that fails to relax properly (Daniels, 2002; Sands, 2007; Visovsky, 2006).

An *esophageal manometry* demonstrates the specific abnormalities of muscle function. A thin tube that measures the pressure generated when the esophageal muscles contract is passed through the client's nose, down the back of the throat, and into the esophagus. This test is used to identify an increased lower esophageal sphincter pressure, incomplete sphincter relaxation when the client swallows, and diminished or absent peristaltic waves in the esophagus. An advantage of manometry is that it can diagnose achalasia in the early stages of the disease (Sands, 2007; Visovsky, 2006).

Antinuclear antibodies can be produced and act against the body's own DNA and nuclear material to cause tissue damage, such as in autoimmune disorders. *Serum ANA testing* is frequently positive in clients with connective tissue diseases such as scleroderma. This test is a fluorescent procedure that assists in differentiating among various connective tissue diseases. Results are reported as a titer. Higher values (greater than 1:320) are more likely to represent true-positive results. A positive result has a 97% sensitivity for scleroderma. If the ANA test is positive, the nuclear staining pattern of the antibodies detected may also be reported, which identifies the intracellular target of the ANA. For example, in a client with diffuse systemic scleroderma, the staining pattern is described as "nucleolar" and an "anticentromere" pattern is highly specific for CREST syndrome (Daniels, 2002; Lane & Gravel, 2002; Sands, 2007; Visovsky, 2006).

The endoscopy, barium swallow, and esophageal manometry require Mrs. Kenton's informed consent. She does not need to sign a consent form to have a blood sample drawn for ANA testing. Mrs. Kenton must remain NPO for at least eight hours prior to each of these diagnostic tests. She should be given instructions to remain NPO for at least eight hours prior to having her barium swallow, esophageal manometry, and ANA blood test; and for at least twelve hours prior to her endoscopy. The HCP may allow her to take medications with a small sip of water (Daniels, 2002).

3. Scleroderma has been ruled out and Mrs. Kenton is diagnosed with achalasia. Discuss the pathophysiology of this disorder, characteristic clinical manifestations, potential complications, and incidence. Achalasia is an esophageal motility disorder that is believed to be caused by a neuromuscular defect in the inner circular muscle layer of the esophagus and loss of the nerve impulses through the esophagus (called denervation), although the exact cause is unknown. The term achalasia means "failure to relax." In the person with achalasia, the lower esophageal sphincter (a ring of muscle between the lower esophagus and the stomach) fails to relax properly and in synchrony when the person swallows, and normal peristalsis of the esophagus is replaced with abnormal muscle contractions. The motility disorder of the esophagus may be a primary esophageal problem (achalasia) or secondary to another systemic disease (such as scleroderma). Achalasia is characterized by chronic and progressive dysphagia (difficulty swallowing). Because individuals usually learn to compensate for their dysphagia by taking smaller bites, eating more slowly, and altering their diet, symptoms may progress for months to a couple of years before the client seeks help. Over time, peristaltic failure and esophageal spasm results in a dilated esophagus. This further impairs the passage of food. Individuals may report epigastric pain and the sensation that food is stuck in their lower esophagus. The client often experiences the regurgitation of swallowed food, especially at night, which can cause coughing and aspiration. Left untreated, the progressive dysphagia results in weight loss. Achalasia is an uncommon disorder that is most often seen in men and women between the ages of 20 and 40 years old but also occurs in children and older adults.

There are no cultural differences in incidence. Approximately 5% to 10% of clients with achalasia develop esophageal squamous cell carcinoma. Other potential complications of untreated achalasia include esophageal candidiasis, lower esophageal diverticula, airway obstruction, and aspiration pneumonia. A genetic basis for the disorder has been considered since there have been cases of familial clustering (Marks & Lee, 2005; Sands, 2007; Visovsky, 2006).

4. What are five additional assessment findings that should be considered to gain a more thorough understanding of the severity of Mrs. Kenton's achalasia? Additional assessment findings to consider in Mrs. Kenton's case include:

- Variability of the dysphagia (intermittent or constant)
- Swallowing ability with liquids versus solids
- Regurgitation/reflux of solids, liquids, or both
- Chest pain (esophageal spasm is often intense and mimics angina)
- Factors that aggravate the symptoms (such as changes in position or changes in diet)
- Nutritional history (dietary habits, food tolerances, responses to foods of differing textures and temperatures)
- Baseline weight prior to symptoms and current weight
- Respiratory symptoms, lung sounds
- Halitosis (foul mouth odor) which is caused by the fermentation and regurgitation of previously ingested food
- History of previous esophageal surgery or trauma
- Treatments tried (medications, home remedies, changes in diet) and degree of success

(Sands, 2007; Visovsky, 2006).

5. Identify three nursing diagnoses for the client with achalasia. List the diagnoses in priority order. Nursing diagnoses for the client with achalasia, in suggested order of priority, include:

- Impaired swallowing related to (r/t) neuromuscular impairment
- Imbalanced nutrition: less than body requirements r/t inability to ingest food
- Acute pain r/t stasis of food in the esophagus
- Risk for aspiration r/t nocturnal regurgitation
- Risk for ineffective coping r/t chronic, progressive disease

(Ackley & Ladwig, 2006).

6. Mild cases of achalasia are treated with medication, diet therapy, and changes in position. Discuss these treatment recommendations. Mild cases of achalasia can be managed with medications to help reduce the lower esophageal sphincter pressure and provide symptom relief. Medications of choice are calcium channel blockers such as nifedipine and verapamil, or a nitrate such as isosorbide dinitrate or sublingual nitroglycerin. Although some clients with achalasia, particularly early in their disease, have improvement in their symptoms with oral medications, for most the relief is only short term. Another therapy option is the direct injection of botulinum toxin type A into the lower esophageal sphincter muscle via endoscopy. Botulinum toxin type A acts by suppressing acetylcholine release, which deprives the distal esophagus with an adequate cholinergic nerve supply by blocking the nerve connections (denervates) and weakens the lower sphincter. The positive effects of this toxin are not sustained however and symptoms often recur within six months. Antacids can provide relief of GERD symptoms, and analgesics may be needed to manage pain (Ignatavicius & Matzko, 2006; Sands, 2007; Visovsky, 2006).

The client should be encouraged to make changes to their diet in response to their symptoms. Diet modification is often effective in easing the pressure and reflux associated with achalasia. Foods that aggravate the symptoms should be avoided. Many clients with achalasia find that semisoft foods (such as mashed potatoes and pudding) and warm foods and liquids are better tolerated. A change in the frequency and size of meals is recommended. Eating four to six smaller meals rather than three large meals helps to facilitate the passage of food and digestive process. Cutting food into smaller pieces, chewing each bite carefully, and taking small amounts of fluid after each bite can ease swallowing (Ignatavicius & Matzko, 2006; Visovsky, 2006).

Changes in the client's position can help relieve symptoms. The client should experiment with different changes in position during and/or after meals to help reduce the sensation of a pressure in the gastrointestinal tract. Some clients have found relief by arching their back while swallowing. The nocturnal reflux of food and liquids into the laryngopharynx and oral cavity is caused by a dilated esophagus and is often prevented if the client sleeps in a semisitting position with the head of the bed elevated. Clients may raise the head of the bed by placing the legs of the bed frame on blocks or may find relief by sleeping in a reclining chair (Visovsky, 2006).

7. Mrs. Kenton has been diagnosed with a moderately severe form of achalasia and will require surgical intervention. Discuss the traditional esophageal dilation procedure and the esophagomyotomy procedure. What are the risks and benefits of each procedure? More severe cases of achalasia are treated with dilation of the lower esophageal sphincter. The traditional method of esophageal dilation is an ambulatory care (outpatient) procedure which involves the passage of progressively larger sizes of esophageal dilators (called bougies) using a catheter equipped with a polyurethane pneumatic balloon. Clients are sedated but awake during this interventional procedure. Most clients (60% to 90%) report an improvement in their swallowing and relief of symptoms. The dilation procedure may need to be repeated in two to three months to sustain its benefits. Large-diameter metal stents may be used for some clients to keep the lumen of the esophagus open for a longer duration.

An esophagomyotomy is a surgical procedure that involves the longitudinal incision (cutting) of the muscle fibers surrounding the lower esophageal sphincter that opens the sphincter and facilitates the passage of food by minimizing the obstruction. Open thoracic and abdominal approaches can be used, but laproscopic surgery has become more common. A success rate of 80% to 90% is reported, but this procedure does not guarantee a permanent cure. The most common and significant adverse effect of a reduction in pressure with an esophagomyotomy is reflux of acid (or GERD). In order to prevent this, a fundoplication may be part of the procedure. A fundoplication takes the portion of the stomach (the fundus) that is proximal to the entry of the esophagus and wraps and sutures the fundus around the lower end of the esophagus and lower esophageal sphincter. The gathering and suturing of one tissue to another is called "plication," which gives the procedure its name. The increased pressure at the lower end of the esophagus created by the placation reduces GERD.

The benefits of traditional esophageal dilation are that it is a less invasive procedure that requires a shorter recovery time. However, the effects of the procedure in relieving the client's symptoms may be short-term and require repeat interventions over the course of the client's lifetime.

The conventional esophagomyotomy is a more complex surgical procedure. When the thoracic or abdominal (open) approach is used, general anesthesia is required and the client must remain hospitalized during the first several days of recovery. Postoperative care of these clients includes managing chest tubes and drains, monitoring the healing of the surgical incision, pain management, and nasogastric feedings. A laproscopic esophagomyotomy is performed using conscious sedation rather than general anesthesia, which offers the benefit of a shorter length of stay and fewer complications as compared to the thoracic or abdominal approach. (Marks & Lee, 2005; Visovsky, 2006)

8. **Mrs. Kenton has a laproscopic esophagomyotomy with fundoplication. At the follow-up appointment with her surgeon, she complains of nausea when she eats. "It is almost like my stomach got used to eating small meals. Now that I am trying to eat normally again, I feel too full and sick to my**

stomach." The surgeon would like Mrs. Kenton to take metoclopramide for a few weeks. Discuss how this medication works, suggested length of therapy, and common adverse effects, and provide the client with reminders about the most effective administration of the medication. Metoclopramide is a GI stimulant. This dopamine antagonist acts by increasing sensitivity to acetylcholine, which increases the muscle tone of the lower esophagus sphincter and increases the motility of the upper GI tract. Gastric emptying time and GI transit time are shortened, which hastens the stomach emptying of solid and liquid meals into the intestines. Metoclopramide decreases stomach acid reflux by strengthening the lower esophagus sphincter. Metoclopramide interferes with the dopamine receptors in the brain. Since dopamine causes nausea, this medication can be an effective antiemetic. Metoclopramide is used on a short-term basis (two to eight weeks) to relieve nausea and other symptoms related to postoperative gastric stasis. Common adverse effects include restlessness, insomnia, sedation, depression, or anxiety. The sedative effect may not be felt for up to two hours after taking a dose. Mrs. Kenton should avoid driving or potentially dangerous activities until the medication effects are realized. Metoclopramide is usually given four times daily. It is very important that the medication be taken thirty minutes before each meal and at bedtime to maximize its therapeutic effect. Since metoclopramide accelerates stomach emptying, it can increase the absorption and effects of other medications. Mrs. Kenton should tell her surgeon if she is taking any other prescription or over-the-counter medications. As well, she should refrain from drinking alcohol while taking this medication since the sedative effects of alcohol can be accelerated when used together with metoclopramide (Spratto & Woods, 2006).

References

Ackley, B., & Ladwig, G. (2006). *Nursing diagnosis handbook: A guide to planning care*. St. Louis, MO: Mosby, Inc.

Daniels, R. (2002). *Delmar's guide to laboratory and diagnostic tests*. Albany, NY: Delmar.

Ignatavicius, D. D., & Matzko, C. K. (2006). Interventions for clients with connective tissue disease and other types of arthritis. In D. Ignatavicius & L. Workman (Eds.), *Medical-surgical nursing: Critical thinking for collaborative care* (pp. 412–413). St. Louis, MO: Elsevier Saunders.

Lane, S. K., & Gravel, J. W. (2002). Clinical utility of common serum rheumatologic tests. *American Family Physician, 65*(6), 1073–1080.

Marek, J. F. (2007). Degenerative disorders. In F. Monahan, J. Sands, M. Neighbors, J. Marek, & C. Green (Eds.), *Phipps' Medical-surgical nursing: Health and illness perspectives* (p. 1567). St. Louis, MO: Mosby Elsevier.

Marks, J. W., & Lee, D. (2005). *Achalasia*. Retrieved August 26, 2006 from www.medicinenet.com.

Sands, J. K. (2007). Mouth and esophagus problems. In F. Monahan, J. Sands, M. Neighbors, J. Marek, & C. Green (Eds.), *Phipps' Medical-surgical nursing: Health and illness perspectives* (pp. 1195–1198). St. Louis, MO: Mosby Elsevier.

Spratto, G. R., & Woods, A. L. (2006). *PDR nurse's drug handbook.* Clifton Park, NY: Thomson Delmar Learning.

Visovsky, C. (2006). Interventions for clients with esophageal problems. In D. Ignatavicius & L. Workman (Eds.), *Medical-surgical nursing: Critical thinking for collaborative care* (pp. 1273–1274). St. Louis, MO: Elsevier Saunders.

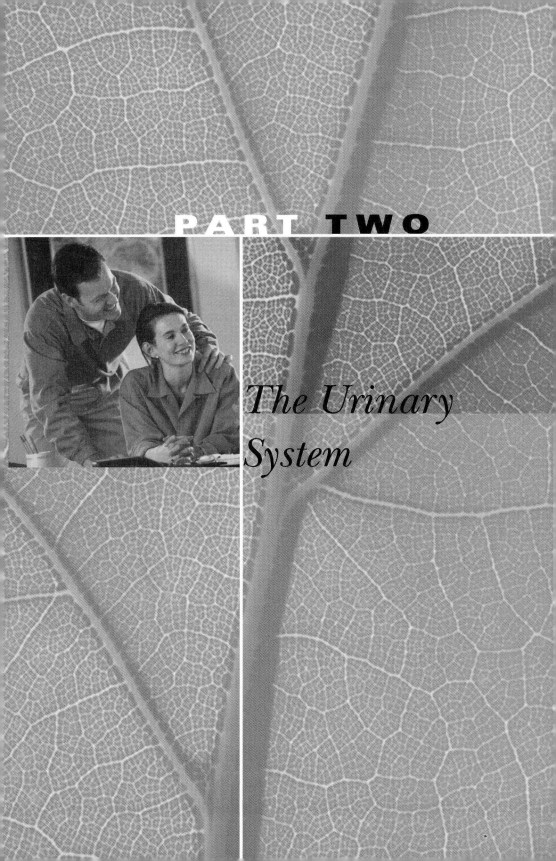

PART TWO

The Urinary System

Mrs. Reese

EASY

GENDER

Female

AGE

27

SETTING

- Hospital

ETHNICITY

- White American

CULTURAL CONSIDERATIONS

PREEXISTING CONDITION

- Urinary tract infection (UTI) three years ago

COEXISTING CONDITION

- Daily Ortho Tri-Cyclen

COMMUNICATION

DISABILITY

SOCIOECONOMIC

- Married; one daughter (12 months old)

SPIRITUAL/RELIGIOUS

PHARMACOLOGIC

- Ketorolac tromethamine (Toradol); ondansetron hydrochloride (Zofran); levofloxacin (Levaquin)

LEGAL

ETHICAL

ALTERNATIVE THERAPY

- Cranberry-based products to prevent UTIs

PRIORITIZATION

DELEGATION

THE URINARY SYSTEM

Level of Difficulty: Easy

Overview: The client in this case has been admitted with acute pyelonephritis. The pathophysiology and risk factors for developing this condition are reviewed. Characteristic clinical manifestations of acute pyelonephritis are discussed. A diagnostic X-ray of the kidneys, ureters, and bladder (KUB) with intravenous pyelography (IVP) is explained. Nursing diagnoses are prioritized, and a plan of care is initiated. Discharge teaching is provided regarding a prescribed antibiotic and prevention of future urinary tract infections.

Client Profile

Mrs. Reese is a 27-year-old woman who had a sudden onset of abdominal pain at 2:00 A.M. Upon arrival in the emergency department, she describes the pain as a constant ache in the lower right quadrant of her abdomen that radiates across the flank to her lower back. She rates her pain as a 9 out of 10 on a 0 to 10 pain scale. She also is complaining of nausea and has vomited three times prior to arrival. She is febrile and complaining of chills.

Case Study

Mrs. Reese's vital signs are blood pressure 118/60, pulse 108, respiratory rate 24, and temperature 104.1°F (40°C). Her oxygen saturation is 100% on room air. The nurse asks Mrs. Reese if she has noticed any recent changes in her voiding, such as burning, frequency, or feeling as if she is unable to empty her bladder completely. The nurse also asks Mrs. Reese if she has had a fever in the days prior to coming to the hospital. Mrs. Reese states, "Now that I think about it, I have been going to the bathroom more often than usual, and it smelled a little funny. The other day I noticed a dull pain in my lower back. I figured it was from picking up my daughter. Yesterday I remember thinking I felt warm, but my daughter was getting into something and I got distracted and never took my temperature."

Upon physical examination, Mrs. Reese's skin is warm, and her face is flushed. Her abdomen is slightly distended and tender on palpation. Her bowel sounds are hypoactive in all four quadrants. She is admitted with a suspected diagnosis of acute pyelonephritis. Mrs. Reese will be hospitalized for a few days. She expresses concern to the nurse stating, "I need to hurry up and get better. My husband works two jobs, and my parents can only stay at my house for a day or two to care for my daughter. I need to get home as soon as possible. My daughter needs me."

Intravenous (IV) fluids are prescribed as ½ normal saline (1/2 NS) at 100 mL per hour. Diagnostic tests include a complete blood count with differential (CBC with diff), comprehensive metabolic panel (CMP), urinalysis with culture and sensitivity (U/A C & S), X-ray of the kidneys, ureters, and bladder (KUB) with intravenous pyelography (IVP), and blood cultures × 2 sites. Medications prescribed include ketorolac tromethamine, ondansetron hydrochloride, and levofloxacin.

Results of the CBC include a white blood cell (WBC) count of 14,200 cells/mm^3. Her CMP results are all within normal limits. The urinalysis reveals the presence of a large amount of occult blood, protein 30 mg/dL, 6–10 WBCs/low power field (LPF), 21–30 red blood cells/LPF, 0–2 WBC casts/high power field, moderate mucous, and a moderate amount of bacteria. The urine culture and sensitivity is positive for *Escherichia coli (E. coli)* bacteria. The KUB with IVP shows normal urinary structures without the presence of stones or obstructions.

Questions

1. While in the emergency department, the nurse asks Mrs. Reese if she has noticed any recent changes in her voiding or a fever in the days prior to hospitalization. Explain how the assessment data relates to Mrs. Reese's admitting diagnosis.

2. Women are more likely to experience a UTI up until the age of 50 years, when the risk is similar in both genders. Briefly explain why women are at an increased risk and why older men experience more UTIs than younger men do.

3. Briefly discuss the pathophysiology of acute pyelonephritis and identify the most common organism causing this infection.

4. Identify the risk factors that placed Mrs. Reese at greater risk for the development of acute pyelonephritis.

5. What are the characteristic clinical manifestations of pyelonephritis?

6. Mrs. Reese has a KUB with IVP. Explain this diagnostic test. How do the results help the heath care provider (HCP) to confirm the admitting diagnosis?

7. Mrs. Reese has no known allergies. She has been prescribed the following medications, ketorolac tromethamine, ondansetron hydrochloride, and levofloxacin. Provide a rationale for why each medication has been included as part of her medical management and any potential contraindication(s) of her taking these medications.

8. The nurse is designing Mrs. Reese's plan of care. Identify three priority nursing diagnoses for inclusion in the plan.

9. The nurse places highest priority on the nursing diagnosis acute pain r/t inflammation and irritation of urinary tract. State an outcome goal appropriate for Mrs. Reese and at least two nursing interventions to help achieve the goal.

10. Two days later, Mrs. Reese is afebrile and her nausea and vomiting have resolved. She is being discharged on an oral antibiotic. Provide the client with education about her prescribed antibiotic and symptoms that warrant notification of her HCP.

11. While the nurse is discontinuing the IV access, Mrs. Reese asks, "My doctor said that there is a chance I could get sick with this infection again. Is there anything I can do to help prevent that?" Offer Mrs. Reese at least five health promotion behaviors to help prevent a UTI and recurrent acute pyelonephritis.

12. Mrs. Reese asks the nurse, "I heard if you drink cranberry juice it can cure a urinary tract infection. Is that true?" How will the nurse respond and what are three other complimentary therapies that the nurse might suggest?

Questions and Suggested Answers

1. While in the emergency department, the nurse asks Mrs. Reese if she has noticed any recent changes in her voiding or a fever in the days prior to hospitalization. Explain how the assessment data relates to Mrs. Reese's admitting diagnosis. The kidneys are susceptible to inflammation caused by bacterial infections in the lower urinary drainage system. UTIs are among the most common bacterial infections. A lower UTI produces altered function at the site of the disease, affecting the bladder (called cystitis) or urethra (urethritis) in women. An infection within the lower urinary tract, especially when left untreated, can spread upward producing altered function in the kidney (pyelonephritis). A UTI alone does not lead to decreased kidney function. However, repeated UTIs (which can cause scar tissue) and complicated UTIs (following invasive urinary procedures) can cause acute pyelonephritis, sepsis, and subsequent kidney failure. To determine if Mrs. Reese had developed a UTI in the days prior to her admission, the nurse assesses for the common clinical manifestations of a UTI. Common manifestations of a UTI include urinary frequency (voiding more often than every two hours), urgency, dysuria (burning), incomplete emptying, cloudy or foul smelling urine, vaginal itching, suprapubic or lower back discomfort, hematuria (blood-tinged urine), fever, and chills (Potter, Weigel, & Green, 2007; Winkelman, 2006).

2. Women are more likely to experience a UTI up until the age of 50 years, when the risk is similar in both genders. Briefly explain why women are at an increased risk and why older men experience more UTIs than younger men do. UTIs occur more frequently in women than in men until after the age of 50 when the incidence in men and women is similar. Women are more likely to develop UTIs than men because of the female anatomy. The female urethra is shorter and closer to the rectum, which increases the chance of bacteria being introduced into the urinary tract from the vagina and rectal area. Men over the age of 50 are at greater risk of developing a UTI because of a natural decrease in prostatic fluid, which contains zinc, an antibacterial agent that provides younger men with protection against UTIs (Potter, Weigel, & Green, 2007).

3. Briefly discuss the pathophysiology of acute pyelonephritis and identify the most common organism causing this infection. Acute pyelonephritis is an active bacterial infection of the upper urinary tract. The infection begins as a lower UTI where the bacteria reach the bladder through the urethra and ascend upward affecting the renal pelvis, tubules, and interstitial tissue of one or both kidneys. Bacteria trigger an inflammatory response, resulting in acute interstitial inflammation, tubular cell necrosis, and possible abscess formation. The kidney becomes inflamed with multiple abscesses (pockets of localized infection) on its surface and within the renal pelvis. The client with a lower UTI may be asymptomatic and the clinical manifestations of kidney involvement may be the first indication of infection. The most common microorganism identified in acute pyelonephritis is *E. coli* (Winkelman, 2006).

4. Identify the risk factors that placed Mrs. Reese at greater risk for the development of acute pyelonephritis. The risk of a UTI and subsequent acute pyelonephritis is greatest among females, in women who are sexually active, and in those with a history of UTIs (Potter, Weigel, & Green, 2007).

5. What are the characteristic clinical manifestations of pyelonephritis? Clients with pyelonephritis usually appear quite ill and complain of nausea, vomiting, and malaise. Clients report pain in their lower abdomen, flank, and lower back (costovertebral angle tenderness) on the affected side, especially on palpation. The pain may be described as colicky. Clients often report frequency, dysuria with a burning sensation, and hematuria. Nocturia also is common. Urine output is usually concentrated and cloudy with an ammonia-like or fishy odor. The client will often have tachycardia, tachypnea, a fever above 102°F (38.8°C), and chills. A CBC reveals leukocytosis (elevated WBCs), and WBCs, WBC casts, protein, and bacteria are present in a urinalysis (Potter, Weigel, & Green, 2007; Winkelman, 2006).

6. Mrs. Reese has a KUB with IVP. Explain this diagnostic test. How do the results help the heath care provider (HCP) to confirm the admitting diagnosis? A KUB is a type of abdominal X-ray that uses a contrast medium, called "intravenous pyelography" or "IVP" dye. The structure and function of the kidneys, ureters, and bladder are examined by measuring the time it takes for the dye to pass through the kidneys, ureters, and into the bladder. During this 45-minute exam, multiple X-rays of the urinary tract are taken while the dye is excreted normally. Any blockage along the tract will be visualized. A KUB provides Mrs. Reese's health care provider with useful information by detecting ureteral and renal calculi (kidney stones), acute renal failure, tumors, kidney disease, chronic pyelonephritis, urinary retention, congenital abnormalities, and trauma. Following this diagnostic test, the nurse should monitor the client for allergic reactions to the IVP contrast medium and encourage fluid intake to facilitate rehydration and excretion of the IVP dye. The nurse should be aware that clients with an allergy to IVP dye, iodine, eggs, or shellfish and those who are pregnant or have a blood urea nitrogen (BUN) greater than 40 mg/dL (impaired kidney function) should not undergo this diagnostic test (Daniels, 2002).

7. Mrs. Reese has no known allergies. She has been prescribed the following medications, ketorolac tromethamine, ondansetron hydrochloride, and levofloxacin. Provide a rationale for why each medication has been included as part of her medical management and any potential contraindication(s) of her taking these medications. *Ketorolac tromethamine* is a nonsteroidal anti-inflammatory medication that possesses anti-inflammatory, analgesic, and antipyretic effects. This medication is prescribed for the short-term management (up to five days) of severe, acute pain that requires analgesia at the opiate level. Its antipyretic effects help to decrease the client's fever. *Ondansetron hydrochloride* is an antiemetic prescribed to reduce nausea and vomiting. *Levofloxacin* is an antibiotic used to treat mild to moderate urinary tract infections due to *E. coli.* Mrs. Reese should be asked if she is breastfeeding her daughter since lactation is a contraindication for each of these medications (Spratto & Woods, 2006).

8. The nurse is designing Mrs. Reese's plan of care. Identify three priority nursing diagnoses for inclusion in the plan. Priority nursing diagnoses for Mrs. Reese include:

- Acute pain (abdomen, flank, back) related to (r/t) inflammation and irritation of urinary tract
- Impaired urinary elimination r/t irritation of urinary tract
- Hyperthermia r/t increased metabolic rate from infection
- Caregiver role strain r/t situational factors
- Ineffective health maintenance r/t deficient knowledge regarding disease, self-care, treatment of disease, prevention of further urinary tract infections
- Risk for activity intolerance r/t malaise, debilitation, and generalized weakness associated with infection
- Risk for urge urinary incontinence r/t irritation of urinary tract

(Ackley & Ladwig, 2006).

9. The nurse places highest priority on the nursing diagnosis acute pain r/t inflammation and irritation of urinary tract. State an outcome goal appropriate for Mrs. Reese and at least two nursing interventions to help achieve the goal. *Outcome goal:* By the second day of medical treatment, the client will report pain is being managed effectively as evidenced by report of pain ≤3 on a 0 to 10 pain scale.

Nursing interventions:

- Assess and document pain level hourly.
- Position the client for comfort.
- Administer ketorolac tromethamine as prescribed to decrease pain.
- Assess degree of pain relief and any adverse effects of ketorolac tromethamine.
- Administer antibiotic levofloxacin as prescribed.
- Increase fluid intake to 2 to 3 liters per day to flush the bladder and decrease the bacterial count.
- Apply heating pad to abdomen, flank, and lower back to relieve discomfort and possible bladder spasms.
- Provide balance between rest and activity.

(Ackley & Ladwig, 2006; Potter, Weigel, & Green, 2007).

10. Two days later, Mrs. Reese is afebrile and her nausea and vomiting have resolved. She is being discharged on an oral antibiotic. Provide the

client with education about her prescribed antibiotic and symptoms that warrant notification of her HCP. Mrs. Reese should be instructed to complete all of her antibiotic medication. Despite the fact that she may feel much better, she should finish her prescription, completing a 10- to 14-day antibiotic course as prescribed by her HCP. This insures the bacteria have been eliminated and helps to prevent the recurrence of infection. Many antibiotics decrease the efficacy of oral contraception. Mrs. Reese should use a second form of birth control, such as condoms or abstinence, while she is taking the antibiotic. A two-week follow-up appointment with her HCP will be scheduled, and a urinalysis with culture and sensitivity will be collected to determine if the infection has resolved. Prior to her follow-up appointment, she should notify her HCP if she develops abdominal, flank, or back pain; fever or chills; urinary frequency or urgency; or if she notices that her urinary output is much less than her fluid intake, which may indicate impaired renal function. In addition antibiotic medication can cause a superinfection. Mrs. Reese should notify her HCP if she experiences a furry overgrowth on her tongue, vaginal itching or discharge, and/or loose or foul-smelling stool (Deglin & Vallerand, 2007; Potter, Weigel, & Green, 2007; Smeltzer & Bare, 2004).

11. While the nurse is discontinuing the IV access, Mrs. Reese asks, "My doctor said that there is a chance I could get sick with this infection again. Is there anything I can do to help prevent that?" Offer Mrs. Reese at least five health promotion behaviors to help prevent a UTI and recurrent acute pyelonephritis. Literature proposes that the development of a UTI "depends on a series of complex interactions that allow bacterial colonization of the periurethral area, bacterial ascent into the urinary bladder, multiplication of bacteria in the urine, tissue invasion, and a resultant immune reaction" (Cohen & Powderly, 2004 as cited in Potter, Weigel, & Green, 2007). Although some research indicates that the risk of developing a UTI is not associated with dietary practices, personal hygiene practices, or tight clothing, many still suggest that individuals consider the following health promotion behaviors in an effort to decrease the risk of infection.

Health promotion behaviors to prevent a UTI include:

- Acidify the urine by drinking cranberry juice or taking ascorbic acid (vitamin C).
- Avoid coffee, tea, colas, and alcohol, which are urinary tract irritants.
- Avoid scented hygiene products (soaps, sanitary products, sprays).
- Avoid tight fitting clothes.
- Clean the perineum and urethral meatus from front to back after a bowel movement.

- Drink an adequate amount of fluid (eight to 10 glasses of fluid per day) to promote voiding and dilution of urine.
- Empty the bladder completely and frequently (every two to three hours) during the day to eliminate bacteria from the bladder and reduce urinary stasis.
- Recognize the symptoms of a UTI early.
- Seek early treatment of a UTI.
- Take showers instead of bubble baths to decrease the risk of bacteria in the bath water from entering the urethra.
- Void after intercourse (postcoital voiding), and wash the perineal area because sexual intercourse can bring organisms up from urethra into the bladder.
- Wear cotton underwear.

(Potter, Weigel, & Green, 2007; Smeltzer & Bare, 2004).

12. Mrs. Reese asks the nurse, "I heard if you drink cranberry juice it can cure a urinary tract infection. Is that true?" How will the nurse respond and what are three other complimentary therapies that the nurse might suggest? Research supports the use of several complimentary therapies for the prevention and treatment of UTIs. Consuming cranberry-based products is one of the more common suggestions. Research indicates that the ingestion of cranberry juice or cranberry products has been effective in preventing UTIs and decreasing the clinical manifestations of a UTI. The active ingredient found in cranberries (as well as in blueberries) is proanthocyanidins. This active ingredient acidifies the urine and inhibits certain urinary pathogens (such as *E. coli*) from adhering to the epithelial cells of the bladder wall. The recommendation is to drink cranberry juice or eat cranberries. Cranberry tablets also are available for dietary supplementation, but the research is less conclusive regarding cranberry tablets. Both cranberry-based products and tablets have been shown to statistically reduce the number of UTIs. Additional examples of complimentary therapies to promote urinary health include vitamin C to acidify the urine, beta-carotene and zinc to support immune function, garlic and celery seed, which are thought to have antibacterial activity, and parsley that is believed to act as an antiseptic in the urinary tract.

(Bernier, 2005; Potter, Weigel, & Green, 2007).

References

Ackley, B., & Ladwig, G. (2006). *Nursing diagnosis handbook: A guide to planning care.* St. Louis, MO: Mosby, Inc.

Bernier, F. (2005). Cranberry-based products in the prevention/treatment of urinary tract infections. In J. Black & J. Hawks (Eds.), *Medical-surgical nursing: Clinical management for positive outcomes* (p. 861). St. Louis, MO: Elsevier.

Cohen, J., & Powderly, G. (Eds.). (2004). *Infectious diseases.* St. Louis, MO: Mosby.

Daniels, R. (2002). *Delmar's guide to laboratory and diagnostic tests.* Albany, NY: Delmar.

Deglin, J. H., & Vallerand, A. H. (2007). *Davis's drug guide for nurses.* Philadelphia, PA: F. A. Davis.

Potter, C. K., Weigel, K. A., & Green, C. J. (2007). Kidney and urinary tract problems. In F. Monahan, J. Sands, M. Neighbors, J. Marek & C. Green (Eds.), *Phipps' medical-surgical nursing: Health and illness perspectives* (pp. 961–968). St. Louis, MO: Mosby Elsevier.

Smeltzer, S., & Bare, B. (2004). Management of patients with urinary disorders. In L. Brunner & D. Suddarth (Eds.), *Textbook of medical-surgical nursing* (pp. 1315–1317). Philadelphia, PA: Lippincott Williams & Wilkins.

Spratto, G. R., & Woods, A. L. (2006). *PDR nurse's drug handbook.* Clifton Park, NY: Thomson Delmar Learning.

Winkelman, C. (2006). Interventions for clients with renal disorders. In D. Ignatavicius & L. Workman (Eds.), *Medical-surgical nursing: Critical thinking for collaborative care* (pp. 1712–1715). St. Louis, MO: Elsevier Saunders.

Mr. Rossi

GENDER

Male

AGE

58

SETTING

- Home

ETHNICITY

- White American

CULTURAL CONSIDERATIONS

PREEXISTING CONDITIONS

- Diabetes mellitus type 2, diabetic nephropathy

COEXISTING CONDITIONS

- End-stage renal disease (ESRD), peritoneal dialysis (PD)

COMMUNICATION

DISABILITY

SOCIOECONOMIC

- Married, two sons (ages 34 and 31 years old), early retirement from the police department due to illness

SPIRITUAL/RELIGIOUS

- Active in the church community

PHARMACOLOGIC

- Calcium carbonate (Tums); rosiglitazone (Avandia); epoetin alfa recombinant (erythropoietin, Epogen, Procrit)

LEGAL

ETHICAL

ALTERNATIVE THERAPY

PRIORITIZATION

- Aseptic technique, renal diet, and fluid restrictions

DELEGATION

- Collaboration with a dietician

THE URINARY SYSTEM

Level of Difficulty: Difficult

Overview: This case requires the nurse to provide the client and his wife with teaching regarding the proper technique for peritoneal dialysis treatments in the home. Potential complications of renal failure and peritoneal dialysis are discussed. The nurse responds to Mrs. Rossi's concerns about her husband's risk of a fracture. Dietary and fluid restrictions are reviewed. The impact of chronic renal failure on quality of life is addressed. Priority nursing diagnoses for the client on peritoneal dialysis are identified.

DIFFICULT

Client Profile

Mr. Rossi is a 58-year-old male diagnosed with diabetic nephropathy 10 years ago. He is now in end-stage renal failure and has recently started continuous ambulatory peritoneal dialysis (CAPD) in his home.

Case Study

On a snowy day in February, the visiting nurse has come to see Mr. Rossi and his wife to reinforce instructions regarding the proper technique for peritoneal dialysis and to assess how the Rossis are coping. When the nurse arrives, Mr. Rossi is resting comfortably in a reclining chair with a bottle of diet cola on the tray table beside his chair. The nurse has concerns about Mr. Rossi's diet, and during the home visit, she observes several behaviors that indicate a need for further teaching.

Questions

1. Briefly discuss how Mr. Rossi's past medical history increased his risk of developing renal failure.

2. Describe the physiologic changes in the kidneys that lead to chronic renal failure (CRF).

3. What is glomerular filtration rate (GFR)? How is GFR measured and what is the normal range in a healthy adult?

4. According to the National Kidney Foundation's five-stage classification system of chronic kidney disease, which stage of chronic kidney disease (CKD) is Mr. Rossi in, and what would you anticipate his GFR to be?

5. Briefly describe the changes in urine output characteristic of ESRD.

6. Briefly explain how peritoneal dialysis clears the body of excess water and waste products of metabolism. Describe three main types of peritoneal dialysis.

7. What are some advantages of peritoneal dialysis as compared with hemodialysis? Discuss why peritoneal dialysis is more favorable for Mr. Rossi than the hemodialysis treatment option.

8. Mrs. Rossi shows the nurse where they have cleared a clean space in their garage to store the supplies for Mr. Rossi's dialysis. What should the nurse remind the Rossis to do before attaching the dialysate to Mr. Rossi's peritoneal catheter?

9. The nurse asks Mrs. Rossi about the last few meals she prepared for her husband. Mrs. Rossi indicates the following meals:

(a) Whole grain cereal with milk, orange juice, and a banana
(b) A roast beef sandwich with cheese and mayonnaise
(c) White bread toast, apple juice, and tea
(d) A peanut butter and jelly sandwich with diet cola

Clarify for Mrs. Rossi which of these meals was the most appropriate for Mr. Rossi regarding his renal diet, and explain your concerns about the other meals she prepared.

Questions (continued)

10. The nurse notices that by the reclining chair where Mr. Rossi sits is a 2-liter bottle of diet cola. Why is the nurse concerned?

11. Who should the visiting nurse arrange to meet with the Rossis to provide additional teaching regarding appropriate food and beverage choices for the client with renal failure?

12. Mrs. Rossi asks the nurse, "Someone at church said I should watch that my husband does not fall. They said he could break his hip very easily because people with bad kidneys have very brittle bones. Is that true?" Help the nurse explain why clients with renal failure develop changes in their bones, and offer some examples of renal osteodystrophy that may develop.

13. Identify five priority nursing diagnoses for Mr. Rossi.

14. The nurse reminds Mr. Rossi that he is at risk of becoming anemic. Briefly explain to Mr. Rossi why he is at risk and what signs and symptoms he should report to the nurse or his health care provider.

15. The nurse notices a napkin on the kitchen table with two Tums tablets on it. When the nurse asks Mr. Rossi if he is taking his Tums with every meal, Mr. Rossi replies, "Sometimes I remember. Sometimes I forget. I figure it is not a problem if I forget once and a while. I do not have any symptoms of heartburn anyway." In lay terminology, how might the nurse explain to Mr. Rossi the importance of taking his prescribed Tums with every meal?

16. Mrs. Rossi calls the visiting nurse to report that "When my husband's solution was drained out of his belly today, I noticed it was cloudy looking and he has a fever of 102°F (38.9°C)." Briefly discuss the common complication of peritoneal dialysis that Mr. Rossi appears to have developed. What should the nurse tell the Rossis to do?

17. Discuss the lifestyle changes imposed upon the client who is on peritoneal dialysis and how these changes may affect the client's quality of life.

Questions and Suggested Answers

1. Briefly discuss how Mr. Rossi's past medical history increased his risk of developing renal failure. Diabetes mellitus is the leading cause of CRF, accounting for more than 30% of CRF clients (Molzahn, 2005). "Diabetic nephropathy is the leading cause of end-stage renal disease in the United States, accounting for approximately 43% of new cases. Twenty percent of all persons with diabetes have nephropathy" (Ulchaker, 2007, p. 1120). Manifestations of renal disease generally appear 10 years or more after the onset of type 1 diabetes mellitus, but may be present at the time of diagnosis in those with type 2 diabetes mellitus. Diabetic nephropathy is marked by glomerular hypertrophy, hyperfiltration, and an elevated glomerular filtration rate. The earliest laboratory abnormality of nephropathy is microscopic amounts of albumin in the urine (microalbuminuria). The microalbuminuria can progress to albuminuria, proteinuria, and eventually ESRD.

2. Describe the physiologic changes in the kidneys that lead to CRF. Gradual deterioration and destruction of nephrons in the kidneys leads to progressive loss of kidney function. As filtration through the kidneys decreases, the clearance of toxins is impaired. The remaining functioning nephrons must filter greater amounts of solutes, causing them to become hypertrophied. The kidneys eventually lose their ability to filter waste and concentrate the urine. The body's attempt to continue to excrete solutes results in the production of an increased volume of dilute urine. In addition the renal tubules lose their ability to reabsorb electrolytes, which results in large amounts of sodium in the urine (called salt wasting), leading to more polyuria (excessive urine output) and placing the client at risk for volume depletion. The ability of the remaining nephrons to function eventually declines, filtration through the kidneys decreases markedly, and the body is no longer capable of ridding itself of urea, creatinine, and other nitrogenous waste products of protein and amino acid metabolism, as well as excess water. The client will develop elevated electrolyte levels (such as hyperkalemia), and elevated blood urea nitrogen (BUN) and serum creatinine, which is a fatal condition called azotemia (or uremia) if not treated with dialysis (Molzahn, 2005).

3. What is GFR? How is GFR measured and what is the normal range in a healthy adult? The process by which the fluid part of the urine is formed is called ultrafiltration. As blood passes through the glomerulus, the pressure of plasma forces fluid across the semipermeable membrane of the glomerulus into Bowman's capsule. Approximately 180 liters of blood filters through the glomerulus each day. Of the total volume, 99% is reabsorbed by the kidneys, resulting in an adult's average daily urine output of 1 to 2 liters per day. This ultrafiltration process is measured as the kidney's GFR. GFR is defined as the amount of glomerular filtrate formed in one minute. The GFR in an adult of average size is approximately 125 mL/minute (or 7.5 L/hour). The average GFR of a female is about 10% less than that of a male, and individuals with a larger body surface will have a greater GFR.

As GFR decreases, the clearance of toxins by the kidneys is reduced and levels of BUN and creatinine increase, leading to azotemia (Weigel & Potter, 2007).

4. According to the National Kidney Foundation's five-stage classification system of CKD, which stage of CKD is Mr. Rossi in, and what would you anticipate his GFR to be? According to the National Kidney Foundation's five-stage classification system, Mr. Rossi is in Stage 5, which is kidney failure. His GFR would likely be less than 15 mL/minute (National Kidney Foundation, 2006).

Stages of Chronic Kidney Disease

Stage	Description	GFR (mL/min/1.73 M²)
1	Kidney damage with normal or increased GFR	Greater than or equal to 90
2	Kidney damage with mildly decreased GFR	60–89
3	Moderately decreased GFR	30–59
4	Severely decreased GFR	15–29
5	Kidney failure	Less than 15 (or dialysis)

5. Briefly describe the changes in urine output characteristic of ESRD. ESRD is irreversible chronic renal failure that develops when the kidneys can no longer function to maintain the body's homeostasis. The clinical manifestations of ESRD are evident throughout the body's systems. Polyuria (excessive urine output) eventually progresses to anuria (suppression of urine formation), and the client no longer has a normal pattern of voiding, and often does not urinate at all (Ehrlich & Schroeder, 2005; Molzahn, 2005).

6. Briefly explain how peritoneal dialysis clears the body of excess water and waste products of metabolism. Describe three main types of peritoneal dialysis. Peritoneal dialysis removes excess fluid and waste products of metabolism by diffusion and osmosis through the client's peritoneal membrane, restoring the body's fluid and electrolyte balance. A concentrated dialysate (1.5 to 3 liters of an electrolyte solution) is introduced into the peritoneal cavity through a permanent peritoneal catheter implanted in the abdomen. The dialysate remains within the peritoneal cavity for a prescribed amount of time (dwell time). The lining of the peritoneal cavity acts as a "filter." While in the peritoneal cavity, waste products of metabolism and electrolytes in the blood flowing through the capillary system of the peritoneal membrane diffuse into the dialysate. By adding a concentration of glucose to the dialysate, the solution becomes hypertonic and, through osmosis, draws excess water from the blood into the dialysate fluid. The dialysate is drained from the peritoneal cavity, removing the excess fluid and waste products with it (Altman, 2004; Molzahn, 2005).

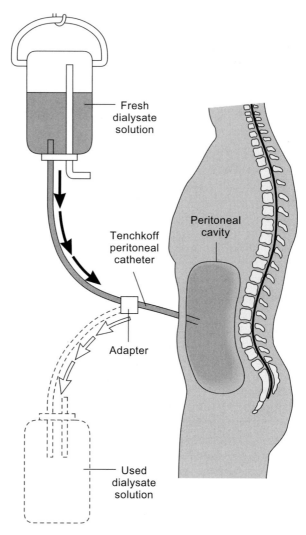

Peritoneal dialysis removes waste through a fluid exchange in the peritoneal cavity

There are three main types of peritoneal dialysis, CAPD, continuous cycling peritoneal dialysis (CCPD), and intermittent peritoneal dialysis. CAPD is ongoing, with the dialysate remaining in the peritoneal cavity for four to eight hours at a time, drained, and then repeated in cycles throughout the day (usually four eight-hour cycles and an eight-hour dwell overnight). CAPD is a daily treatment regimen. Clients can continue to participate in their daily activities while the dialysate is dwelling within their abdomen. The empty dialysate bag is folded and carried in a pouch or pocket until the dialysate is drained by gravity flow. Other clients discon-nect the system after instilling the dialysate and attach a protective cap to the end of the dialysis catheter until a new sterile bag is attached to drain the dialysate solution. CCPD (also called automated peritoneal dialysis) uses a machine (called a cycler) to cycle the dialysate in either continuous or intermittent cycles, or only while the client sleeps at night. The client receiving intermittent peritoneal dialysis allows the dialysate to remain in the peritoneal cavity for a longer period of time (usually 10 to 14 hours). Intermittent peritoneal dialysis is performed three to four times a week, or the client may be treated by performing the dialysis treatments for 8 to 12 hours each night with no daytime dwells (Altman, 2004; Ehrlich & Schroeder, 2005; Molzahn, 2005).

7. What are some advantages of peritoneal dialysis as compared with hemodialysis? Discuss why peritoneal dialysis is more favorable for Mr. Rossi than the hemodialysis treatment option. Peritoneal dialysis is often prescribed for clients who cannot tolerate hemodialysis or in cases where hemodialysis is not readily available or accessible. An advantage of peritoneal dialysis is the increased independence of being able to do the dialysis treatments at home or at work and to remain ambulatory dur-ing the treatments. Conventional hemodialysis takes three to four hours, whereas each manual peritoneal exchange takes only about 30 to 40 min-utes. In addition, because peritoneal dialysis is often a continuous process, it more closely resembles normal kidney function, and the body is better able to maintain homeostasis. Peritoneal dialysis clients also enjoy fewer dietary and fluid restrictions than the client treated with hemodialysis. Some health care providers prescribe peritoneal dialysis for clients with diabetes mellitus because it reduces the client's risk of retinal hemorrhage associated with the use of heparin during hemodialysis. As well, blood glucose control is well achieved by adding insulin to the dialysate solution (Altman, 2004; Molzahn, 2005).

8. Mrs. Rossi shows the nurse where they have cleared a clean space in their garage to store the supplies for Mr. Rossi's dialysis. What should the nurse remind the Rossis to do before attaching the dialysate to Mr. Rossi's peritoneal catheter? To avoid discomfort, the dialysate solution should be at body temperature before introducing it into the client's peritoneal cavity. In the winter, the Rossis should bring a few bags of dialysate into their house to warm before using. Many bags of dialysate come in a pro-tective outer wrapper that is safe for microwave heating. Bags of solution should not be heated in a microwave oven if they do not have a microwave approved wrapper, or if the protective wrapper has been removed, since doing so can change the chemical makeup of the solution. If necessary, a special heating device (such as an aquathermia pad) can be ordered for the Rossis to use to warm each bag of dialysate solution (Altman, 2004; NIDDK, 2006).

9. **The nurse asks Mrs. Rossi about the last few meals she prepared for her husband. Mrs. Rossi indicates the following meals:**

   (a) Whole grain cereal with milk, orange juice, and a banana
   (b) A roast beef sandwich with cheese and mayonnaise
   (c) White bread toast, apple juice, and tea
   (d) A peanut butter and jelly sandwich with diet cola

Clarify for Mrs. Rossi which of these meals was the most appropriate for Mr. Rossi regarding his renal diet, and explain your concerns about the other meals she prepared. Clients with renal failure should limit foods high in phosphorous, potassium, and sodium. Milk and dairy products, whole grains, beans, deli meats, peanut butter, nuts, chocolate, and colas, for example, are high in phosphorus. Potassium is in beverages such as tea, coffee, and orange juice, as well as in bananas. Canned vegetables or soups and many seasonings are very high in sodium. The most appropriate meal for Mr. Rossi was (c) white bread toast, apple juice, and tea. The nurse should explain to Mrs. Rossi that the whole grain cereal with milk is high in phosphorus and orange juice and banana are both high in potassium. The last two meals, which included a roast beef sandwich with cheese and mayonnaise and the peanut butter and jelly sandwich with diet cola, are very high in phosphorus (National Kidney Foundation, 2006).

10. The nurse notices that by the reclining chair where Mr. Rossi sits is a 2-liter bottle of diet cola. Why is the nurse concerned? Since renal failure clients are hyperphosphatemic, they should not drink beverages that contain phosphorus, such as dark colas. In addition, renal failure clients must limit their fluid intake. While the prescribed daily fluid restriction can vary between clients, approximately 1000 mL per day is the recommended fluid allowance. Fluids are any food or beverage that is liquid at room temperature. Therefore, in addition to beverages such as water, tea, coffee, juice, and ice, foods such as popsicles, ice cream, gelatin, and soups are all examples of fluids in one's diet. A 2-liter bottle of cola is 2000 mL of fluid. If Mr. Rossi has been advised to limit his fluid intake to 1000 mL per day and he drinks an entire 2-liter bottle of cola in a day, the cola is double his daily fluid allowance (National Kidney Foundation, 2006).

11. Who should the visiting nurse arrange to meet with the Rossis to provide additional teaching regarding appropriate food and beverage choices for the client with renal failure? The nurse should arrange for a dietician to meet with the Rossis to provide additional teaching regarding appropriate food and beverage choices. The nurse might suggest that one (or both) of Mr. Rossi's sons be present during the teaching in order to educate the family about appropriate dietary choices for Mr. Rossi and to increase the likelihood of compliance with the dietician's recommendations.

12. Mrs. Rossi asks the nurse, "Someone at church said I should watch that my husband does not fall. They said he could break his hip very easily because people with bad kidneys have very brittle bones. Is that true?" Help the nurse explain why clients with renal failure develop changes in their bones and offer some examples of renal osteodystrophy that may develop. The nurse might explain, "Your friend at church is correct. Individuals with kidney disease are at greater risk of injury from a fall because of changes in their bones from the electrolyte imbalances that occur with renal failure. The person with kidney failure is often hypocalcemic, which means they have low levels of calcium in their blood. Clients with kidney failure also have high levels of phosphate in their blood. Because calcium and phosphate are inversely related, a high phosphate level leads to an even lower calcium level. In addition, as renal failure progresses, the kidneys can no longer convert vitamin D to its active form. When the body is faced with these imbalances, it responds by stimulating a gland, called the parathyroid gland, to secrete a hormone that facilitates phosphate excretion from the body and increases the levels of calcium by drawing calcium from the bone. Although this effort is the body's way of trying to help compensate for these electrolyte imbalances, as a result, many clients (up to 90%) often develop adverse changes in their bones. Some of the conditions that can develop include osteomalacia (softening of the bone), osteitis fibrosa (inflammation of the bone), osteoporosis (porous bones with loss of bone density), and osteosclerosis (abnormal hardening of the bone). If your husband were to develop any of these conditions, he would be at increased risk of fracturing a bone, especially if he were to fall" (Molzahn, 2005).

13. Identify five priority nursing diagnoses for Mr. Rossi. Priority nursing diagnoses for Mr. Rossi include:

- Risk for infection (peritoneal) related to (r/t) invasive procedure, presence of catheter, and dialysate
- Deficient knowledge r/t treatment procedure, self-care with peritoneal dialysis, and dietary restrictions
- Risk for fluid volume excess r/t retention of dialysate
- Risk for ineffective breathing pattern r/t pressure from dialysate
- Risk for injury r/t hypo-/hyperglycemia, bone changes, neuropathy, and hemodynamic changes
- Risk for ineffective coping r/t disability requiring change in lifestyle
- Risk for powerlessness r/t chronic condition

(Ackley & Ladwig, 2006).

14. The nurse reminds Mr. Rossi that he is at risk of becoming anemic. Briefly explain to Mr. Rossi why he is at risk and what signs and symptoms he should report to the nurse or his health care provider. The primary hematologic effect of renal failure is anemia (Molzahn, 2005). Anemia is common in clients with renal disease because the kidneys are no longer able to produce erythropoietin, which is a hormone essential for red blood cell production. Mr. Rossi should inform the nurse (or his health care provider) if he notices fatigue, weakness, pallor (paleness of the skin), or an intolerance to cold. Mrs. Rossi should monitor her husband for an increasing need to rest or take naps (fatigue), becoming short of breath, weakness, and for indications that he is experiencing cold intolerance, such as requesting more blankets or raising the thermostat in the house. Mr. Rossi has been prescribed epoetin alfa recombinant (erythropoietin). This medication stimulates erythropoiesis (the production of red blood cells) and is commonly prescribed for the treatment of anemia associated with chronic renal failure.

15. The nurse notices a napkin on the kitchen table with two calcium carbonate (Tums) tablets on it. When the nurse asks Mr. Rossi if he is taking his Tums with every meal, Mr. Rossi replies, "Sometimes I remember. Sometimes I forget. I figure it is not a problem if I forget once and a while. I do not have any symptoms of heartburn anyway." In lay terminology, how might the nurse explain to Mr. Rossi the importance of taking his prescribed Tums with every meal? "Because your kidneys do not function anymore, your body cannot get rid of excess electrolytes. When the level of these electrolytes increases, they have negative effects on your body. Phosphorus is one of these electrolytes, which in high levels, can affect your bones, as we discussed earlier. When your health care provider prescribed Tums for you, it was not to treat or prevent heartburn. The calcium in Tums tablets acts as a phosphate binder that attracts phosphorus and helps to excrete the excess phosphorus from your body."

16. Mrs. Rossi calls the visiting nurse to report that "When my husband's solution was drained out of his belly today, I noticed it was cloudy looking and he has a fever of 102°F (38.9°C)." Briefly discuss the common complication of peritoneal dialysis that Mr. Rossi appears to have developed. What should the nurse tell the Rossis to do? Mr. Rossi appears to have developed peritonitis. Peritonitis is a complication of peritoneal dialysis that usually occurs as a result of inadequate aseptic technique during handling of the dialysis catheter, tubing, and/or dialysate solution. Contamination allows bacteria to enter the peritoneal cavity, resulting in an infection. Clinical manifestations of peritonitis that clients often report include cloudy dialysate output, fever, abdominal pain, rebound abdominal tenderness, nausea or vomiting, redness around the peritoneal catheter insertion site, and complaints of malaise. Meticulous aseptic technique is paramount to help prevent peritonitis since this infection can cause scarring, making future peritoneal dialysis impossible (Molzahn, 2005).

Peritonitis requires immediate intervention. The nurse should tell Mrs. Rossi to notify Mr. Rossi's health care provider and arrange for admission into the hospital for further assessment and medical treatment.

17. Discuss the lifestyle changes imposed upon the client who is on peritoneal dialysis and how these changes may affect the client's quality of life. Common stressors of living with a chronic and life-threatening illness include powerlessness, changes in body image, and changes in sexuality. Mr. Rossi is likely to experience a sense of a loss of control over the illness and the treatment needed to sustain life. Peritoneal dialysis, while more convenient because it does not require three times weekly traveling to a dialysis center, is an intrusive therapy that invades the home with medical equipment and supplies and presents the risk of feeling as if the safe haven of home, free from the reminders of the illness, are gone. There are changes in body image with the peritoneal catheter and drainage bag connected to the body during cycles. Sexuality is often affected since there is a night-time cycle, which can interfere with the comfort and ease of sexual activity; many renal failure clients develop impotence. There is often a change in the dynamics of the couple's relationship and a loss of role identity. As in this case, Mrs. Rossi has become a care provider, as well as a spouse and mother, and Mr. Rossi's illness has necessitated early retirement and a loss of his role as breadwinner for the family. Being retired may pose a financial strain on the client and his wife if he does not have adequate health care insurance to cover the cost of supplies and home care. Retirement savings formerly set for their future may need to be utilized earlier than anticipated for Mr. Rossi's care and treatment needs, depleting future savings. Each client will react to these lifestyle changes differently. The nurse should acknowledge these changes and the potential stressors that they present. The nurse can help the Rossis prepare and cope by helping them to recall past coping mechanisms that were effective in overcoming a significant life stressor, and identifying family, friends, and members of their church who can serve as a support network for them. Developing a therapeutic alliance with the couple will help facilitate honest and open discussion of their concerns and fears about how their lives will be impacted by the peritoneal dialysis treatments (Molzahn, 2005).

References

Ackley, B., & Ladwig, G. (2006). *Nursing diagnosis handbook: A guide to planning care.* St. Louis, MO: Mosby.

Altman, G. B. (2004). Administering peritoneal dialysis. In G. B. Altman (Ed.), *Delmar's fundamental & advanced nursing skills* (pp. 833–840). Clifton Park, NY: Thomson Delmar Learning.

Ehrlich, A., & Schroeder, C. L. (2005). *Medical terminology for health professions* (pp. 252–259). Clifton Park, NY: Thomson Delmar Learning.

Molzahn, A. E. (2005). Management of clients with renal failure. In *Black & Hawks' Medical-surgical nursing: Clinical management for positive outcomes* (pp. 949–958; 961–968). St. Louis, MO: Elsevier.

National Institute of Diabetes and Digestive and Kidney Diseases (NIDDK). (2006). Equipment and supplies for PD. *Treatment methods for kidney failure: Peritoneal dialysis*. Retrieved January 17, 2007, from www.kidney.niddk.nih.gov.

National Kidney Foundation. (2006). Nutrition and peritoneal dialysis. *Kidney disease outcomes quality initiative*. Retrieved January 17, 2007, from www.kidney.org.

Ulchaker, M. M. (2007). Diabetes mellitus and hypoglycemia. In F. Monahan, J. Sands, M. Neighbors, J. Marek, & C. Green (Eds.), *Phipps' Medical-surgical nursing: Health and illness perspectives* (pp. 1120–1121). St. Louis, MO: Mosby Elsevier.

Weigel, K. A., & Potter, C. K. (2007). Assessment of the renal system. In F. Monahan, J. Sands, M. Neighbors, J. Marek, & C. Green (Eds.), *Phipps' Medical-surgical nursing: Health and illness perspectives* (pp. 945–946). St. Louis, MO: Mosby Elsevier.

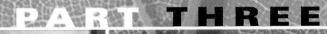

PART THREE

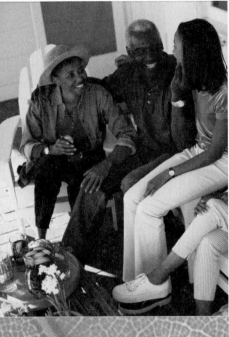

The Respiratory System

CASE STUDY 1

Mr. Yang

GENDER

Male

AGE

90

SETTING

- Hospital

ETHNICITY

- Hmong

CULTURAL CONSIDERATIONS

- Language barrier
- Appropriate greetings
- Eye contact
- Touch

PREEXISTING CONDITION

COEXISTING CONDITION

COMMUNICATION

- Speaks green Hmong (also called Hmoob)
- Nonverbal communication

DISABILITY

SOCIOECONOMIC

- Married

SPIRITUAL/RELIGIOUS

PHARMACOLOGIC

LEGAL

- Use of a medical interpreter

ETHICAL

- Use of a medical interpreter

ALTERNATIVE THERAPY

PRIORITIZATION

- Intervention when a chest tube is dislodged

DELEGATION

- Collaboration with certified nursing assistant

THE RESPIRATORY SYSTEM

Level of Difficulty: Moderate

Overview: The nurse must care for the client with a hemothorax. The appropriate setup of a chest drainage system is reviewed. The nurse must respond when the chest tube becomes dislodged. Priority nursing diagnoses are identified, and outcome goals written. Cultural beliefs to consider while caring for a Hmong client are addressed, and the role of a medical interpreter explained.

Client Profile

Mr. Yang is a 90-year-old man who fell on the ice while walking to his mailbox this afternoon. Upon arrival, the nurse observes that Mr. Yang is grimacing and guarding his left side. His vital signs are blood pressure 132/80, heart rate 96, respiratory rate 16 with shallow breathing, and temperature 98.4°F (36.9°C). His oxygen saturation is 96% on room air. Physical assessment findings include increased pain on inspiration and tenderness when gently palpating the left side of his thorax. A chest X-ray reveals that the client has fractured his six and seventh ribs on the left side and has a left lung hemothorax. Fortunately Mr. Yang's spleen has not been injured as a result of the trauma. Pain medication is prescribed, and a chest tube is inserted. The health care provider prescribes oxygen 2 liters by nasal cannula as needed for oxygen saturation below 92%. Mr. Yang is admitted to the hospital.

Case Study

The next day, the nurse assigned to Mr. Yang's care is concerned because she does not speak Hmong. When the nurse enters Mr. Yang's room, she greets him warmly with a smile and introduces herself. The client's wife is present in the room. The nurse extends her hand to shake Mrs. Yang's hand, but Mrs. Yang averts her eyes shyly and looks to her husband. The nurse turns her attention back to Mr. Yang and assesses the dressing covering the chest tube insertion site. The dressing is dry and intact. The chest tube drainage system is functioning normally. The canister has 700 mL of bloody drainage noted since admission as indicated by markings on the outside of the drainage container.

Questions

1. Mr. Yang is diagnosed with a hemothorax. Briefly explain what this is and what has likely caused the hemothorax in the client's case.

2. Briefly discuss the challenges of developing a nurse-client relationship when a language barrier exists between the client and nurse.

3. The nurse would like a medical interpreter to assist in gathering client assessment data and collaborating with the client to plan his care for the day. Briefly explain the difference between a medical "interpreter" and a medical "translator." Discuss the resources available to the nurse when he/she feels an interpreter is needed. What should the nurse document in the client's record regarding the use of an interpreter?

4. Discuss the nurse's primary concerns for the client with a rib fracture and hemothorax, and the appropriate interventions to prevent these complication(s).

Questions (continued)

5. Identify three priority nursing diagnoses for this client. Write at least one outcome goal for each diagnosis.

6. A chest drainage system contains three chambers. Identify each chamber.

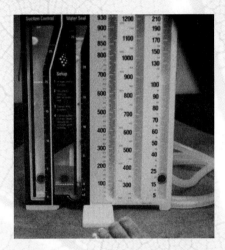

7. Explain how the nurse sets up a water seal and the function of a water seal. Next, explain how the nurse establishes chest tube suction and the function of the suction.

8. The certified nursing assistant working with the nurse anxiously reports, "Come quick, Mr. Yang's chest tube has fallen out!" The nurse finds that the chest tube is on the floor and that the dressing has partially fallen off. What should the nurse do?

9. Discuss the nonverbal cues the nurse should monitor indicating that Mr. Yang is in pain.

10. Provide an explanation for Mrs. Yang's response when greeted by the nurse.

11. The nurse expresses to a colleague that she is concerned she will offend the Yangs because she is not familiar with their culture and health care beliefs. The colleague states, "I remember learning in nursing school that you should not touch the head of a Hmong person, especially not the head of a child. And do not tell them their children or grandchildren are cute." Discuss the cultural interpretation of touching a Hmong client's head (or that of their children), and why the nurse should refrain from complimenting the child.

12. It is the end of an eight-hour shift and the nurse is checking the chest drainage system to determine the amount of drainage during their shift of care. The last mark made by the nurse on the previous shift is at 675 mL. The level of fluid in the drainage collection chamber is now at 800 mL. The nurse uses a marker to mark the current level and indicates the time and date of the measurement. How much drainage does the nurse document on the client's intake and output record, and should the nurse call to notify the health care provider (HCP) of the output?

Questions and Suggested Answers

1. Mr. Yang is diagnosed with a hemothorax. Briefly explain what this is and what has likely caused the hemothorax in the client's case. A hemothorax results when there is blood between the lung and thin serous membrane that surrounds the lung (pleura), impeding lung expansion and causing respiratory distress. If a fractured rib is displaced or splintered, it can cause a penetrating injury that penetrates the pleura and/or lung, resulting in a hemothorax (blood in the pleural cavity). Ribs four through nine are more likely to be fractured in a chest injury because they are not well protected by the chest muscles (Dennison, 2007; Frisch & Altman, 2004; Strauss, 2007).

2. **Briefly discuss the challenges of developing a nurse-client relationship when a language barrier exists between the client and nurse.** When caring for a client who is non-English speaking or has limited English proficiency, there are professional, ethical, and legal considerations. Effective communication between a client and caregiver is essential for the provision of safe and appropriate care, as well as demonstrating respect, appreciation for diversity, and empowering the client to make informed health care decisions. Nurses have a responsibility to serve as a client advocate. The lack of effective verbal communication between the nurse and client can result in misunderstandings, misinterpretation of data, noncompliance with treatment suggestions, failure to address client needs, and an inability to assess symptoms accurately. The inability to understand the nurse can invoke fear and frustration for the client and family members. Nurses experience frustration as they struggle to understand what the client is trying to convey. Potential legal and ethical concerns exist when clients are deprived of quality health care, timely interventions, or receive incorrect information because of a language barrier. The nurse should facilitate effective communication while maintaining client confidentiality. For example the nurse can use a medical interpreter to facilitate effective and accurate communication.

3. **The nurse would like a medical interpreter to assist in gathering client assessment data and collaborating with the client to plan his care for the day. Briefly explain the difference between a medical "interpreter" and a medical "translator." Discuss the resources available to the nurse when he/she feels an interpreter is needed. What should the nurse document in the client's record regarding the use of an interpreter?** Medical interpreters and translators enable cross-cultural communication between clients and health care providers. While the terms "interpreter" and "translator" are often used interchangeably, there is a difference between the two regarding the role of the professional interpreter versus that of a translator. *Interpreters* convert one spoken language into another and facilitate communication between clients and their health care providers. *Translators* primarily convert client materials and informational brochures into a desired language. The Hmong have their own language, which is called Hmoob (Hmong in English). The Hmong language has many dialects. Most speak either white or green Hmong. Since Hmong was not a written language until the late 1960s, it has few medical terms and is often conveyed using metaphors. An interpreter with knowledge of the Hmong culture is critical to understanding what the Hmong client is trying to communicate. Medical interpreters who speak the languages common to the geographic region are employed by health care facilities to assist staff and clients in a timely fashion. Language assistance is also often available through community volunteer networks, telephone language lines, and private interpreter services. Legally an interpreter should be available to facilitate effective communication for limited English proficiency clients receiving health care services. Title VI of the Civil Rights Act of 1964 (also known as the Hill-Burton Act) requires every HCP and health care facility that receives any federal financial assistance (such as Medicare and Medicaid) to provide free interpreter services to clients with limited English proficiency. Whenever possible the same interpreter should be used for each client interaction. When an interpreter is used, the nurse should address all questions and information directly to the client. The nurse should confirm that the interpreter understands what the nurse is asking or trying to convey to the client. Caution should be taken when using community volunteers since clients may have concerns about confidentiality if the interpreter is a volunteer from the client's community. Hmong clients value their privacy and often share information only among certain family members. The privacy rules of the Health Insurance Portability and Accountability Act of 1996 (HIPAA) and staff commitment to honor the client's privacy should be communicated to the client. As well, interpreters of the same gender as the client are preferred to minimize the risk of ineffective communication secondary to gender mismatch (Bureau of Labor Statistics, U.S. Department of Labor, 2005; Children's Hospitals and Clinics of Minnesota, 2003; HHS, 2003; Minnesota Medical Association, 2004).

The nurse should document in the client's record (chart) that the client is non-English speaking and indicate that the client's primary language is Hmong. The name and contact information for the interpreter, as well as the client's consent for the use of an interpreter, should be documented in the client's record. If the client is offered interpreter services but declines, this should be documented (HHS, 2003; Minnesota Medical Association, 2004; Zator Estes, 2006).

4. Discuss the nurse's primary concerns for the client with a rib fracture and hemothorax and appropriate interventions to prevent these complication(s). The nurse's primary concern is that the client could experience hypovolemia as a result of the blood loss from a severe hemothorax. An adult client with a small amount of blood (<300 mL) in the pleural space may not have clinical manifestations and often does not require treatment since the blood will spontaneously reabsorb. On the other hand, a severe hemothorax (≥1500 mL) can be life threatening. In an older adult, such as Mr. Yang, clinical manifestations may be noted with smaller amounts of blood loss, and treatment may be required. The nurse monitors the client's chest drainage system for the output and notifies the HCP if the drainage is greater than 100 mL per hour. In the older adult, the HCP may request that the nurse report drainage of greater than 50 mL per hour. The nurse assesses the client for respiratory distress, shock, and a mediastinal shift. A mediastinal shift is detected by assessing for the shift of the trachea away from midline toward the client's unaffected side (in this case the client's right). This shift indicates the collapse of the lung from a tension pneumothorax (White, 2005).

The acute pain of a rib fracture can result in the client's inability to breathe deeply. This can result in the stasis of secretions, atelectasis (collapse of alveolar sacs), and respiratory distress. In the elderly client, multiple rib fractures increase the incidence of developing pneumonia. The nurse should assess the client's breathing and airway status frequently. If the client experiences shortness of breath or chest pain, the HCP should be notified immediately. The nurse should provide analgesia as prescribed to relieve the client's pain and collaborate with the HCP if the client's pain is not being managed effectively with the current treatment regimen. Positioning is an important intervention for facilitating comfort and improving the client's breathing effort. The client should be in a Fowler's or semi-Fowler's position. Providing the client with instructions on the proper use of an incentive spirometer and encouraging deep-breathing exercises increases lung expansion, keeps alveoli open, helps remove mucous secretions, and strengthens respiratory muscles. Adequate hydration will help liquefy secretions and cough, and deep breathing exercises are encouraged every one to two hours while awake to mobilize secretions. The client's vital signs should be monitored closely, and the HCP notified of any significant changes, especially if the client becomes febrile (Dennison, 2007; Strauss, 2007).

5. Identify three priority nursing diagnoses for this client. Write at least one outcome goal for each diagnosis. Priority diagnoses and suggested outcome goals for this client include:

1. Acute pain related to (r/t) presence of chest tube, injury, movement, and deep breathing as evidenced by (aeb) shallow breathing, grimacing, guarding, and tenderness on palpation
   - Client will use a pain rating scale to identify current pain intensity and determine comfort goal/level by (specify).
   - Client will report that pain management regimen relieves pain to a satisfactory level with acceptable and manageable adverse effects by (specify).
   - Client will perform activities of daily living with reported acceptable level of pain by (specify).
   - Client will describe at least one nonpharmacological method that can be used to help control pain by (specify).
2. Risk for deficient fluid volume r/t active fluid volume loss (blood in pleural space) aeb chest x-ray
   - Client will maintain blood pressure, heart rate, and body temperature within normal limits by (specify).
   - Client will maintain elastic skin turgor, moist mucous membranes, and orientation to person, place, and time throughout hospitalization.
   - Client will remain free of clinical manifestations of respiratory distress, shock, and pneumothorax throughout hospitalization.
3. Risk for ineffective breathing pattern r/t pain and asymmetrical lung expansion secondary to fractured ribs aeb chest X-ray, shallow breathing, and acute pain
   - Client will report ability to breathe comfortably by (specify).
   - Client will not experience respiratory distress throughout hospitalization.
   - Client will demonstrate a breathing pattern that supports oxygen saturation within the client's normal parameters throughout hospitalization.
4. Risk for infection r/t hemothorax and inadequate primary defenses (presence of invasive chest tube) aeb trauma, possible stasis of secretions and tissue destruction
   - Client will remain free from symptoms of infection throughout hospitalization.
   - Client will remain afebrile throughout hospitalization.
   - Client will maintain white blood cell count and differential within normal limits throughout hospitalization.

(Ackley & Ladwig, 2006).

6. A chest drainage system contains three chambers. Identify each chamber.

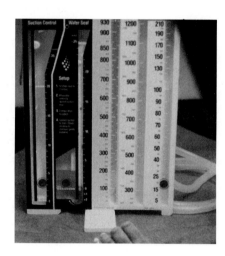

The three chambers of a chest tube drainage system (from left to right) are the suction control chamber, water seal chamber, and fluid/drainage collection chamber.

7. Explain how the nurse sets up a water seal and the function of a water seal. Next, explain how the nurse establishes chest tube suction and the function of the suction. A *water seal* is established by pouring a measured amount of sterile water or saline through a funnel into the designated water seal chamber as instructed in the chest drainage system manufacturer's instructions. The water seal allows air from the pleural space to pass through the fluid in the water seal chamber and bubble out through a vent to the atmosphere, but not return to the client. This mechanism prevents air from entering the pleural cavity and causing a pneumothorax, which can collapse the lung. If wall suction is prescribed, the nurse fills the *suction control* chamber to the prescribed level of fluid (sterile water). Usually 20 cm of fluid is indicated. The nurse then attaches one end of the suction tubing to the suction port on the drainage system (as labeled on the system and indicated in the manufacturer's instructions) and the other end of the tubing to the suction source in the client's room (wall suction). The wall suction should be turned up until there is gentle bubbling in the suction control chamber. Suction control on the chest drainage system provides additional suction to increase the drainage of fluid (or air) from the pleural space. The nurse should document the type of chest drainage system used and the centimeter level of fluid in the suction control chamber (Frisch & Altman, 2004; Strauss, 2007).

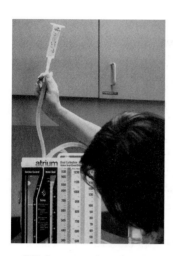

Fill the appropriate chamber with sterile water or saline

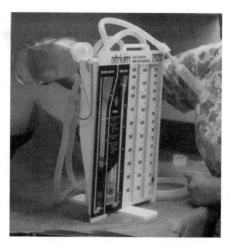

If suction has been prescribed, fill the suction control chamber to the prescribed level of fluid

8. The certified nursing assistant working with the nurse anxiously reports, "Come quick, Mr. Yang's chest tube has fallen out!" The nurse finds that the chest tube is on the floor and that the dressing has partially fallen off. What should the nurse do? Fluid drains from a hemothorax into the fluid collection chamber through a six-foot long flexible tube. All connections between the tubing are airtight. If a connection breaks, or the tube becomes dislodged, there is a high risk of allowing air to move into the pleural space. Emergency items including Vaseline gauze and tape should be available at the client's bedside to be used if the chest tube becomes dislodged or disconnected. The dressing over the insertion site should be removed, and the insertion site covered immediately with an occlusive Vaseline gauze dressing that is secured to the client with tape on three sides of the dressing. The Vaseline gauze establishes a one-way "valve" in which air can exit the pleural space upon exhalation but through which environmental (ambient) air cannot enter. Taping only three sides prevents a tension pneumothorax, a potentially life-threatening condition that occurs when air in the pleural space becomes trapped, creating positive intrapleural pressure that causes the lung to collapse. The nurse should notify the HCP immediately so that the chest tube can be reinserted and a new chest drainage system established (Strauss, 2007).

9. Discuss the nonverbal cues the nurse should monitor indicating that Mr. Yang is in pain. There is much more to listening and communicating than hearing or speaking words. Communication does not need to be elaborate. A few simple words can convey an entire thought or feeling. Learning a few essential words in the client's primary language can facilitate an understanding of common needs. Message boards with pictures of objects and symbols that the client can point to work well also. Hand gestures are capable of conveying a message. Using "sign language" with hand gestures can help to indicate what the nurse would like the client to do or inform the client of what the nurse intends to do next. Nonverbal expression (or body language) is very telling. The nurse must use critical thinking skills to interpret what the client's nonverbal behavior and expressions are "saying." Nonverbal cues that can indicate a person is in pain include guarding an area; assuming a fetal or side-lying position; facial grimacing; wincing; changes in vital signs such as an increase in blood pressure, heart rate, or respiratory rate; inability to deep breathe; diaphoresis; and pupil dilation. Clients in pain may have a loss of appetite, changes in sleep pattern, muscle tension/rigidity, tearfulness/crying, and can often indicate a level of pain on a pain scale such as the Wong-Baker Faces Pain Rating Scale. The nurse should use caution when interpreting what is observed and clarify observations with the client. It is important to recognize that not everyone of a particular culture will conform to a set of expected behaviors. Perceptions and expressions of pain vary widely. Transculturally, nonverbal communication varies widely. Facial expressions and touch often allow the nurse to express care, concern, and comfort, thus helping to develop a therapeutic relationship. With Mr. Yang, however, the nurse should keep in mind that some members of the Hmong culture may not like to be touched on the head and may consider direct eye contact inappropriate and rude (Ackley & Ladwig, 2006; Children's Hospitals and Clinics of Minnesota, 2003; Daniels, 2004; Hmong Cultural Center, 2000; Zator Estes, 2006).

10. Provide an explanation for Mrs. Yang's response when greeted by the nurse. While a smile is considered a sign of greeting and welcome in the Hmong culture, looking an individual in the eye can be considered rude. When speaking to a Hmong person, he or she may not look directly at you or make eye contact. They may look down or away. Shaking an individual's hand during a greeting is a new concept to the traditional Hmong person, especially among women. Traditional Hmong men and women do not usually shake hands with a female. Verbal expressions of welcome are the traditionally accepted greeting. As well, the male is considered the head of the family and should be addressed first. Particularly in elders, decisions regarding health care are made by the men and may be done so according to the advice of a religious leader (shaman) or a clan leader, whom is determined by ancestral lineage (Children's Hospitals and Clinics of Minnesota, 2003; Hmong Cultural Center, 2000).

**11. The nurse expresses to a colleague that she is concerned she will offend the Yangs because she is not familiar with their culture and healthcare beliefs. The colleague states, "I remember learning in nursing school that you should not touch the head of a Hmong person, especially not the head of a child. And do not tell them their children or grandchildren are cute." Discuss the cultural interpretation of touching a Hmong client's head (or that of their children), and why the nurse should refrain from complimenting the child. Most traditional Hmong elders, especially men, do not like a stranger to touch their head. A common belief in the Hmong culture is that the head is considered sacred because the soul lives there. Touching (or patting) the head, especially the head of a child, is considered inappropriate because the gesture may startle the soul from the body. In addition the nurse should not make a comment that a child is "cute." Such compliments in the Hmong culture are not considered favorable. Some believe that if an evil spirit overhears such comments, that spirit will take the child's soul. It is important to recognize that not everyone of a particular culture or religion will conform to a set of expected behaviors. However, a client's cultural and religious beliefs are an important consideration in providing holistic nursing care. If the nurse is unsure, he/she should clarify Mr. Yang's personal beliefs, practices, and preferences with the help of the medical interpreter (Children's Hospitals and Clinics of Minnesota, 2003; Hmong Cultural Center, 2000).

12. It is the end of an eight-hour shift and the nurse is checking the chest drainage system to determine the amount of drainage during their shift of care. The last mark made by the nurse on the previous shift is at 675 mL. The level of fluid in the drainage collection chamber is now at 800 mL. The nurse uses a marker to mark the current level and indicates the time and date of the measurement. How much drainage does the nurse document on the client's intake and output record and should the nurse call to notify the HCP of the output? The nurse documents 125 mL of output from the chest tube on the client's intake and output record. To determine this amount, the nurse subtracts the previous drainage total (675 mL) from the current drainage total (800 mL) to determine the amount of drainage during this shift (125 mL). There is no need to notify the HCP of the output unless the HCP has requested that the nurse do so. The client has had 125 mL of drainage in eight hours (approximately 15 to 16 mL per hour). The nurse would notify the HCP if the client's output were greater (50 to 100 mL) per hour (Johnson & Tang, 2004).

References

Ackley, B., & Ladwig, G. (2006). *Nursing diagnosis handbook: A guide to planning care*. St. Louis, MO: Mosby

Bureau of Labor Statistics, U.S. Department of Labor. (2005). *Occupational outlook handbook, 2006–07 edition: Interpreters and translators*. Retrieved June 24, 2006, from ww.bls.gov.

Children's Hospitals and Clinics of Minnesota. (2003). *Hmong culture and medical traditions*. Retrieved February 18, 2007, from www.xpedio02.childrenshc.org.

Daniels, R. (2004). The nurse-client relationship. In *Nursing fundamentals of nursing: Caring & clinical decision making* (pp. 75–76, 79). Clifton Park, NY: Thomson Learning.

Dennison, P. D. (2007). Lower airway problems. In F. Monahan, J. Sands, M. Neighbors, J. Marek, & C. Green (Eds.), *Phipps' Medical-surgical nursing: Health and illness perspectives* (p. 666). St. Louis, MO: Mosby Elsevier.

Frisch, S., & Altman, G. B. (2004). *Preparing the chest drainage system*. In G. B. Altman (Ed.), *Delmar's fundamental & advanced nursing skills* (pp. 934–937). Clifton Park, NY: Thomson Learning.

Hmong Cultural Center. (2000). *Etiquette for interacting with the Hmong*. Retrieved February 18, 2007, from www.hmongcenter.org.

Johnson, K., & Tang, H. (2004). *Measuring the output from a chest drainage system*. In G. B. Altman (Ed.), *Delmar's fundamental & advanced nursing skills* (pp. 953–955). Clifton Park, NY: Thomson Learning.

Minnesota Medical Association. (2004). *A physician's guide to language interpreter services*. Retrieved June 25, 2006, from www.mmaonline.net.

Strauss, B. (2007). Lower airway dysfunction: Nursing management. In R. Daniels, L. H. Nicoll, & L. J. Nosek (Eds.), *Contemporary medical-surgical nursing* (pp. 1082–1087). St. Louis, MO: Mosby Elsevier.

United States Department of Health and Human Services (HHS). (2003). *HSS publishes new guidelines on language service for people with limited English proficiency*. Retrieved June 25, 2006, from www.hhs.gov.

White, A. H. (2005). Management of clients with acute pulmonary disorders. In *Black & Hawks' Medical-surgical nursing: Clinical management for positive outcomes* (pp. 1905–1906). St. Louis, MO: Elsevier.

Zator Estes, M.E. (2006). Cultural assessment. In *Health assessment & physical examination* (p. 126). Clifton Park, NY: Thomson Delmar Learning.

CASE STUDY 2

Mrs. Harriet

GENDER

Female

AGE

68

SETTING

- Hospital

ETHNICITY

- Black American

CULTURAL CONSIDERATIONS

PREEXISTING CONDITION

- Allergy to erythromycin and aspirin

COEXISTING CONDITION

- Obesity

COMMUNICATION

DISABILITY

SOCIOECONOMIC

- Retired
- Lives at home with her husband
- Volunteers as a receptionist at a local adult community center
- Smokes a half of a pack of cigarettes per day
- Positive tobacco use for 54 years

SPIRITUAL/RELIGIOUS

PHARMACOLOGIC

- Dextromethorphan hydrobromide (Robitussin Maximum Strength); isoniazid (INH, Nydrazid); ceftriaxone sodium (Rocephin); erythromycin; azithromycin (Zithromax); albuterol (Proventil, Ventolin); acetaminophen (Tylenol)

LEGAL

ETHICAL

ALTERNATIVE THERAPY

PRIORITIZATION

- Respiratory isolation until diagnosis of tuberculosis is ruled out

DELEGATION

- Smoking cessation and weight loss programs

THE RESPIRATORY SYSTEM

Level of Difficulty: Difficult

Overview: This case requires the nurse to recognize the clinical manifestations of bronchitis and pneumonia. The possibility of exposure to tuberculosis is also considered, and Mantoux testing is discussed. The client's risk factors for pneumonia and lifestyle considerations to help prevent pneumonia in the future are reviewed. Rationales for the health care provider's (HCP) prescribed diagnostic tests and the treatment plan are provided. The client's arterial blood gases (ABGs) are analyzed. Teaching a client the proper use of an incentive spirometer is reviewed.

Client Profile

Mrs. Harriet is a 68-year-old woman who is alert and oriented. She presents to the emergency department with complaints of chest tightness, shortness of breath, cough, and congestion. She states, "I have been having these symptoms for three days now. I have been taking Maximum Strength Robitussin for my cough but it has not helped very much. When I woke up this morning, I felt very weak so I came in to be checked out." Her vital signs are blood pressure 110/70, pulse 94, respiratory rate of 28, and a temperature of 102.7°F (39.3°C). Her oxygen saturation on room air is 92%. She is placed on 2 liters (L) of oxygen by nasal cannula. The HCP prescribes a 12-lead electrocardiogram (ECG, EKG) and chest X-ray (CXR). Laboratory tests prescribed include complete blood count (CBC), basic metabolic panel (BMP), brain natriuretic peptide (B-type natriuretic peptide assay or BNP), total creatine kinase (CK, CPK), creatine kinase-MB (CPK-MB), and troponin. The HCP will also assess blood cultures × 2, ABGs on room air, sputum culture and sensitivity (C&S), and asks that the client have a Mantoux (tuberculin, purified protein derivative, or PPD) test.

Case Study

Mrs. Harriet's ECG shows normal sinus rhythm (NSR) with a heart rate of 98 beats per minute. The CXR reveals a right lower lobe (RLL) infiltrate. Laboratory tests include the following results: white blood cell count (WBC) 12,200 cells/mm^3, 72% seg neutrophils with a left shift of 11% bands, and a BNP of 50.9 pg/mL. ABGs on room air are pH 7.44, partial pressure of carbon dioxide (PaCO$_2$) 39 mmHg, bicarbonate (HCO$_3^-$) 26.9 mEq/L, partial pressure of oxygen (PaO$_2$) 58 mmHg, and oxygen saturation (SaO$_2$) of 92%. Results of the sputum culture show *Streptoccus pneumoniae*. The CPK, CPK-MB, and troponin are all within normal limits. Mrs. Harriet is five feet three inches tall and weighs 224 pounds (101.8 kg). On assessment, the nurse hears expiratory wheezes and rhonchi bilaterally with diminished lung sounds in the right base. Her thoracic (chest) expansion is equal but slightly decreased on inspiration. Accessory muscle retraction is not noted, and she does not exhibit central cyanosis. Capillary refill of the client's nail beds is four seconds.

Mrs. Harriet is admitted with acute bronchitis and pneumonia. The HCP prescribes oxygen via nasal cannula to keep the client's oxygen saturation ≥95%, ceftriaxone sodium, erythromycin, albuterol, acetaminophen every four to six hours as needed, bed rest, an 1800-calorie diet, increased oral (PO) fluid intake to 2 to 4 liters per day, coughing and deep breathing exercises, and use of an incentive spirometer (IS).

Questions

1. Discuss additional assessment data that would be helpful in gaining a more thorough understanding of Mrs. Harriet's symptoms.

2. Discuss the causes, pathophysiology, and symptoms of acute bronchitis.

3. Discuss the pathophysiology and causes of pneumonia in general.

4. Compare the defining characteristics of *community-acquired pneumonia, hospital-acquired pneumonia,* and *viral pneumonia.*

5. Discuss the factors that place Mrs. Harriet at greater risk for the development of pneumonia.

6. Mrs. Harriet asks the nurse to explain what the HCP saw on her chest X-ray. She asks, "The doctor said something about a 'trate' he saw on my lung. What did he mean by that?" How would the nurse explain what an infiltrate is?

7. Briefly explain the pathophysiology, and identify at least five clinical manifestations of the respiratory diagnosis that is being ruled out for Mrs. Harriet by administering the Mantoux test.

8. While awaiting test results to confirm if Mrs. Harriet has TB, what precautions should be taken when assigning her to a room and providing nursing care?

9. Discuss the measurement of induration that would indicate a positive Mantoux test for Mrs. Harriet. If she tested positive for exposure to TB but did not have assessment findings consistent with active disease, what medication could be prescribed, and what is the benefit of this treatment?

10. The nurse asks Mrs. Harriet if she has been using her incentive spirometer.

Mrs. Harriet states, "I tried to use it a couple of times but I think it is broken. When I blow into it, the ball does not go up like I was told it should." How should the nurse intervene?

11. Briefly discuss the significance of each of the following laboratory results: (a) WBC 12,200 cells/mm^3, (b) 72% seg neutrophils (c) left shift of 11% bands, (d) BNP 50.9 pg/mL, (e) results of the sputum culture show *S. pneumoniae,* (f) CPK within normal limits, (g) CPK-MB within normal limits, and (h) troponin within normal limits.

12. Analyze Mrs. Harriet's ABG results. Determine whether each value is high, low, or within normal limits; interpret the acid-base balance; determine if there is compensation; and indicate whether the client has hypoxemia.

13. The nurse calls the HCP to request a change in the medications that have been prescribed for Mrs. Harriet. Discuss which medication the nurse is concerned is unsafe for this client.

14. Provide a rationale for each of the following prescribed components of Mrs. Harriet's treatment plan: oxygen to keep the client's oxygen saturation ≥95%, ceftriaxone sodium, albuterol, acetaminophen, bed rest, 1800-calorie diet, increased oral (PO) fluid intake to 2 to 4 liters per day, coughing and deep breathing exercises, and use of an incentive spirometer.

15. Mrs. Harriet was taking dextromethorphan at home to help manage her cough. The HCP did not prescribe continued use of the dextromethorphan during hospitalization. Explain this omission.

16. If it was learned that Mrs. Harriet has a past medical history of chronic obstructive lung disease (COPD), how would the

Questions (continued)

HCP's prescription that oxygen be delivered to keep the client's oxygen saturation ≥95% be changed?

17. Identify three priority nursing diagnoses that should be included on Mrs. Harriet's plan of care.

18. You are the nurse providing discharge teaching to Mrs. Harriet. Briefly discuss what you will recommend to her regarding seeking follow-up care, lifestyle considerations, and how to help prevent pneumonia in the future.

Questions and Suggested Answers

1. Discuss additional assessment data that would be helpful in gaining a more thorough understanding of Mrs. Harriet's symptoms. Other symptoms to assess include rhinitis (profuse nasal discharge, also called coryza), chills, back and muscle pain (myalgia), headache, and a sore throat, which are indicative of an upper respiratory tract infection that often accompanies or precedes bronchitis. The nurse should ask if Mrs. Harriet's cough is productive or nonproductive and assess the amount, color, and consistency of the sputum. Mrs. Harriet's nail beds and lips may be pale. Clients with bronchitis often have pleuritic chest pain. The nurse would assess for pleuritic chest pain by asking Mrs. Harriet if her chest pain increases with inspiration. She may exhibit a general tension of her facial or shoulder muscles since pain, fatigue, and shortness of breath can promote anxiety. Clients with bronchitis and/or pneumonia often have increased tactile fremitus on assessment. Tactile (or vocal) fremitus is the palpable vibration of the chest wall (most commonly using the ulnar aspect of the hand) produced when the client says "99" or "1, 2, 3." Diseases that involve consolidation, such as bronchitis and pneumonia, often result in increased tactile fremitus in the affected area because solids conduct sound better than air. A patient with a large chest wall, or who is obese, such as Mrs. Harriet, may not have as prominent an increase in tactile fremitus since the sound waves are dampened as they pass through a greater distance (Zator Estes, 2006). Assessment of voice sounds also helps to determine if the lungs are filled with air, fluid, or are solid. Bronchophony, egophony, and whispered pectoriloquy are three variations of the same assessment technique to auscultate the transmission of the client's spoken word. Consolidation in the lung, such as pneumonia, will produce a clear transmission of the voice sounds since sound is transmitted well through a fluid medium. For example, the client with pneumonia will often have clear transmission of "99" or "1, 2, 3" while performing bronchophony or whispered pectoriloquy; and the transformation of the spoken "ee" to an "ay" sound while performing egophony. Percussion over the affected lobe of the right lung will be dull. Tracheal position should be midline, although there may be a slight shift to the affected (right) side (Zator Estes, 2006). Asking Mrs. Harriet about her fluid intake in the past 24 to 72 hours as well as assessing her serum blood urea nitrogen (BUN) and creatinine, sodium, skin turgor, and orthostatic (postural) vital signs can help detect dehydration. In addition, Mrs. Harriet should be asked if she received the influenza vaccine this year or the pneumococcal (pneumonia polysaccharide) vaccine within the past five years. It would be helpful to know if she is aware of any adults who visit the community center who have been diagnosed with pneumonia or have exhibited symptoms of a respiratory infection recently. The nurse is aware that Mrs. Harriet is a tobacco smoker. Mrs. Harriet should also be asked about exposure to the fumes of chemical agents, dust, or air pollution. Mrs. Harriet should be asked of she has recently taken an antibiotic for any reason since this may obscure identification of the causative bacteria and may increase the chance that she has an antimicrobial resistance (Dennison, 2007; Workman, 2006).

2. Discuss the causes, pathophysiology, and symptoms of acute bronchitis. Acute bronchitis is an inflammation of the bronchi. Often the inflammation also involves the trachea, making the diagnosis "tracheobronchitis" also accurate for the client with acute bronchitis. Acute bronchitis is most common in clients with chronic lung disease, but it also occurs in the client with an upper respiratory tract infection. Acute bronchitis in the client without underlying lung disease is communicable to others. Acute bronchitis is most often viral, but bacteria such as *S. pneumoniae* and *Haemophilus influenzae* also cause bronchitis. Physical or chemical agents such as tobacco, dust, fumes, and air pollution also trigger acute bronchitis. The incidence of bronchitis increases in the spring and late winter. The respiratory tract of a healthy individual is usually able to destroy inhaled microbes through its defense mechanisms. However, when these defense mechanisms are weakened, bacteria that are normally contained within the nose and pharynx may colonize in the trachea and bronchi. Blood flow to the affected area increases in response to the inflammatory response, causing the increased production of pulmonary secretions. As a result, the client experiences a painful productive cough, low-grade fever, malaise, and chest pain resulting from the inflammation of the tracheal wall and repeated coughing. Wheezes and rhonchi are common when assessing lung sounds. Symptoms may last one to four weeks. Pneumonia should be suspected if the client with acute bronchitis has a worsening of symptoms, high fever, shortness of breath, pleuritic chest pain, tachypnea (increased respiratory rate), crackles, or consolidation visible on a chest X-ray (Dennison, 2007, Workman, 2006).

3. Discuss the pathophysiology and causes of pneumonia in general. The seventh leading causes of death from an infectious agent, pneumonia is an acute inflammation of lung tissue caused by infection with bacteria, viruses, or other organisms (American Lung Association, 2006; Schmitt, 2004). Infection results from the inhalation of an infectious agent or the transport of an infectious agent to the lungs via the bloodstream. People develop pneumonia when their body's immune system is unable to combat invading organisms from the environment, from invasive medical devices or supplies, or from other people. The highest incidence of pneumonia in adults occurs in older adults, those residing in long-term care facilities, hospitalized clients, and individuals on mechanical ventilation. Pneumonia is an excess of fluid in the lungs that results from inflammation of the interstitial spaces, alveoli, and often the bronchioles. White blood cells migrate to the area of infection and cause local capillary leak, edema, and exudates. These fluids collect in and around the alveoli and the alveolar walls thicken. These changes reduce gas exchange and lead to hypoxemia. Red blood cells and fibrin also move into the alveoli. The capillary leak facilitates the spread of the infection to other areas of the lung. Fibrin and edema cause the lung to stiffen, which reduces compliance and decreases the vital capacity of the lung. The alveoli can collapse (called atelectasis), which reduces the lung's ability to oxygenate the blood that moves through the collapsed alveoli. This causes a decreased arterial oxygen tension leading to an insufficient amount of oxygen in the blood (hypoxemia). Pneumonia can be lobar with consolidation (solidification or lack of air spaces) in a segment or entire lobe of the lung. Diffusely scattered patches may also develop around the bronchi (bronchopneumonia). Pneumonia is caused by viruses, bacteria, mycoplasmas, fungi, rickettsiae, protozoa, and helminthes (worms). Dramatic shifts in antimicrobial resistance patterns have resulted in significant changes in the pathogens that cause bacterial pneumonia. Noninfectious causes include radiation treatment, inhalation of noxious fumes or chemicals, and the aspiration of food, fluid, or vomitus. Pneumonia is classified as either community-acquired pneumonia or hospital-acquired pneumonia (HAP or nosocomial pneumonia). Classification is determined by where the person was exposed to the infectious agent that caused the infection (American Lung Association, 2006; Dennison, 2007; Schmitt, 2004; Workman, 2006).

4. Compare the defining characteristics of *community-acquired pneumonia*, *hospital-acquired pneumonia*, and *viral pneumonia*. Individuals who are not hospitalized or residing in a long-term care facility within 14 days of the onset of their acute infection are diagnosed with *community-acquired pneumonia*. CAP is more common than HAP and occurs most frequently in late fall and winter as a complication of influenza. CAP affects healthy individuals, but most often (70% of cases) it affects those with preexisting conditions or infections such as chronic obstructive pulmonary disease (COPD), diabetes mellitus, or heart failure. Also at increased risk are those with impaired immunity, such as with acquired immune deficiency syndrome (AIDS), cancer, or an organ transplant. CAP is common and is associated with significant morbidity and mortality rates that range from 1% in outpatients to 30% in those requiring hospitalization. The most commonly identified pathogen in CAP, and most frequent cause of fatal CAP, is *S. pneumoniae* (American Lung Association, 2006; Schmitt, 2004). The onset of bacterial pneumonia can be sudden or gradual. The clinical manifestations of CAP include fever, chills (rigors), sweats, productive or nonproductive cough, a change in the color of the sputum, chest discomfort, and shortness of breath (Dennison, 2007; Schmitt, 2004; Workman, 2006).

HAP is acquired 48 hours or more after hospitalization. HAP is the "second most common nosocomial infection in the United States and the leading cause of death from nosocomial infections. Nearly 1% of clients admitted to the hospital develop pneumonia, and nearly one-third of these die. Up to 60% of clients in intensive care units (ICUs) develop pneumonia" (Dennison, 2007, p. 624). The majority of HAP infections are caused by gram-negative aerobes such as *Staphylococcus aureus, Pseudomonas aeruginosa, Enterobacter,* and *Klebsiella pneumonia.* HAP develops following the aspiration of bacteria into the lower respiratory tract and colonization when clients have impaired defenses or an underlying disease, such as COPD, heart failure, stroke, or malignancy (Dennison, 2007; Workman, 2006).

Viral pneumonia accounts for approximately 50% of all cases of pneumonia and 8% of the cases of pneumonia in adults. Viral pneumonia illness is usually less severe than bacterial pneumonia. Different viruses are responsible and vary with the age distribution of the population and the season. Influenza virus accounts for 50% or more of the cases, and respiratory syncytial virus (RSV) is increasingly recognized as another cause, but primarily in the very young. Symptoms of viral pneumonia are similar to the symptoms of influenza (flu) with individuals often experiencing fever, headache, muscle pain, a nonproductive cough, weakness, and increasing dyspnea (American Lung Association, 2006; Dennison, 2007).

5. Discuss the factors that place Mrs. Harriet at greater risk for the development of pneumonia. Several factors are of concern and may have increased Mrs. Harriet's risk of developing pneumonia. Mrs. Harriet is 68 years old. Advanced age increases the risk that an adult will develop pneumonia. The highest rate of pneumonia is seen in those 65 and older (American Lung Association, 2006). Mrs. Harriet volunteers as a receptionist at a local adult community center, which exposes her to many people and thus an increased bacterial exposure and risk of transmission of respiratory diseases. As well, she smokes a half of a pack of cigarettes per day and has a long history of tobacco use (54 years). Tobacco use is a risk factor associated with community-acquired pneumonia. Another consideration is that she is retired. Perhaps she does not have adequate health care insurance coverage as a retired adult, which could result in less frequent HCP examinations and opportunities for receiving annual vaccinations. Pneumonia and influenza vaccines are covered by Medicare, as well as some state and private insurance companies (American Lung Association, 2006). She does work at an adult community center, and perhaps this affords her an opportunity to obtain information about participation in community-sponsored vaccination clinics if in fact her health care coverage is not adequate.

6. Mrs. Harriet asks the nurse to explain what the health care provider saw on her chest X-ray. She asks, "The doctor said something about a 'trate' he saw on my lung. What did he mean by that?" How would the nurse explain what an infiltrate is? The term "infiltrate" is used to describe an accumulation of substances in a tissue not normal to that area or in amounts in excess of normal findings. The infiltrate visualized in the right lower lobe of the lung on Mrs. Harriet's chest X-ray is the result of local capillary leak, edema, and exudates. This indicates the area of the infection in her lung.

7. Briefly explain the pathophysiology and identify at least five clinical manifestations of the respiratory diagnosis that is being ruled out for Mrs. Harriet by administering the Mantoux test. A diagnosis of tuberculosis (TB) should be considered for an individual who presents with a persistent cough, shortness of breath, fever, pallor, chills, night sweats, hemoptysis (blood-stained sputum), anorexia, weight loss, and/or chest pain. TB is a highly communicable infectious disease caused by the *Mycobacterium tuberculosis* (or tubercle bacillus) organism. Each year there are approximately 8 million new cases of TB and 3 million deaths attributed to TB (Jarahzadeh & Sutjita, 2003). Individuals most at risk are those with AIDS, immigrants, and individuals of low-economic status (Dennison, 2007). TB infection occurs when an individual with no previous exposure to TB inhales a sufficient number of the tubercle bacillus organism into their alveoli. The organism is transmitted via aerosolization (airborne route) when a person with active TB infection coughs, sneezes, or laughs, for example. As the body's natural defense mechanism, inflammation then occurs within the alveoli (parenchyma). The inflammatory process and subsequent cellular reaction result in the formation of a small, firm white nodule called a primary tubercle. Cells gather around the center of this nodule in the lung, and the outer portion becomes fibrosed. Blood vessels are compressed, and nutrition of the tubercle is impaired, causing necrosis at the center of the tubercle. This area of the lung becomes walled off and gradually becomes an area of soft necrosis, which can become calcified or liquefy. If a liquefied material forms, the person may cough up the liquefied necrosis, leaving a cavity or hole in the parenchyma of the lung. This cavitation is visible on a chest X-ray (Dennison, 2007; Workman, 2006).

Most people who are exposed to TB and develop the infection will have a positive Mantoux test, but do not develop an active form of the disease. These individuals will have a visible calcified nodule known as a "Ghon tubercle" or "primary complex" on a chest X-ray. These individuals are now sensitized to the tubercle bacillus and will always test positive when the Mantoux test is administered since there will be an antigen-antibody reaction when they receive an injection of the purified protein derivative (PPD) antigen (Dennison, 2007).

8. While awaiting test results to confirm if Mrs. Harriet has TB, what precautions should be taken when assigning her to a room and providing nursing care? Clients suspected of having tuberculosis are assigned to a private respiratory (acid fast bacilli or AFB) isolation room and placed on droplet and airborne precautions. Droplet precautions protect those providing care from infections transmitted by large-particle droplets generated during coughing, sneezing, or speaking and from aerosol-generating procedures such as suctioning. Organisms transmitted by this method travel approximately three feet from the client and settle onto surfaces where they can no longer be inhaled. Airborne precautions reduce the transmission of organisms in dust particles and in the airborne droplet nuclei of evaporated droplets. The respiratory isolation room should be maintained at negative pressure relative to the hallway to prevent the client's room air from flowing into the hallway when the door is open. Negative-pressure rooms ventilate the air in the client's room directly to the outside with frequent air exchanges (six to 12 exchanges per hour) avoiding the spread of infectious particles to others on the nursing unit. In addition, high-efficiency particulate air (HEPA) filtration systems and ultraviolet germicidal irradiation (UVGI) lights can be used in the isolation room to reduce the concentration of infectious TB droplets. All health care workers entering Mrs. Harriet's room should use NIOSH-certified (National Institute for Occupational Safety and Health) personal protective equipment called particulate respirators (also called N-95 HEPA filter respirators). These masks filter droplet nuclei and are fitted to each HCP to insure a proper fit and maximum protection. TB is not spread by handling the client's bed sheets, furniture, eating utensils, or personal belongings. HCPs should be screened annually for TB infection and disease. Those who are in frequent contact with clients infected with TB should be tested more often (every six months) (ALA, 2006; York, 2007).

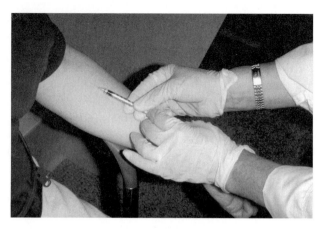

Administrating the Mantoux skin test

9. Discuss the measurement of induration that would indicate a positive Mantoux test for Mrs. Harriet. If she tested positive for exposure to TB but did not have assessment findings consistent with active disease, what medication could be prescribed and what is the benefit of this treatment? The Mantoux test (also called the tuberculin or PPD skin test) evaluates the body's cell-mediated immune function and determines the body's sensitivity to infectious agents. A positive reaction is manifested by a hardened or raised area (induration) at the site of the intradermal injection 48 to 72 hours following administration of the test and indicates that the client has developed antibodies to the agent. Singh, Sutton, & Woodcock (2002) suggest assessing the test at 72 hours to help decrease the risk of a false-negative result when read after only 48 hours. Induration of ≥15 mm is positive for clients in low-risk groups with no known risk factors for TB. Induration of ≥10 mm is considered positive for clients in high-risk groups. A high-risk group includes children under four years of age, recent immigrants, injection drug users, those with illnesses that place them at risk (e.g., diabetes, chronic renal failure, and cancer) and residents or employees of high-risk settings, including prisons, long-term care facilities, and hospitals. Induration of ≥5 mm is positive for individuals at greatest risk, including those with human immunodeficiency virus, organ transplant, recent contact with a person with TB, or a chest X-ray that reveals fibrotic changes consistent with prior TB. For individuals with no known risk factors for TB, such as Mrs. Harriet, an area of induration of 15 mm or more is significant for a past or present TB infection. An induration of 5 to 14 mm for Mrs. Harriet is not likely indicative of infection, but retesting may be suggested to confirm. An area of 4 mm or less (or no induration at all) is a negative result. A negative Mantoux test should be repeated if it is determined that Mrs. Harriet has been exposed to someone with TB (perhaps at the community center). If warranted, the test is often repeated in four to six weeks since it can take that long for the Mantoux test to convert to positive. A positive skin test reaction must be evaluated further by assessing clinical symptoms and the findings of a chest X-ray and acid fast bacillus sputum culture to confirm active TB disease (Dennison, 2007; York, 2007).

If Mrs. Harriet tested positive for tuberculosis exposure, then she has been infected with *M. tuberculosis* and will harbor this organism in her lung for the remainder of her life. The organism remains walled-off in a resting state within the lung. Although minimal (one out of 10 persons), the risk is that when she is under physical or emotional stress in the future, this organism can become active and multiply and cause active TB disease. Isoniazid is an antitubercular drug that interferes with lipid and nucleic acid metabolism of growing bacteria. Isoniazid can be prescribed prophylactically to decrease her risk of developing active disease in the future. Isoniazid kills actively growing organisms in the extracellular environment and inhibits the growth of the dormant *M. tuberculosis* organism. This protection is believed to last a person's lifetime (Dennison, 2007; Spratto & Woods, 2006).

10. The nurse asks Mrs. Harriet if she has been using her incentive spirometer. Mrs. Harriet states, "I tried to use it a couple of times but I think it is broken. When I blow into it, the ball does not go up like I was told it should." How should the nurse intervene? The nurse should provide additional teaching. Mrs. Harriet is not using the incentive spirometer (IS) correctly. She is exhaling into the IS instead of inhaling. The nurse should review the steps for using the IS correctly and ask Mrs. Harriet to demonstrate proper use of the IS to assess her level of comprehension of the instructions and ability to use the IS effectively. The steps for using the IS include:

1. Take a normal breath and exhale.
2. Hold the IS upright and seal her mouth and lips completely around the IS mouthpiece.
3. Take a slow, deep breath in (as if sucking through a straw) to elevate the ball or plastic bar within the plastic chamber/tube.
4. Hold her inspiration for at least three seconds.
5. Simultaneously, she should measure the amount of inspired air volume using the calibrated plastic tube.
6. Remove the mouthpiece and exhale normally.
7. Take several normal breaths.
8. Repeat these steps up to ten times per session every hour while awake.

Mrs. Harriet should splint and cough after incentive effort to expel sputum and then wash her hands to help prevent the transmission of bacteria to others (Altman, 2004).

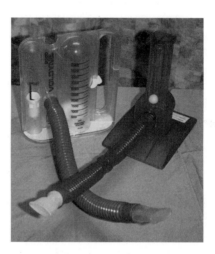

Incentive spirometer

11. Briefly discuss the significance of each of the following laboratory results: (a) WBC 12,200 cells/mm³, (b) 72% seg neutrophils, (c) left shift of 11% bands, (d) BNP 50.9 pg/mL, (e) results of the sputum culture show S. pneumoniae, (f) CPK within normal limits, (g) CPK-MB within normal limits, and (h) troponin within normal limits.

(a) *WBC 12,200 cells/mm³:* White blood cells (WBCs; leukocytes) encapsulate organisms and destroy them. The body uses WBCs to fight infection. An elevated WBC count (leukocytosis), resulting from the inflammatory process, is a common finding in the client with an acute infection such as pneumonia.

(b) *72% seg neutrophils:* There are five different types of WBCs: neutrophils, eosinophils, basophils, lymphocytes, and monocytes. Neutrophils are the primary defense against bacterial infection. There are two types of neutrophils: segmented neutrophils (segs) and band neutrophils (bands). The normal range for segs is 54% to 62%. Elevated segs indicate infection.

(c) *Left shift of 11% bands:* There are two types of neutrophils: segmented neutrophils (segs) and band neutrophils (bands). Bands are immature neutrophils that multiply quickly in the presence of acute infection. The normal range for bands is 3% to 5%. Elevated bands indicate acute infection. An increased number of band cells is called a "shift to the left" or "left shift." This terminology originated in reference to the traditional diagram of neutrophil maturation that shows the stem cell on the left of the diagram with progressive stages of maturation moving toward the right, ending with a fully mature neutrophil on the right side of the diagram. A shift to the left indicates that there are more immature cells present in the blood than normally occurs (Smeltzer & Bare, 2004).

(d) *BNP 50.9 pg/mL:* Also called B-type natriuretic peptide assay or proBNP, the brain natriuretic peptide is a cardiac biomarker. It is prescribed to help diagnose heart failure and to grade the severity of heart failure. A high BNP level is a good predictor of increased risk of death or subsequent heart attack in patients with acute coronary syndromes. Concentrations of 80 pg/mL or greater accurately diagnose heart failure. However, standard reference values are dependent on many factors, including age, gender, and test method. Levels correlate with the severity of heart failure. A BNP is useful for distinguishing heart failure from pulmonary disease.

(e) *Results of the sputum culture show* S. pneumoniae: *S. pneumoniae* is a gram-positive organism. It is the organism causing Mrs. Harriet's respiratory infections. This information helps the HCP to select an appropriate anti-infective medication to treat the infection.

(f) *CPK within normal limits:* CPK (CK, creatine kinase) is an enzyme contained in the heart muscle, skeletal muscle, and the brain. When the heart muscle is damaged, such as in a myocardial infarction, CPK is released into the blood. Creatine kinase is composed of three isoenzymes: CK-MB (heart muscle), CK-MM (skeletal muscle), and CK-BB (brain).

(g) *CPK-MB* within normal limits: CPK-MB (creatine kinase-MB) is a cardiac isoenzyme released specifically from the cardiac muscle and indicating cardiac muscle damage.

(h) *Troponin* within normal limits: Troponin is an inhibitory protein found primarily in cardiac muscle. Troponin is a good indicator of myocardial injury because it is released as early as one hour after relatively small amounts of cardiac injury and will remain elevated for two weeks postcardiac injury.

CPK, CPK-MB, and troponin values all within normal limits indicate that Mrs. Harriet has not had any acute cardiac muscle injury (myocardial infarction) within the past few days that could be causing her symptoms.

(Chernecky & Berger, 2004; Daniels, 2002; Workman, 2006)

12. Analyze Mrs. Harriet's ABG results. Determine whether each value is high, low, or within normal limits; interpret the acid-base balance; determine if there is compensation; and indicate whether the client has

hypoxemia. ABGs help to determine Mrs. Harriet's baseline arterial oxygen and carbon dioxide levels and help to determine her need for supplemental oxygen. Several ABGs may be necessary to understand the client's acid/base balance, and the nurse must look at the whole picture of the client's status to make an accurate assessment. Mrs. Harriet's ABGs on room air are pH 7.44, partial pressure of carbon dioxide ($PaCO_2$) 39 mmHg, bicarbonate (HCO_3^-) 26.9 mEq/L, partial pressure of oxygen (PaO_2) 58 mmHg, and SaO_2 of 92%.

- pH of 7.44 is within the normal limits of 7.35 to 7.45.
- $PaCO_2$ of 39 mmHg is within the normal limits of 35 to 45 mmHg.
- HCO_3^- of 26.9 mEq/L is slightly elevated above the normal limits of 22 to 26 mEq/L.
- PaO_2 of 58 mmHg is below the normal limits of 75 to 100 mmHg.
- SaO_2 of 92% is below the normal limits of 95% to 100%.

Interpretation: Partially compensated respiratory alkalosis with moderate hypoxemia (Chernecky & Berger, 2004; Daniels, 2002)

13. **The nurse calls the HCP to request a change in the medications that have been prescribed for Mrs. Harriet. Discuss which medication the nurse is concerned is unsafe for this client.** Erythromycin is an antibiotic (or macrolide) recommended for the treatment of CAP, especially if there is concern that the client has *Mycoplasma, Chlamydia,* or *Legionella.* However, this is not an appropriate option for Mrs. Harriet since she has an allergy to erythromycin. Recognizing this potential risk to Mrs. Harriet's safety, the nurse should not administer the erythromycin and should notify the HCP to ask that a different medication be prescribed (Spratto & Woods, 2006; Workman, 2006).

14. **Provide a rationale for each of the following prescribed components of Mrs. Harriet's treatment plan: oxygen to keep the client's oxygen saturation ≥95%, ceftriaxone sodium, albuterol, acetaminophen, bed rest, 1800-calorie diet, increased oral (PO) fluid intake to 2 to 4 liters per day, coughing and deep breathing exercises, and use of an incentive spirometer.** *Oxygen* is administered by nasal cannula or mask to maintain an adequate oxygen saturation and is often indicated when the partial pressure of oxygen (PaO_2) is less than 60 mmHg (which is the case for Mrs. Harriet). Oxygen should be delivered at the lowest concentration needed to achieve the desired pulse oximetry saturation. In this case, the desired oxygen saturation is ≥95%.

Ceftriaxone sodium is a third-generation cephalosporin. This anti-infective is prescribed to treat lower respiratory tract infections caused by *S. pneumoniae,* which is the causative organism as indicated by Mrs. Harriet's sputum culture result. The choice of initial antibiotic therapy for the client with CAP has a direct effect on survival. Initiating therapy with the correct antibiotic within eight hours or less is the ideal treatment approach (Dennison, 2007). The choice of antibiotic is reconsidered if results of a culture and sensitivity indicate that therapy should be modified to address the bacteria's specific sensitivity or resistance.

Albuterol is an inhaled beta-2-agonist that has been prescribed to help decrease Mrs. Harriet's symptoms of expiratory wheezing and rhonchi heard on assessment. Albuterol is a sympathomimetic that stimulates the beta-2 receptors of the bronchi which leads to bronchodilation. It is effective in the treatment of bronchospasm due to reversible obstructive airway disease and acute attacks of bronchospasm. An inhaled bronchodilator should be administered using a metered-dose inhaler with a spacer device to enhance safe and effective delivery of the medication to the lungs.

Acetaminophen is a mild analgesic-antipyretic medication prescribed to help decrease the client's level of discomfort and decrease the client's fever. Aspirin may also be prescribed for a client; however, this is contraindicated in Mrs. Harriet's case because she is allergic to aspirin.

Bed rest has been prescribed to conserve Mrs. Harriet's energy since recovery from pneumonia requires rest and gradual resumption of activities.

An 1800-calorie diet has been prescribed because an adequate and balanced diet facilitates recovery from bacterial infections. Smaller, more frequent meals may be better tolerated than three large meals depending on Mrs. Harriet's level of fatigue.

Increasing the client's PO fluid intake to 2 to 4 liters per day helps to decrease her risk of dehydration, which can cause thick, tenacious sputum production. Increasing her intake of fluids will also help to decrease the viscosity of pulmonary secretions and help her to expectorate the secretions more easily.

The nurse teaches the client effective *coughing and deep breathing exercises* (called the huff cough technique) to help promote airway clearance by expelling airway secretions. The client is instructed to inspire deeply and hold the breath for a few seconds. Mrs. Harriet should hold a pillow over her chest (splinting) to minimize discomfort and then cough forcefully two or three times with her mouth open. She repeats this exercise several times and then rests. This controlled cough and forced expiration technique promotes movement of the mucus along the pulmonary tree from the lower respiratory tract to the upper tract for expectoration. Mrs. Harriet should do this exercise at least every two hours.

An *incentive spirometer* (also referred to as sustained maximal inspiration) is a deep-breathing exerciser that increases lung expansion, keeps alveoli open, helps remove mucous secretions, and strengthens respiratory muscles. Use of an incentive spirometer can help prevent or reverse atelectasis (alveolar collapse) (Altman, 2004; Dennison, 2007; Workman, 2006).

15. Mrs. Harriet was taking dextromethorphan at home to help manage her cough. The HCP did not prescribe continued use of the dextromethorphan during hospitalization. Explain this omission. Dextromethorphan is a common ingredient in over-the-counter antitussives that helps relieve the nonproductive cough caused by a cold or inhaled irritant. Dextromethorphan has a direct effect on the cough center in the medulla, which suppresses the cough reflex. Coughing is necessary, however, to clear the secretions caused by infection. This medication can cause bronchial secretions to become more viscous and result in the client having difficulty expectorating them. Upon arrival to the emergency department, Mrs. Harriet noted, "I have been taking Robitussin for my cough but it has not helped very much." In addition, it has been determined that her pneumonia is bacterial and not viral. For these reasons, the continued use of dextromethorphan as part of Mrs. Harriet's treatment plan will not offer relief of her symptoms (Deglin & Vallerand, 2005; Spratto & Woods, 2006).

16. If it was learned that Mrs. Harriet has a past medical history of chronic obstructive lung disease (COPD), how would the HCP's prescription that oxygen be delivered to keep the client's oxygen saturation ≥95% be changed? In patients without COPD, increased levels of carbon dioxide (CO_2) in the blood act as a stimulus to breathe. For a client with COPD, however, the opposite is true. It is a decrease in blood oxygenation (hypoxemia) and an increase in CO_2 levels that stimulates respiration. The respiratory system of a client with COPD adjusts to a state of oxygenation-perfusion mismatch and compensates to create a new "balance." Increasing the flow of oxygen (over 2 liters per minute) causes increased oxygenation and suppresses a COPD client's drive to breathe. While a higher level of oxygen will increase a client's oxygen saturation level in the short term, doing so causes the client to breathe at a slower rate. This oxygen-induced hypoventilation, which can cause a toxic increase of CO_2 in the body, is prevented by administering oxygen at low rates (usually 1 to 3 liters per minute).

As well, the normal oxygen saturation values for a client without COPD are between 95% to 100% on room air. The baseline oxygen saturation for a client with COPD is lower, with oxygen saturation above 89% considered within normal limits (Smeltzer & Bare, 2004).

17. Identify three priority nursing diagnoses that should be included on Mrs. Harriet's plan of care. Priority nursing diagnoses for Mrs. Harriet's care include:

- Impaired gas exchange related to (r/t) decreased functional lung tissue, effects of alveolar-capillary membrane changes
- Ineffective airway clearance r/t inflammation and increased, thickened tracheobronchial secretions, fatigue, and chest discomfort

- Hyperthermia r/t dehydration, increased metabolic rate, illness
- Acute pain r/t effects of inflammation and coughing
- Activity intolerance r/t imbalance between oxygen supply and demand
- Deficient knowledge (diagnoses, risk factors, treatment) r/t lack of exposure, unfamiliarity with information resources
- Risk for deficient fluid volume r/t fever, infection, increased metabolic rate, and possibly inadequate intake of fluids
- Risk for infection (sepsis)

(Ackley & Ladwig, 2006; Dennison, 2007; Workman, 2006).

18. You are the nurse providing discharge teaching to Mrs. Harriet. Briefly discuss what you will recommend to her regarding seeking follow-up care, lifestyle considerations, and how to help prevent pneumonia in the future. The purpose of any medications prescribed at the time of discharge should be reviewed and proper administration and adverse effects discussed. The course of antibiotic (anti-infective) therapy is often seven to 10 days for the client with uncomplicated CAP. Mrs. Harriet should be instructed to <u>finish</u> all of her antibiotic medications as prescribed, even if her symptoms have resolved and she feels better. She should notify her primary HCP if her symptoms fail to resolve and she experiences chills, fever, a persistent cough, dyspnea, wheezing, increased sputum production, hemoptysis (bloody sputum), increased chest discomfort, or fatigue.

Cigarette smoke is irritating to the respiratory tract and a risk factor for respiratory disease. Mrs. Harriet should be given information about smoking cessation programs. In conjunction with a comprehensive behavioral smoking cessation program, the HCP could prescribe a transdermal system (such as Nicoderm SQ) to help her stop smoking while providing relief of nicotine withdrawal symptoms. Medication safety should be addressed, and Mrs. Harriet should be made aware of the risk of myocardial infarction if she continues to smoke while wearing the transdermal nicotine patch. Mrs. Harriet is five feet three inches tall and weighs 224 pounds (101.8 kg). Her body mass index (BMI) is 39.7, and a BMI of 30 or higher is considered obese (NHLBI, 2006). Obesity increases Mrs. Harriet's risk of respiratory and cardiovascular disease. A nutritionist could work with her to discuss healthier food choices and eating habits and work to develop a safe weight loss program, helping to promote better health and prevention of illness in the future.

To help prevent a second pneumonia, Mrs. Harriet should receive an annual influenza vaccination (unless contraindicated) and the pneumococcal vaccine with revaccination every five years as recommended by her health care provider. The pneumococcal vaccine protects against 23 types of pneumococcal bacteria and is effective in approximately 60% to 80%

of healthy adults (American Lung Association, 2006; Schmitt, 2004). She should avoid crowded public areas during flu and holiday seasons. She should avoid pollutants such as tobacco, dust, smoke, toxic chemicals, and gases. Adequate rest and sleep as well as a well-balanced diet with a sufficient amount of nonalcoholic fluids each day is recommended. Most important, Mrs. Harriet should practice proper and frequent hand washing. This will be especially important when she works as a receptionist at the community center where she is at greatest risk of exposure to bacteria and transmission of infection to and from others.

References

Ackley, B., & Ladwig, G. (2006). *Nursing diagnosis handbook: A guide to planning care*. St. Louis, MO: Mosby.

Altman, G. B. (2004). Assisting a client with an incentive spirometer. In G. B. Altman (Ed.), *Delmar's fundamental & advanced nursing skills* (pp. 897–901). Clifton Park, NY: Thomson Delmar Learning

American Lung Association. (2006). *Pneumonia fact sheet*. Retrieved August 21, 2006, from www.lungusa.org.

American Lung Association (ALA). (2006). *Tuberculosis and health care workers*. Retrieved September 26, 2006, from www.lungusa.org.

Chernecky, C. C., & Berger, B. J. (2004). *Laboratory tests and diagnostic procedures*. Philadelphia, PA: Elsevier.

Daniels, R. (2002). *Delmar's guide to laboratory and diagnostic tests*. Albany, NY: Delmar.

Deglin, J. H., & Vallerand, A. H. (2005). *Davis's drug guide for nurses (9th ed.)* (pp. 291–293). Philadelphia, PA: F. A. Davis.

Dennison, P. D. (2007). Lower airway problems. In F. Monahan, J. Sands, M. Neighbors, J. Marek, & C. Green (Eds.), *Phipps' Medical-surgical nursing: Health and illness perspectives* (pp. 621–638). St. Louis, MO: Mosby Elsevier.

Jarahzadeh, M., & Sutjita, M. (2003). Respiratory tract infections. *Topics in Emergency Medicine, 25* (2), 134–138.

National Institutes of Health, National Heart, Lung, and Blood Institute (NHLBI) (2006). *Calculate your body mass index*. Retrieved July 17, 2006, from www.nhlbisupport.com.

Schmitt, A. K. (2004). Community-acquired pneumonia. *The Cleveland Clinic Foundation*. Retrieved August 21, 2006, from www.clevelandclinicmeded.com.

Singh, D., Sutton, C., & Woodcock, A. (2002). Tuberculin test measurement: Variability due to the time of reading. *Chest, 122* (4), 1299–1301.

Smeltzer, S., & Bare, B. (2004). Assessment and management of patients with hematologic disorders. In L. Brunner & D. Suddarth (Eds.), *Textbook of medical-surgical nursing* (pp. 868, 872). Philadelphia, PA: Lippincott Williams & Wilkins.

Smeltzer, S., & Bare, B. (2004). Management of patients with chronic obstructive pulmonary disease. In L. Brunner & D. Suddarth (Eds.), *Textbook of medical-surgical nursing* (pp. 568–598). Philadelphia, PA: Lippincott Williams & Wilkins.

Spratto, G. R., & Woods, A. L. (2006). *PDR nurse's drug handbook*. Clifton Park, NY: Thomson Delmar Learning.

Workman, M. L. (2006). Interventions for clients with infectious problems of the lower respiratory tract. In D. Ignatavicius & L. Workman (Eds.), *Medical-surgical nursing: Critical thinking for collaborative care* (pp. 633–639). St. Louis, MO: Elsevier.

York, N. (2007). Management of clients with parenchymal and pleural disorders. In J. Black & J. Hawks (Eds.), *Medical-surgical nursing: Clinical management for positive outcomes* (pp. 1844–1849). St. Louis, MO: Elsevier.

Zator Estes, M. E. (Ed.). (2006). *Health assessment & physical examination (3rd ed.)* (pp. 463–465, 472–475). Clifton Park, NY: Thomson Delmar Learning.

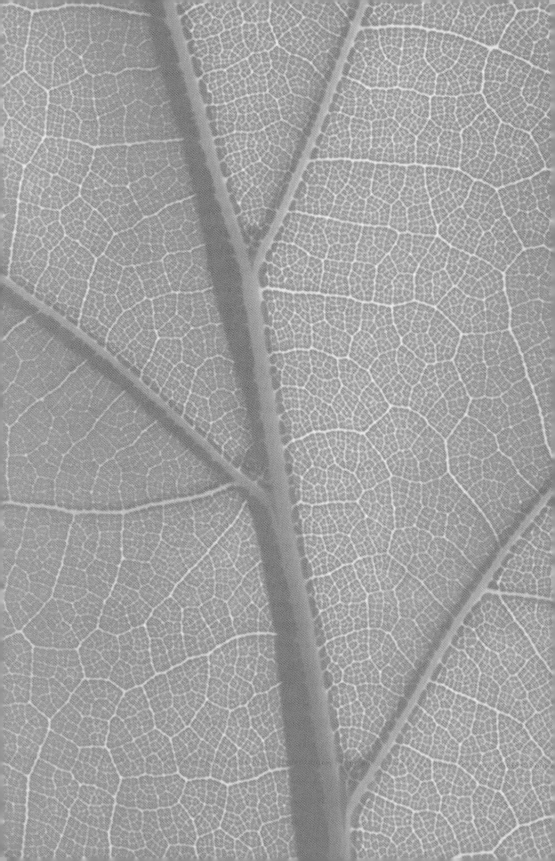

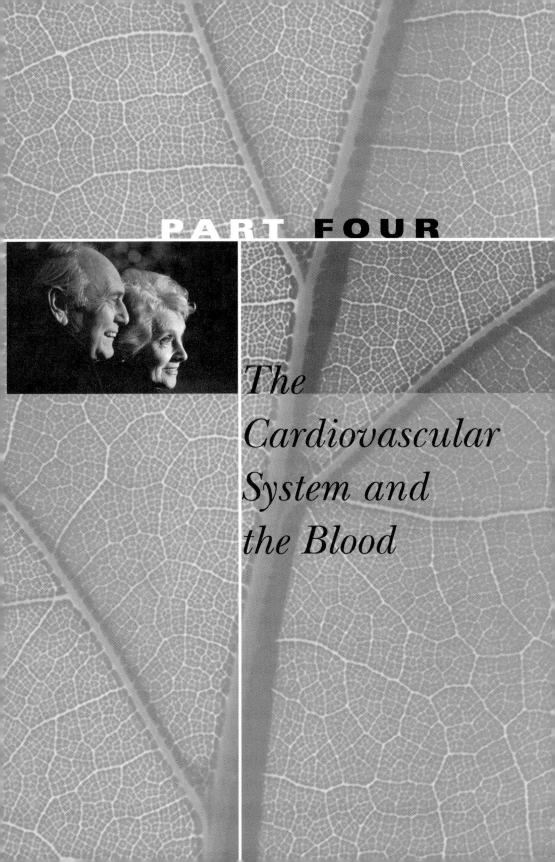

PART FOUR

The Cardiovascular System and the Blood

Mr. Cowen

GENDER

Male

AGE

50

SETTING

- Primary Care

ETHNICITY

- Black American

CULTURAL CONSIDERATIONS

PREEXISTING CONDITION

- Appendectomy at 16 years of age

COEXISTING CONDITIONS

- Height 5 feet 9 inches, weight 225 pounds
- No known drug allergies (NKDA)

COMMUNICATION

DISABILITY

SOCIOECONOMIC

- Employed as a customer service representative for a computer software company in Florida
- Sedentary lifestyle

SPIRITUAL/RELIGIOUS

PHARMACOLOGIC

- Hydrochlorothiazide (HCTZ)

LEGAL

ETHICAL

ALTERNATIVE THERAPY

PRIORITIZATION

DELEGATION

- Collaboration with dietician

THE CARDIOVASCULAR SYSTEM AND THE BLOOD

Level of Difficulty: Easy

Overview: The client is newly diagnosed with hypertension (HTN). The Seventh Report of the Joint National Committee on Prevention, Detection, Evaluation, and Treatment of High Blood Pressure (JNV VII) classification system for HTN is reviewed. The nurse considers the client's modifiable and nonmodifiable risk factors in order to establish a teaching plan to educate the client about appropriate lifestyle modification. The Dietary Approaches to Stop Hypertension (DASH) diet is discussed, and the client's compliance with the diet evaluated. Appropriate nursing diagnoses are identified and instruction regarding a newly prescribed medication is provided.

Client Profile

Mr. Cowen's employer sponsored a free blood pressure (BP) screening program for its employees. Mr. Cowen's BP is 160/90 mm Hg when measured with a large BP cuff. The nurse observes that the client is overweight. The nurse assesses the client for risk factors for hypertension and learns that Mr. Cowen sits at a desk all day answering telephone calls from customers with questions about the use of the company's computer software. He does not exercise regularly and admits that he does not follow a special diet stating, "My wife is a great cook. I'll eat anything she puts in front of me. At night I like to have a snack while I watch television." The client denies tobacco and recreational drug use and reports drinking "socially." "I have four or five beers on the weekend watching the football game." Mr. Cowen does not take any prescription medication or herbal supplements but reports taking "Tylenol on occasion when I have a headache." The nurse records Mr. Cowen's BP and gives the client the reading materials with instructions to make an appointment with his primary health care provider (HCP) as soon as possible for a more thorough assessment and to discuss treatment options.

Case Study

Mr. Cowen calls his primary HCP to schedule an appointment. Prior to the appointment, Mr. Cowen goes to a local laboratory and has a series of blood tests drawn as prescribed by the HCP.

At his appointment with the HCP, the nurse weighs Mr. Cowen. He is 5 feet 9 inches tall and weighs 225 pounds. Mr. Cowen's BP is 166/92 mm Hg with a large cuff in the right arm and 168/96 mm Hg in the left arm. His heart rate is 84 beats per minute with a regular rhythm, respiratory rate is 18, and he is afebrile. His total cholesterol is 260 mg/dL. During the health history and assessment, the HCP learns that Mr. Cowen drinks at least four six-ounce cups of regular coffee per day, and that his father has coronary artery disease and HTN. Mr. Cowen denies feeling stress because of his job, relationship with his wife and family, or other factors. "I am a pretty laid-back guy. I am not worked up or excited about much. I leave the worrying to my wife." The HCP notes that Mr. Cowen carries the majority of his weight in his upper body. He has an increased amount of subcutaneous fat around his waist and in his abdomen.

The HCP prescribes hydrochlorothiazide daily for the client and asks the nurse to provide Mr. and Mrs. Cowen with instructions regarding the medication and lifestyle modifications. A follow-up appointment is scheduled for one month.

Questions

1. Briefly explain what the systolic and diastolic BP readings indicate.

2. According to the Seventh Report of the JNV VII, what is the definition of prehypertension, stage 1 HTN, and stage 2 HTN? Describe primary and secondary HTN. Based on Mr. Cowen's clinical manifestations and history, how would you classify his HTN, and does he have primary or secondary HTN?

3. Generate at least five questions the nurse should ask the client in order to assess for the possible symptoms of HTN.

4. Identify Mr. Cowen's risk factors for HTN. Indicate which of the client's risk factors are nonmodifiable and which are modifiable.

5. Mr. Cowen asks the nurse, "Is my cholesterol really that bad? What should my numbers be?" How should the nurse respond?

6. The HCP prescribes hydrochlorothiazide for Mr. Cowen. Discuss the benefits of monotherapy with hydrochlorothiazide to treat the client's HTN.

7. The nurse is providing Mr. Cowen with instructions regarding his newly prescribed hydrochlorothiazide. What are the most common adverse effects of hydrochlorothiazide that Mr. Cowen should monitor, and what should Mr. Cowen do if he forgets to take his daily dose of medication as prescribed?

8. The nurse warns Mr. Cowen not to discontinue the medication abruptly. Briefly explain why the nurse offers this precaution.

9. The nurse is providing Mr. and Mrs. Cowen with instructions regarding lifestyle modifications to help reduce the client's HTN. Identify at least two points of discussion the nurse will include in the teaching plan.

10. In priority order, identify five nursing diagnoses the nurse should include in Mr. Cowen's plan of care.

11. One month later, Mr. Cowen returns for a follow-up appointment with his HCP. His BP is 138/82. The nurse congratulates Mr. Cowen on his success and asks him about his compliance with the DASH diet. He states, "I don't like it, but I am following it like you said. My wife has been keeping a close eye on me, and everything that I eat. She walks with me every night to give me the push I need to exercise." To confirm his compliance with the DASH diet, the nurse asks him to recall his last three meals and any snacks. Which meal or snack is least compliant with the DASH diet, and what alternative(s) can the nurse suggest?

Breakfast: a bowl of whole grain cereal with low-fat milk, a banana, and a glass of orange juice

Lunch: roast beef sandwich on white bread with mayonnaise and a soft drink

Dinner: fish, cooked vegetable, brown rice, and a glass of low-fat milk

Snack: a toasted slice of bread with grape jelly

Questions and Suggested Answers

1. **Briefly explain what the systolic and diastolic BP readings indicate.** BP is the product of the body's cardiac output and peripheral resistance. Arteries expand during systole and contract during diastole. These two

distinct pressure phases are represented by a measure of the client's BP in millimeters of mercury (mm Hg). A client's systolic blood pressure (SBP) is the measurement of the maximal pressure exerted against the arterial walls when the myocardial fibers contract and tighten to eject blood from the ventricles (the heart beat, or systole). The SBP is a reflection of the client's cardiac output and in a healthy adult is ≤120 mm Hg. The diastolic blood pressure (DBP) measures the pressure remaining in the arterial system during the period of relaxation after the heart has pumped (the heart at rest, or diastole). The DBP is a reflection of the client's peripheral vascular resistance and is ≤80 mm Hg in the healthy adult (Delaune & Ladner, 2006).

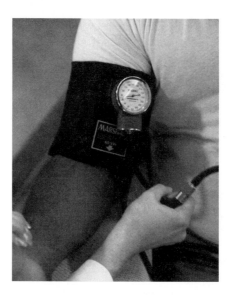

2. According to the Seventh Report of the JNV VII, what is the definition of prehypertension, Stage 1 HTN, and Stage 2 HTN? Describe primary and secondary HTN. Based on Mr. Cowen's clinical manifestations and history, how would you classify his HTN, and does he have primary or secondary HTN? Primary HTN is also called "essential" or "idiopathic" HTN. Approximately 90% to 95% of clients are diagnosed with primary HTN, which develops from an unknown cause. Clients with secondary HTN have developed high blood pressure as a result of (or secondary to) another disease or condition, such as renal artery stenosis, thyroid dysfunction, or pregnancy (Denison, 2007). Based on Mr. Cowen's clinical manifestations and history, he has developed primary HTN classified as Stage 2. When a client's SBP falls into one classification (Stage 2 in Mr. Cowen's case) and the DBP falls into another (Stage 1 in Mr. Cowen's case), the client's disease

JNV VII Classification of Blood Pressure in Adults

Classification	Systolic Pressure	Diastolic Pressure
Normal	Less than or equal to 120 mm Hg	Less than or equal to 80 mm Hg
Prehypertension	120–139 mm Hg	80–90 mm Hg
Stage 1 hypertension	140–159 mm Hg	90–99 mm Hg
Stage 2 hypertension	Greater than or equal to 160 mm Hg	Greater than or equal to 100 mg Hg

Denison, D. (2007). Hypertension: Nursing management. In R. Daniels, L. H. Nicoll, & L. J. Nosek (Eds.), *Contemporary medical-surgical nursing*. St. Louis, MO: Mosby Elsevier.

is classified according to the highest category. The higher the client's BP, the greater his health risk is (Maxwell-Thompson & Reid, 2007; National Institutes of Health, National Heart, Lung, and Blood Institute [NHLBI], 2006; Smeltzer, Bare, Hinkle, & Cheever, 2006).

3. **Generate at least five questions the nurse should ask the client in order to assess for the possible symptoms of HTN.** HTN is often referred to as the "silent killer" because most clients do not have symptoms. In clients with severely elevated BP, however, there can be an increased workload on the heart and damage to blood vessels and target organs. These changes can manifest as secondary symptoms of HTN. To assess the client for secondary symptoms, the nurse should ask Mr. Cowen if he has experienced:

- Angina
- Blurred vision
- Dizziness
- Dyspnea
- Fatigue
- Headaches
- Numbness or tingling in his hands or feet
- Palpitations
- Rapid heart rate, especially with exertion
- Spontaneous nosebleed

Headaches are one of the more common symptoms and are most often described as a throbbing pain located in the back of the head that is present upon waking and lasts for only a few hours, even when the client does not treat the headache with an analgesic (Denison, 2007; Maxwell-Thompson & Reid, 2007).

4.　Identify Mr. Cowen's risk factors for HTN. Indicate which of the client's risk factors are nonmodifiable and which are modifiable.　Mr. Cowen's risk factors include:

- Age (nonmodifiable)
  Primary HTN appears between 30 and 50 years of age.
- Alcohol use (modifiable)
  Excessive alcohol intake contributes to the development of HTN. The risk is increased when the client consumes three or more alcoholic beverages a day, which exceeds Mr. Cowen's four to five beers a week. Because alcohol intake poses a risk for HTN, Mr. Cowen should be encouraged to continue to consume alcohol in moderation.
- Body shape (modifiable)
  Upper body obesity and increased waist circumference (referred to as an apple shape) is associated with an increased risk of HTN.
- Caffeine intake (modifiable)

Caffeine increases BP. Although the body often adapts to this increase, studies have shown that decreasing one's intake of caffeine can lower BP.

- Ethnicity (black American) (nonmodifiable)
  HTN is more prevalent in black Americans than in any other ethnic group in the United States. HTN in black Americans tends to develop at an earlier age, be more pronounced, and progress more rapidly. In adults over the age of 18 years, 32% of black Americans versus 23% of Caucasians have HTN. Although the reason is not understood, the highest incidence of HTN in the United States is among black Americans who live in southeastern states (such as Florida).
- Family history (nonmodifiable)
  When one parent has HTN, the client has a 25% chance of developing HTN during his lifetime. If both parents have HTN, his risk increases to 60%.
- Gender (nonmodifiable)
  Among young and middle age adults, men are more likely to develop HTN. However, after 55 years of age, when most women are postmenopausal, women become more likely than men to develop HTN.
- Hypercholesterolemia/Dyslipidemia (modifiable)
  Elevated levels of cholesterol cause atherosclerosic changes in blood vessels that lead to high BP.
- Obese (modifiable)
  There is a correlation between increased body weight and body mass index and an increase in BP.

- Physical inactivity (modifiable)
  Regular physical activity strengthens the heart muscle and lowers BP.
- Dietary intake (modifiable)
  The typical American diet is calorie-rich, nutrient-poor, and often characterized by an increased intake of saturated fat and salt (sodium). While not every client with a poor diet develops HTN, increased fat intake contributes to hyperlipidemia and a diet high in salt can cause sodium and fluid retention, which elevates BP.

(Denison, 2007; Maxwell-Thompson & Reid, 2007)

5. Mr. Cowen asks the nurse, "Is my cholesterol really that bad? What should my numbers be?" How should the nurse respond? The normal range for total cholesterol in a healthy male varies in the literature. Chernecky and Berger (2004) indicate that the total cholesterol in a healthy male adult between 50 to 54 years of age is 158 to 277 mg/dL. The normal range of total cholesterol for black American men is approximately 10% higher. Daniels (2002) cites a range of 150 to 200 mg/dL for the normal total cholesterol in an adult. To minimize the client's risk of the comorbidities associated with hypercholesterolemia and HTN (such as cerebrovascular, cardiac, vascular, and renal disease), maintaining a total cholesterol in the lower range of normal is strongly recommended. Mr. Cowen's total cholesterol of 260 mg/dL is elevated, and health promotion interventions should be initiated to lower this value to 200 mg/dL or less.

6. The HCP prescribes hydrochlorothiazide for Mr. Cowen. Discuss the benefits of monotherapy with hydrochlorothiazide to treat the client's HTN. The treatment recommendation for the client diagnosed with Stage 2 HTN is lifestyle modification in addition to a prescribed antihypertensive medication. The first choice of pharmacological therapy is a thiazide diuretic such as hydrochlorothiazide, which lowers BP by decreasing the volume of circulating blood through the excretion of water. Hydrochlorothiazide is an effective first-line therapy for black Americans because this group of clients tends to have higher levels of intracellular sodium. Benefits of monotherapy include an increased likelihood of compliance with therapy and less adverse effects and interactions with other medications (Denison, 2007; Maxwell-Thompson & Reid, 2007).

7. The nurse is providing Mr. Cowen with instructions regarding his newly prescribed hydrochlorothiazide. What are the most common adverse effects of hydrochlorothiazide that Mr. Cowen should monitor, and what should Mr. Cowen do if he forgets to take his daily dose of medication as prescribed? The most common adverse effects of hydrochlorothiazide are hypokalemia (abnormally low potassium level in the blood), hyperuricemia (excess of uric acid in the blood), and orthostatic hypotension. Mr. Cowen should monitor for muscle weakness, cramps, palpitations, and dizziness and notify his HCP if these occur. He should be instructed to rise from a lying or sitting position slowly to prevent orthostatic changes. Mrs. Cowen can be taught how to assess her husband's BP using a manual or electronic blood pressure cuff. Mr. Cowen's daily BP should be recorded and reviewed at their follow-up appointment(s). Low BP readings and/or symptoms of orthostatic hypotension should be reported to the HCP. To facilitate compliance with the medication regimen and help prevent hypokalemia, Mr. Cowen should take his dose of medication at the same time every day with a glass of orange juice. He should include potassium-rich foods in his diet, such as fruits, legumes, and whole grains. To help prevent frequent awakening at night and a disruption in his sleep cycle due to nocturia, the client should take his medication in the morning. If he forgets to take his medication in the morning, he should take the medication as soon as he remembers, but skip the missed dose if he does not remember to take the medication that day and resume his therapy by taking his dose the next morning. He should not take double doses. It is important that the client return for his follow-up appointments with the HCP and obtain laboratory work as prescribed to monitor the effects of the medication and detect any adverse effects (Deglin & Vallerand, 2007; Maxwell-Thompson & Reid, 2007; Spratto & Woods, 2006).

8. The nurse warns Mr. Cowen not to discontinue the medication abruptly. Briefly explain why the nurse offers this precaution. Clients who abruptly discontinue antihypertensive medication therapy often experience a rapid increase in BP. This phenomenon is called rebound hypertension (Denison, 2007).

9. The nurse is providing Mr. and Mrs. Cowen with instructions regarding lifestyle modifications to help reduce the client's HTN. Identify at least two points of discussion the nurse will include in the teaching plan. Lifestyle modifications can help reduce a client's blood pressure. Limiting one's *dietary, sodium, caffeine, and alcohol intake; weight reduction; and regular exercise* are lifestyle modifications that reduce BP, promote health, and decrease the client's risk of developing secondary medical conditions. Some clients may be referred to a dietician to help educate them about appropriate meal choices and provide ongoing assessment and support to encourage compliance with recommendations and a safe reduction in weight.

Dietary intake: The Seventh Report of the JNV VII recommends dietary approaches to reduce HTN. The DASH diet is high in whole grains, fish, poultry, fruits, vegetables, and fat-free or low-fat dairy products. Following the guidelines of the DASH plan limits the client's intake of fat, saturated fat, and cholesterol, while providing ample amounts of fiber, protein, potassium, calcium, and magnesium. Dietary modification according to the DASH diet has been shown to reduce a client's BP by 8 to 14 mm Hg, with BP reductions noted within two weeks of starting the DASH plan. Combining the DASH eating plan with a reduced sodium intake results in the maximum benefit and lowers the client's BP more effectively (Denison, 2007; Maxwell-Thompson & Reid, 2007; NHLBI, 2006).

Sodium intake: There is a positive correlation between an individual's sodium intake and their BP. An adult needs only one-fourth of a teaspoon (or 500 mg) of sodium in their diet each day. Many foods and commercially prepared meals contain sodium, making it easy for an adult in the United States to consume an average of 4000 to 6000 mg of sodium a day. Black Americans are at greater risk since they are predisposed to having low renin activity. Having a decreased amount of renin, an enzyme that plays a role in regulating BP, makes these clients more sensitive to the cardiovascular effects of sodium and places them at risk for fluid retention and subsequent HTN. A sodium-restricted diet can be prescribed as a mild (2000 to 3000 mg), moderate (1000 mg), strict (500 mg), or severe (250 mg) restriction. Placing the client on a sodium restriction can help reduce a client's BP by 2 to 8 mm Hg (Denison, 2007; Halas, 2004; Maxwell-Thompson & Reid, 2007; NHLBI, 2006).

Caffeine intake: Caffeine is found in a variety of foods and beverages, including coffee, tea, soft drinks, and chocolate. Clients with HTN should limit their caffeine intake to approximately 200 mg per day. Mr. Cowen reports consuming at least four six-ounce cups of coffee each day. Each six-ounce cup of brewed or drip coffee contains 103 mg of caffeine. Mr. Cowen should be advised to decrease his coffee intake by half (to two cups per day). He should be advised to taper the amount of coffee he drinks over a couple of weeks to help reduce the likelihood of withdrawal headaches that can occur with a sudden decrease in caffeine intake (Denison, 2007).

Alcohol intake: The calories in alcohol do not contain nutritional value. An excessive consumption of alcohol increases BP. Some literature proposes that two glasses of alcohol (especially red wine) each day can have a protective effect on the heart. However, the recommended consumption of alcohol is limited to no more than 1 ounce of alcohol a day. This is equivalent to 24 ounces of beer, 10 ounces of wine, or 3 ounces of liquor daily. Mr. Cowen should be encouraged to decrease his alcohol consumption (Denison, 2007; Maxwell-Thompson & Reid, 2007).

Weight reduction: Weight loss is shown to reduce BP by 5 to 20 mm Hg per 10 kilograms (22 pounds) (Denison, 2007; Maxwell-Thompson & Reid, 2007). A client's BMI is the measure of body fat based on the individual's height and weight. Maintaining a healthy BMI helps to reduce the client's BP. The ideal BMI for an adult Mr. Cowen's height (5 feet 9 inches) is between 18.5 and 24.9 kg/m^2. Given Mr. Cowen's weight of 225 pounds, his current BMI is 33.2 kg/m^2. A BMI $\geq$30 kg/m^2 is classified as obese. If he were to reduce his weight to 200 pounds, he would still be considered overweight (a BMI of 29.5 kg/m^2). However, reducing his weight to 170 pounds would move him closer to the normal BMI range at 25.1 kg/m^2 (NHLBI, 2007). An individual's abdominal fat is associated with an increased risk of HTN. A waist circumference of greater than 40 inches in men increases the risk of HTN. Changing his diet and getting regular exercise can help Mr. Cowen lose weight and attain a healthy BMI.

Regular exercise: Clients who are physically capable of participating in aerobic exercise are encouraged to engage in a moderate amount of physical activity for at least 30 minutes a day on at least four days of the week. Exercise contributes to a stronger, more efficient heart muscle and opens blood vessels to allow more nutrients and oxygen to flow through body tissues and organs. These changes help to lower BP by 4 to 9 mm Hg. Regular exercise contributes to weight loss and a decreased risk of heart disease and stroke. If a HCP's assessment reveals no need for limitations, appropriate exercises the nurse can suggest include walking, climbing stairs, bicycling, swimming, and organized sports activities. Clients should begin with a lower level of intensity and gradually increase the intensity of the exercise program and the duration (from 15 to 30 minutes) as their body becomes more conditioned. The nurse should remind clients of the importance of safety equipment for certain activities such as a helmet for bicycling (Denison, 2007; Maxwell-Thompson & Reid, 2007).

10. In priority order, identify five nursing diagnoses the nurse should include in Mr. Cowen's plan of care. Priority nursing diagnoses for Mr. Cowen's plan of care include:

- Altered health maintenance related to (r/t) lack of knowledge of pathology, complications, and management of HTN
- Deficient knowledge (HTN) r/t lack of exposure and unfamiliarity with information resources regarding relationship between diet and exercise and disease process
- Imbalanced nutrition: More than body requirements r/t caloric intake exceeding energy expenditure
- Sedentary lifestyle r/t deficient knowledge of health benefits of physical exercise, lack of motivation, and lack of interest
- Risk for noncompliance r/t adverse effects of treatments and lack of understanding regarding importance of controlling HTN
- Risk for ineffective therapeutic regimen management r/t noncompliance with treatment

- Risk for ineffective coping r/t effects of chronic illness and major changes in lifestyle
- Risk for deficient fluid volume r/t adverse effects of prescribed medication
- Risk for altered sleep pattern r/t therapeutic effects of prescribed medication
- Risk for activity intolerance r/t sedentary lifestyle

(Ackley & Ladwig, 2006).

11. One month later, Mr. Cowen returns for a follow-up appointment with his HCP. His blood pressure is 138/82. The nurse congratulates Mr. Cowen on his success and asks him about his compliance with the DASH diet. He states, "I don't like it, but I am following it like you said. My wife has been keeping a close eye on me, and everything that I eat. She walks with me every night to give me the push I need to exercise." To confirm his compliance with the DASH diet, the nurse asks him to recall his last three meals and any snacks. Which meal or snack is least compliant with the DASH diet, and what alternative(s) can the nurse suggest?

> **Breakfast: a bowl of whole grain cereal with low-fat milk, a banana and a glass of orange juice**
> **Lunch: roast beef sandwich on white bread with mayonnaise and a soft drink**
> **Dinner: fish, cooked vegetable, brown rice and a glass of low-fat milk**
> **Snack: a toasted slice of bread with grape jelly**

Mr. Cowen's lunch choice is least compliant with the DASH diet. The nurse should suggest that Mr. Cowen use whole grain breads (such as wheat) for sandwiches, limit his intake of processed deli meats, which are high in sodium, and use low-fat mayonnaise. He should limit his intake of soft drinks since these beverages are high in sodium and caffeine. If Mr. Cowen does drink soft drinks, he should choose diet soft drinks.

References

Ackley, B., & Ladwig, G. (2006). *Nursing diagnosis handbook: A guide to planning care.* St. Louis, MO: Mosby.

Chernecky, C.C., & Berger, B. J. (2004). *Laboratory tests and diagnostic procedures* (pp. 369–372). Philadelphia, PA: Elsevier.

Daniels, R. (2002). *Delmar's guide to laboratory and diagnostic tests* (pp. 215–217). Clifton Park, NY: Thomson Delmar Learning.

Delaune, S. C., & Ladner, P. K. (2006). *Fundamentals of nursing: Standards & practice.* (p. 510). Clifton Park, NY: Thomson Delmar Learning.

Deglin, J. H., & Vallerand, A. H. (2005). *Davis's drug guide for nurses (9th ed.)* (pp. 409–411). Philadelphia, PA: F.A. Davis.

Denison, D. (2007). Hypertension: Nursing management. In R. Daniels, L. H. Nicoll, & L. J. Nosek (Eds.), *Contemporary medical-surgical nursing* (pp. 907–926). St. Louis, MO: Mosby Elsevier.

Halas, M. (2004). Nutrition. In Daniels, R. (Ed.), *Nursing fundamentals: Caring & clinical decision making* (p. 1027). Clifton Park, NY: Delmar Learning.

Maxwell-Thompson, C. L., & Reid, K. B. (2007). Vascular problems. In F. Monahan, J. Sands, M. Neighbors, J. Marek, & C. Green (Eds.), *Phipps' Medical-surgical nursing: Health and illness perspectives* (pp. 857–868). St. Louis, MO: Mosby Elsevier.

National Institutes of Health, National Heart, Lung, and Blood Institute (NHLBI). (2006). *Your guide to lowering your blood pressure with DASH.* Retrieved February 10, 2007, from www.nhlbi.nih.gov.

National Institutes of Health, National Heart, Lung, and Blood Institute (NHLBI). (2007). *Calculate your body mass index.* Retrieved February 14, 2007, from www.nhlbisupport.com.

Smeltzer, S. C., Bare, B.G., Hinkle, J. L., & Cheever, K. H. (2006). Assessment and management of patients with hypertension. In Brunner & Suddarth's textbook of medical-surgical nursing (pp. 1020–1034). Philadelphia, PA: Lippincott, Williams & Wilkins.

Spratto, G. R., & Woods, A. L. (2006). *PDR nurse's drug handbook* (pp. 633–634). Clifton Park, NY: Thomson Delmar Learning.

CASE STUDY 2

Mr. McCann

GENDER

Male

AGE

60

SETTING

- Hospital

ETHNICITY

- White American

CULTURAL CONSIDERATIONS

PREEXISTING CONDITION

- Frequent sinus infections

COEXISTING CONDITION

- Cholecystitis, leukocytosis

COMMUNICATION

DISABILITY

SOCIOECONOMIC

- Retired firefighter
- Married, two children (ages 36 and 33)

SPIRITUAL/RELIGIOUS

PHARMACOLOGIC

- Levofloxacin (Levaquin); metronidazole (Flagyl); chlorambucil (Leukeran); cyclophosphamide (Cytoxan); prednisone; fludarabine phosphate (Fludara); alemtuzumab (Campath); rituximab (Rituxan)

LEGAL

ETHICAL

ALTERNATIVE THERAPY

PRIORITIZATION

- Support for the client (and family) diagnosed with a chronic illness

DELEGATION

THE CARDIOVASCULAR SYSTEM AND THE BLOOD

Level of Difficulty: Difficult

Overview: The client in this case is hospitalized with cholecystitis. Although this acute illness resolves, laboratory tests reveal that the client has a chronic form of leukemia. The pathophysiology and clinical manifestations of cholecystitis are reviewed. The client's new diagnosis of chronic lymphocytic leukemia (CLL) is discussed with a focus on clinical manifestations, laboratory testing, standard treatment in the early stage of CLL, and treatment options for the future. Appropriate nursing diagnoses for the client with a chronic illness are identified. Client education regarding reducing his risk of infection is presented, and the impact of a chronic illness on the client and family considered.

DIFFICULT

Client Profile

Mr. McCann is a 60-year-old man who had not been feeling well for five days. He complained of intermittent stomach cramps, fever, headache, and malaise. His past medical history includes frequent sinus infections. Mr. McCann has noticed that "in the past few years, my sinus infections have been much more frequent and the infection lasts twice as long before I feel any better." He assumed his elevated temperature, headache, and malaise were the early manifestations of another sinus infection and disregarded his gastrointestinal symptoms as insignificant. He had an appointment with his primary care provider (PCP) scheduled for the next day to be examined. That evening, however, Mr. McCann was awakened by severe abdominal cramps. Mr. McCann's wife drove him to the emergency department, and he was admitted with a possible acute cholecystitis and leukocytosis. His temperature was 103°F (39.4°C) and his white blood cell count (WBC) on admission was 35,900 cells/mm^3 with a shift to the left.

Case Study

A gallbladder sonogram revealed a stone within the gallbladder with sludge present. Mr. McCann was treated with intravenous levofloxacin and metronidazole for acute cholecystitis. During his four-day hospital stay, his WBC remained elevated and on the day of discharge was 25,900 cells/mm^3. On physical examination, he did not have lymphadenopathy or splenomegaly. Additional diagnostic testing performed during Mr. McCann's hospitalization included a negative mononucleosis screen, negative hepatitis profile, urinalysis within normal limits, and a colonoscopy that was within normal limits. A laproscopic cholecystectomy is the recommended treatment. However, before Mr. McCann has this procedure, the health care provider (HCP) would like to evaluate the leukocytosis further to be sure the cholecystitis is the only cause of the elevated WBC. Mr. McCann is discharged home with a prescription to take an oral antibiotic twice a day for 10 days to complete a 14-day course of antibiotics. In one week, he is scheduled to have a complete blood count (CBC) with differential and comprehensive metabolic panel (CMP).

Results of the follow-up CBC reveal a WBC of 30,500 cells/mm^3. Concerned that Mr. McCann's chronic leukocytosis is indicative of an underlying hematological malignancy, the HCP refers him to an oncologist. Flow cytometry testing prescribed by the oncologist reveals that Mr. McCann has chronic lymphocytic leukemia that is currently in stage 0.

Questions

1. Mr. McCann was hospitalized for acute cholecystitis. Briefly explain the pathophysiology of acute cholecystitis. Which individuals are at greatest risk for cholecystitis?

2. Discuss the common clinical manifestations of acute cholecystitis.

3. Briefly discuss what leukocytosis is and what causes this change in blood values. Include in your discussion the normal lab values and critical lab values related to leukocytosis.

4. Explain what is meant by a "shift to the left" in Mr. McCann's WBC differential.

5. A laproscopic cholecystectomy is postponed to evaluate the client's leukocytosis further. What is the most likely complication of delaying the surgical procedure, and what recommendations can the nurse suggest to decrease the risk of complications until surgery?

6. Explain how the different types of leukemia are classified and briefly discuss the pathophysiology of CLL.

7. What is the incidence of CLL, and who is at greatest risk for this chronic disease?

8. Briefly discuss the presenting clinical manifestations of the client with CLL.

9. Mr. McCann is diagnosed with stage 0 CLL. What are the characteristics of this stage? Based on the diagnosis of stage 0, what medical treatment will likely be prescribed for Mr. McCann?

10. In disbelief, Mr. McCann asks, "I can't believe I have cancer. What caused this and what is my prognosis?" Discuss the etiology and prognosis for a client diagnosed with CLL.

11. Mrs. McCann asks the nurse, "I understand that at this stage my husband does not need treatment, but what will happen if this leukemia gets worse? What can be done for him then?" What treatment options will be considered when Mr. McCann's CLL advances?

12. Prioritize three nursing diagnoses appropriate for Mr. McCann's plan of care at this stage of his chronic illness.

13. Identify three components of a teaching plan to educate Mr. McCann about ways that he can reduce his risk of infection.

14. Discuss the fear, uncertainty, and risk for depression when diagnosed with a life-threatening, chronic illness. What is the potential impact of a chronic illness on the individual's quality of life and the family dynamic?

15. Identify at least five nursing interventions to address Mr. McCann's coping needs. Include a referral to at least one community resource.

Questions and Suggested Answers

1. Mr. McCann was hospitalized for acute cholecystitis. Briefly explain the pathophysiology of acute cholecystitis. Which individuals are at greatest risk for cholecystitis? Cholelithiasis is the most common disorder of the biliary system. It is the formation of stones in the gallbladder. Acute cholecystitis is the inflammation precipitated by the presence of these stones. "Bile is primarily composed of water plus conjugated bilirubin, organic and inorganic ions, small amounts of proteins, and three lipids: bile salts, lecithin, and cholesterol" (Good & Sands, 2007, p. 1286). Most gallstones (80% of cases) are composed of cholesterol. When the concentrations of these three lipids are balanced, cholesterol is held in solution. However, if this balance is not maintained, the cholesterol can precipitate. The exact cause is unknown, but it is believed that the imbalance in bile components leads to supersaturation and crystallization. Gastrointestinal and gallbladder motility are thought to play a role since most healthy adults experience episodes of supersaturation of the bile throughout their lifetime without developing stones. Supersaturation of the bile with cholesterol impairs gallbladder motility contributing to stasis and the formation of soft, yellowish green stones that range in size from 1 mm to 2½ cm. The formation of a stone is a steady process that may take years. A person may develop one stone or form multiple stones (Good & Sands, 2007).

Gallbladder disease is one of the most common gastrointestinal health problems, affecting more than 20 million Americans each year. This disease is more common in Caucasians, Hispanics, and Native Americans. It is less common in black Americans. Cholelithiasis is two to three times more likely to occur in women than in men, and the incidence increases with age. In addition to age, gender, and ethnicity, individuals at greater risk are those with hypercholesterolemia, diseases of the ileum, pregnancy, women taking oral contraceptives, and those who are obese or have experienced rapid weight loss (Good & Sands, 2007; Lee, Chiang, & Santen, 2006).

2. Discuss the common clinical manifestations of acute cholecystitis. Gallstones obstruct the cystic duct, and the presence of the stone(s) in the biliary tract or the passage of the stone(s) causes edema and spasm. In acute cholelithiasis, the gallbladder is enlarged, tense, and inflamed. Spasm of the gallbladder and transient obstruction cause biliary colic, the most common clinical manifestation in 70% to 80% of cases. The client experiences an acute sharp pain in the upper abdomen or epigastric area. In acute cholecystitis, the intensity of the pain steadily increases over a period of several hours. The pain may awaken the client from sleep and may be described as a pain that is localized in the right upper quadrant of the abdomen that radiates to the shoulder or back. Palpating the abdomen often causes a severe increase in pain and temporary inspiratory arrest (positive Murphy's sign). Diaphoresis, chills and fever, as well as nausea and vomiting may occur. Laboratory results usually reveal leukocytosis with a left shift, and elevated bilirubin and amylase levels. The episode of acute cholelcystitis most often resolves within four days. Almost half of the clients with acute cholecystitis develop a secondary bacterial infection within a few days of the acute attack. If the individual has not done so already, the symptoms of the secondary infection prompt the client to seek evaluation (Good & Sands, 2007).

3. Briefly discuss what leukocytosis is and what causes this change in blood values. Include in your discussion the normal lab values and critical lab values related to leukocytosis. Leukocytosis refers to an increased level of WBCs in circulation. Normal findings are a WBC count that is between 4100 and 10,800 cells/mm^3. An elevated level most often indicates infection from bacteria, trauma, or tissue injury. Leukocytosis is a normal response to the increased need for WBCs in the body such as when the body is fighting an acute infection. Moderate to severe inflammatory responses can produce the systemic clinical manifestations of an increased body temperature, increased erythrocyte sedimentation rate, and increased WBCs. The body fights infection by using WBCs (or leukocytes) to encapsulate and destroy organisms. Leukocytosis develops "when leukopoietins, agents released from damaged cells and from WBCs accumulating at the inflammatory site, are carried by the circulation to the bone marrow, where WBCs are produced" (Green, 2007, p. 430). The leukopoietins signal the release of mature neutrophils that have been held in reserve in the bone marrow. As a result, the WBC count in the peripheral circulation rises to above 10,000 cells/mm^3. A WBC value above 30,000 cells/mm^3 is considered a critical value. As the infection resolves, the level of WBCs in circulation should decrease. If there is a prolonged or increasing elevation, the client should be evaluated since a significant cause of persistent leukocytosis is malignancy (Daniels, 2002).

4. Explain what is meant by a "shift to the left" in Mr. McCann's WBC differential. There are two types of neutrophils: segmented neutrophils (segs) and band neutrophils (bands). Bands are immature neutrophils that multiply quickly in the presence of acute infection. The normal range for bands is 3% to 5%. Elevated bands indicate acute infection. An increased number of band cells is referred to as a "shift to the left" or "left shift." This terminology originated in reference to the traditional diagram of neutrophil maturation that shows the stem cell on the left of the diagram with progressive stages of maturation moving toward the right, ending with a fully mature neutrophil on the right side of the diagram. A shift to the left indicates that there are more immature cells present in the blood than normally occurs (Smeltzer & Bare, 2004).

5. A laproscopic cholecystectomy is postponed to evaluate the client's leukocytosis further. What is the most likely complication of delaying the surgical procedure, and what recommendations can the nurse suggest to decrease the risk of complications until surgery? The most likely complication of nonsurgical management of cholecystitis is recurrence. Recurrence of gallbladder disease can result in sepsis and peritonitis. These infections can present life-threatening complications. Strategies the nurse can suggest to help prevent gallstone disease include regular exercise; eating a low fat, low-carbohydrate diet; and eating small meals. Research also suggests that the consumption of nuts can help to lower a person's risk of sympto-matic gallbladder disease. Nuts are primarily composed of unsaturated fats and are a good source of dietary fiber. Dietary fiber helps lower triglyceride levels and enhances gastrointestinal motility, which helps to reduce bile acid and prevent supersaturation. One study found that those who ate five or more ounces of peanuts, peanut butter, or other types of nuts each week had a lower risk of symptomatic gallstone disease. Other studies have proposed that drinking caffeinated coffee also offers protection against cholecystitis (Tsai et al., 2004 as cited in Good & Sands, 2007).

6.   Explain how the different types of leukemia are classified and briefly discuss the pathophysiology of CLL. Leukemia is a broad term used to describe the classification of four kinds of disease. The four kinds of leuke-mia are classified according to the stem cell line that is involved, either lym-phoid or myeloid, and based on the time it takes for clinical manifestations to evolve, either acute or chronic. An individual with leukemia is diagnosed with either acute lymphoblastic (or lymphocytic) leukemia (ALL), acute myelogenous leukemia (AML), chronic lymphoblastic leukemia (CLL), or chronic myelogenous leukemia (CML). Leukemia is either acute or chronic based on the progression of cell differentiation. The lymphoblastic leukemias are caused by cancerous changes in the lymphocytes. CLL is a malignant disorder of the hematologic system that involves the bone mar-row and lymph nodes. It is characterized by the uncontrolled proliferation of blood cells that originate in bone marrow (hematopoietic cells). These cells include leukocytes, myelocytes, and their precursors. There also may be proliferation of cells in the liver and spleen. CLL is a type of cancer in which the bone marrow produces too many lymphocytes. Three types of lymphocytes, B cells, T cells, and natural killer (NK) cells, develop as a result. Most CLL clients have a B cell type of leukemia. The lymphocytes produced in the client with CLL are not able to fight infection effectively, and their increased accumulation in the blood and bone marrow leaves little room for healthy WBCs, red blood cells (RBCs), and platelets. The excessive production of abnormal cells in the bone marrow interferes with the normal bone marrow production of stem (immature) cells that develop into the mature blood cells of RBCs, WBCs, and platelets and results in the development of immature WBCs, thrombocytopenia (decreased platelets), and anemia. When there is immaturity of the WBCs, the individual is immu-nocompromised and has an increased susceptibility for developing infec-tions. These changes cause decreased synthesis of immunoglobulins and reduce antibody response. In CLL, mature blood cells are affected, and cell growth progresses slowly. Although the cells are abnormal, they can still carry out some degree of normal cell function. Therefore, CLL progresses over a period of months to many years (often two to 10 years) (Garrigues, 2007; National Cancer Institute, 2006; Smeltzer & Bare, 2004).

7. What is the incidence of CLL, and who is at greatest risk for this chronic disease? Approximately 8000 to 10,000 people in the United States are diagnosed with CLL each year (National Cancer Institute, 2006). The peak incidence of CLL occurs in clients between 50 and 70 years old and increases with age. It is rare that a person is diagnosed before the age of 45. CLL is more common in men than in women and affects predominantly Caucasian men. A family history of CLL or another cancer of the lymphatic system increases the risk of developing CLL. Those with relatives who are Russian Jewish or Eastern European Jewish have been found to be at increased risk (Garrigues, 2007; National Cancer Institute, 2006).

8. Briefly discuss the presenting clinical manifestations of the client with CLL. Many clients with CLL are asymptomatic and diagnosed incidentally during a routine physical examination or during the course of treatment for another disease. The client with symptomatic CLL often presents with vague flulike symptoms. The client may complain of fevers and sweating (especially at night). Other clinical manifestations include fatigue, weakness, shortness of breath with physical activity, anorexia, and weight loss. Since clients with CLL have defects in their cell-mediated immune system, repeat infections are common, especially of the skin, lungs, and kidneys. Upon physical examination, lymphadenopathy is often noted, and an enlarged spleen (splenomegaly) and liver (hepatomegaly) may be palpated. Some clients experience painful lymphadenopathy. The client may have pruritic vesicular skin lesions. An increased WBC (lymphocyte) count will always be present and may be extremely elevated (20,000 to 200,000 cells/mm^3). Thrombocytopenia and anemia are often diagnosed in clients in the later stages of CLL (Garrigues, 2007; Newton, 2005).

9. Mr. McCann is diagnosed with stage 0 CLL. What are the characteristics of this stage? Based on the diagnosis of stage 0, what medical treatment will likely be prescribed for Mr. McCann? Mr. McCann has been diagnosed with stage 0 CLL. This means that he has an elevated WBC count of greater than 15,000 cells/mm^3 without lymphadenopathy, hepatosplenomegaly, anemia, or thrombocytopenia. Treatment in the early stages of CLL has not been shown to increase survival. Most clients in stage 0 do well without treatment, especially when they are asymptomatic. Therefore, the standard treatment for the client with stage 0 CLL is watchful waiting. The term "watchful waiting" refers to observation by the HCP that involves closely monitoring the client's condition without giving any treatment until clinical manifestations appear or change. During watchful waiting, any problems caused by the CLL, such as an infection, are treated. The HCP will treat Mr. McCann for his frequent sinus infections with antibiotics. Treatment options for clients with CLL are considered when clinical manifestations become severe and/or there is indication of disease progression manifested by lymphadenopathy, drenching night sweats, anemia, thrombocytopenia, and/or enlargement of the spleen or liver. Routine physical examinations, laboratory testing, and client education about symptoms to report are important elements of the watchful waiting treatment plan (Cleveland Clinic, 2003b; Garrigues, 2007; National Cancer Institute, 2006; Smeltzer & Bare, 2004).

10. In disbelief, Mr. McCann asks, "I can't believe I have cancer. What caused this and what is my prognosis?" Discuss the etiology and prognosis for a client diagnosed with CLL. The specific etiology of CLL is unknown, although genetic factors are believed to be involved in its development. Unlike the other three types of leukemia, CLL is not thought to be associated with the possible risk factors of overexposure to environmental irradiation (such as the atomic bomb at Hiroshima) or radiation for cancer treatment, exposure to chemicals (such as benzene) and drugs, or environmental factors. Genetic factors are thought to play a role in the development of CLL. A genetic factor is believed to alter the nuclear deoxyribonucleic acid (DNA) rendering cells unable to mature and respond to normal regulatory mechanisms. The change in the DNA gives the CLL cell a growth and survival advantage that results in uncontrolled growth of CLL cells in the bone marrow, leading to an increased concentration in the blood. This injury to the DNA is not present at birth, and it is not yet understood what causes the change in the DNA of CLL clients. CLL is thought to have a possible genetic predisposition with a high incidence of CLL reported in some families. The average survival time for those with CLL ranges from 15 years (early stage) to two and a half years (late stage). Complications of the abnormal depression of the cellular elements of the blood (pancytopenia), including hemorrhage and infection, represent the major cause of death (Garrigues, 2007; Leukemia-Lymphoma Society, 2006a; National Cancer Institute, 2006; Newton, 2005; Smeltzer & Bare, 2004, Visovsky, 2006).

11. Mrs. McCann asks the nurse, "I understand that at this stage my husband does not need treatment, but what will happen if this leukemia gets worse? What can be done for him then?" What treatment options will be considered when Mr. McCann's CLL advances? Treatment is considered when the client has symptoms of advanced stages of CLL, including painful lymphadenopathy, drenching night sweats, anemia, thrombocytopenia, and/or enlargement of the spleen or liver. The goal of therapy in the advanced stages is palliation or control of undesired clinical manifestations. Local radiation to the spleen may be prescribed to reduce the complications of hemolytic anemia, which results from autoimmune nature of CLL and hypogammaglobulinemia, which increases the susceptibility to infection. Select clients with advanced CLL have their spleen surgically removed (splenectomy). When treatment is needed, antibiotics, RBC transfusions, and injections of gamma-globulin concentrates may be prescribed. As well, chemotherapy with chlorambucil (Leukeran) or cyclophosphamide (Cytoxan) is often prescribed to stop the growth of the cancer cells by killing the cells or interfering with cell division. Chemotherapy is usually administered for two weeks of every month. If the client should develop anemia (usually seen in stage III) or thrombocytopenia (usually seen in stage IV), daily oral prednisone is prescribed in addition to chemotherapy. The prednisone has a lymphocytolytic effect that stimulates the production of RBCs and platelets. Other medications that have proven successful in the palliative treatment of CLL include fludarabine (Fludara), alemtuzumab (Campath), and rituximab (Rituxan). Bone marrow and stem cell transplantation are under clinical investigation. Treatment is not curative but can put a client's CLL in remission (Cleveland Clinic, 2003b; Garrigues, 2007; National Cancer Institute, 2006; Newton, 2005).

12. Prioritize three nursing diagnoses appropriate for Mr. McCann's plan of care at this stage of his chronic illness. Appropriate diagnoses for Mr. McCann following diagnosis of CLL include:

- Ineffective protection related to (r/t) abnormal blood profile
- Risk for infection r/t ineffective immune system
- Deficient knowledge (disease, management of disease) r/t lack of exposure and unfamiliarity with information resources
- Fear r/t threat to well-being
- Anxiety r/t threat to or change in health status and quality of life
- Grieving r/t actual loss of physical health
- Risk for ineffective coping r/t personal vulnerability in situational crisis
- Risk for interrupted family processes r/t shift in health status of a family member and situational transition
- Risk for fatigue r/t physiological effects of disease state
- Anticipatory grieving r/t potential loss of quality of life and shortened life span
- Risk for hopelessness r/t loss of control and chronic illness
- Risk for powerlessness r/t chronic illness
- Risk for spiritual distress r/t physical illness and test of spiritual beliefs

(Ackley & Ladwig, 2006)

13. Identify three components of a teaching plan to educate Mr. McCann about ways that he can reduce his risk of infection. A teaching plan should include the following items of explanation and discussion to help strengthen Mr. McCann's immune system and reduce his risk of infection:

- Avoid changing pet litter boxes or wear gloves when changing litter.
- Avoid contact with persons with upper respiratory infections.
- Avoid crowds and large gatherings of people who might be ill.
- Avoid excessive stress.
- Avoid live or attenuated vaccines.
- Avoid travel to areas of the world with poor sanitation or less than adequate health care facilities.
- Bathe daily using an antimicrobial soap.
- Do not share eating utensils or cups.
- Do not share personal toiletry articles (toothbrushes, washcloths, deodorant).
- Eat a balanced diet, emphasizing proteins, fatty acids, and vitamins. Avoid foods at high risk of containing bacteria (e.g., salads, raw fruits and vegetables, and undercooked meat).
- Get the proper amount of sleep and balance activity with periods of rest.
- Monitor weight loss, which could be a predictor of protein calorie malnutrition.
- Notify the HCP immediately if symptoms of an infection, fever (temperature greater than 100°F or 38°C), chills, or night sweats are developed.
- Wash dishes and eating utensils using hot water or in a dishwasher.
- Wash hands well before eating, after touching a pet, after using the toilet, after shaking hands, or when returning home after an outing.
- Vaccination with the influenza virus vaccine and the meningococcal polysaccharide (Pneumovax) vaccine (Ackley & Ladwig, 2006; Visovsky, 2006).

14. Discuss the fear, uncertainty, and risk for depression when diagnosed with a life-threatening, chronic illness. What is the potential impact of a chronic illness on the individual's quality of life and the family dynamic?

Fear

Being diagnosed with a life-threatening illness such as leukemia can be extremely frightening. Many individuals experience shock, disbelief, and anger. The person fears the unknown. Aware that, in time, they will experience physical changes and a progressive onset of clinical manifestations, anticipation is accompanied by fear of when and to what extent the disease will advance. The person may also fear the social stigma of the disease, and the reaction of family, friends, and colleagues. Initially denial and avoidance may be protective. The goal becomes the day-to-day management of the illness with an effort to regain a sense of control over one's sense of fear, which can be daunting.

Uncertainty

When diagnosed with a life-threatening illness, it is easy to become preoccupied with dying, yet many individuals live for many years after their diagnosis. Nevertheless the uncertainty of a chronic illness is pervasive. Nothing is as it once was, and an individual's definition of what is "normal" in their life no longer exists. A chronic illness is rarely curable and often persists indefinitely. The course of an illness varies for each individual. Often there is an unpredictable cycle of exacerbations of symptoms and periods of remission.

Quality of life

People diagnosed with chronic illnesses must adjust to the demands of the illness, as well as to treatments for the condition. The illness may affect a person's mobility and independence, and change the way a person lives, sees himself, and/or relates to others. For individuals with a chronic condition, the need to adjust to a new view of oneself begins at the time of diagnosis. Denial, anger, and frustration are common when clients first learn that they must deal with something painful and unexpected. Many people pass through several stages before they begin to accept their new role as a person living with a chronic illness. Treatment may be long and complicated and can change often to achieve optimal effectiveness. Some individuals feel sicker during treatment than they did when diagnosed. It is difficult to be optimistic and hopeful when there are many days when the person does not feel well. Complying with the dietary and medical management of an illness may become stressful and exhausting and often means an increased financial burden. If employed, the chronic illness itself, or its management, may interfere with the person's ability to maintain this role. There are physical, social, and emotional impacts on a person's quality of life when faced with the day-to-day challenges of a chronic illness. The person may have trouble eating, sleeping, and concentrating. It is common for people coping with a life-threatening, chronic illness to feel powerless and have a bad day or even a bad week now and then. It is important that the person try to remain positive and learn coping strategies to do so and to be mindful that, with treatment, there will often be more good days than bad ones. It is important that the person stay involved and live as "normally" and productively as possible. The person should plan social activities for the days when he feels well and participate in activities he finds enjoyable.

Retaining a sense of "self" beyond the diagnosis will help to restore a sense of serenity and well-being.

Depression

Ongoing sadness, fatigue, disinterest, and lack of motivation may be related to the adverse effects of medication or complications of the illness. However, for many, these symptoms represent depression. Depression is one of the most common complications of chronic illness. The risk of getting depression is generally 10% to 25% for women and 5% to 12% for men. However, those with chronic illnesses face a much higher risk of between 25% and 33%. Depression and illness may occur together because the physical changes associated with the illness trigger the depression, and the individual has a psychological reaction to the hardships posed by the illness. Depression often makes people withdraw into social isolation. Depression is not a failure to cope, but rather it indicates a disruption in the body's neuro-chemistry treated with medicine, psychotherapy, or a combination of both.

Effect on the family dynamic

Few experiences are as devastating as learning that a loved one has a life-threatening illness. Hospitalization and treatment disrupts normal family routines. Each member of the family will react in a different manner and will choose different coping strategies. Some avoid discussing the illness, whereas others seek as much information as they can gather through reading, computer Internet resources, and health care professionals. It is important to recognize that the individual and each member of the family will cope with the diagnosis in a different way and at a different pace. As well, there may be family members or friends who are unable to accept or discuss the illness. The individual may choose not to tell his family or friends about the diagnosis. Some people feel that their illness is something that they should handle themselves and that involving their family places a burden on family. Individuals will often withhold sharing their diagnosis in an effort to protect their loved ones from worry. However, friends and family often will sense that the person is not well; and as survivorship rates increase, the person may struggle with keeping the "secret" for a long time. Individuals often find that an open exchange with their family and friends is an important step in accepting the diagnosis and enables a support system. Family members can serve an important role in providing support and comfort to their loved one as well as an extra set of ears during follow-up appointments with the HCP. With the client's permission and in accordance with the Health Insurance Portability and Accountability Act (HIPAA) guidelines, family members can accompany the client during treatment visits or follow-up appointments. During these visits the client may be overwhelmed with emotion and perhaps pain or discomfort. As well, an individual faced with a stressful situation often has the capacity to absorb only as much information as they are ready to accept. The gradual absorption of information allows the client to continue to function without the overwhelming anxiety that results from devastating news. Often the client hears only part of what the HCP says, and some of the terms used by the HCP may not be understood. Family members accompanying their loved one can listen more carefully, take notes, clarify unclear information, and ask the HCP questions that the client may forget to ask. Family members also can help navigate the health care system and manage complex treatment regimens when the individual lacks the energy to do so.

The person's spouse and children may need to take over additional roles and responsibilities, especially during the treatment phase. If a couple is used to sharing financial and household responsibilities, the spouse may now be the only breadwinner and homemaker. Children may need to assume additional responsibilities or children who live a distance away may feel guilt about not being closer and able to assist with responsibilities. The individual living with the illness often struggles with the loss of their traditional roles. It is important to preserve as much of the person's role as possible and include him in activities and family decisions. At some point along the illness trajectory, it may become necessary to obtain outside assistance in caring for the individual. All these role changes will require a period of adjustment and acceptance for the entire family. Emotional outbursts are common, and recognizing each other's need for an opportunity to express and release their emotions will help strengthen communication. Some families find support in individual or group counseling and peer support groups. The individual may have a desire to put their affairs in order. The family should not mistake this as giving up, but as an effort to attend to the details of life. The person may ask their spouse for help in reviewing insurance policies and updating health care proxies and wills.

(Cleveland Clinic, 2003a; Leukemia-Lymphoma Society, 2006b)

15. Identify at least five nursing interventions to address Mr. McCann's coping needs. Include a referral to at least one community resource. Nursing interventions to address the coping needs of Mr. McCann include:

- Assess how much information the client desires regarding his illness, its treatment, and potential complications.
- Explain diagnostic procedures.
- Provide emotional support to both the client and the family.

- Offer support to enhance spiritual well-being.
- Assist the client in role restructuring of normal family functioning as needed.
- Refer to community resources.
  - The American Cancer Society and Leukemia and Lymphoma Society are community resources available to provide additional information and support for Mr. McCann and his family as they begin to cope with this chronic illness and its impact. The American Cancer Society can help the McCann's to identify local resources through the American Cancer Society Web site at www.cancer.org. Information from the Leukemia and Lymphoma Society is accessible at www.leukemia-lymphoma.org.

References

Ackley, B., & Ladwig, G. (2006). *Nursing diagnosis handbook: A guide to planning care*. St. Louis, MO: Mosby.

Cleveland Clinic. (2003a). *Chronic illness and depression*. Retrieved May 21, 2006, from http://www.clevelandclinic.org.

Cleveland Clinic. (2003b). *Chronic lymphocytic leukemia*. Retrieved October 7, 2006, from http://www.clevelandclinic.org.

Daniels, R. (2002). *Delmar's guide to laboratory and diagnostic tests*. Albany, NY: Delmar.

Garrigues, A. L. (2007). Hematologic problems. In F. Monahan, J. Sands, M. Neighbors, J. Marek, & C. Green (Eds.), *Phipps' medical-surgical nursing: Health and illness perspectives* (pp. 928–933). St. Louis, MO: Mosby Elsevier.

Good, E. W., & Sands, J. K. (2007). Gallbladder and exocrine pancreatic problems. In F. Monahan, J. Sands, M. Neighbors, J. Marek, & C. Green (Eds.), *Phipps' medical-surgical nursing: Health and illness perspectives* (pp. 1285–1289). St. Louis, MO: Mosby Elsevier.

Green, C. J. (2007). Assessment of the immune system. In F. Monahan, J. Sands, M. Neighbors, J. Marek, & C. Green (Eds.), *Phipps' medical-surgical nursing: Health and illness perspectives* (pp. 424–432). St. Louis, MO: Mosby Elsevier.

Lee, F., Chiang, W., & Santen, S. (2006). *Cholelithiasis*. Retrieved October 7, 2006, from http://www.emedicine.com.

Leukemia-Lymphoma Society. (2006a). *Chronic lymphocytic leukemia*. Retrieved October 7, 2006, from http://www.leukemia-lymphoma.org.

Leukemia-Lymphoma Society. (2006b). *CLL: A guide for patients and familes*. Retrieved October 7, 2006, from http://www.leukemia-lymphoma.org.

National Cancer Institute. (2006). *Chronic lymphocytic leukemia: Treatment*. Retrieved October 7, 2006, from http://www.cancer.gov.

Newton, S. (2005). Management of clients with leukemia and lymphoma. In J. Black & J. Hawks (Eds.), *Medical-surgical nursing: Clinical management for positive outcomes* (pp. 2401–2411). St. Louis, MO: Elsevier.

Smeltzer, S., & Bare, B. (2004). Assessment and management of patients with hematologic disorders. In L. Brunner & D. Suddarth (Eds.), *Textbook of medical-surgical nursing* (pp. 872, 896–897, 901–905). Philadelphia, PA: Lippincott Williams & Wilkins.

Tsai, C. J., Leitzmann, M. F., Hu, F. B., Willett, W. C., & Giovannucci, E. L. (2004). Frequent nut consumption and decreased risk of cholecystectomy in women. *American Journal of Clinical Nutrition* 80 (1), 76–81.

Visovsky, C. (2006). Interventions for clients with hematologic problems. In D. Ignatavicius & L. Workman (Eds.), *Medical-surgical nursing: Critical thinking for collaborative care* (pp. 897–908). St. Louis, MO: Elsevier.

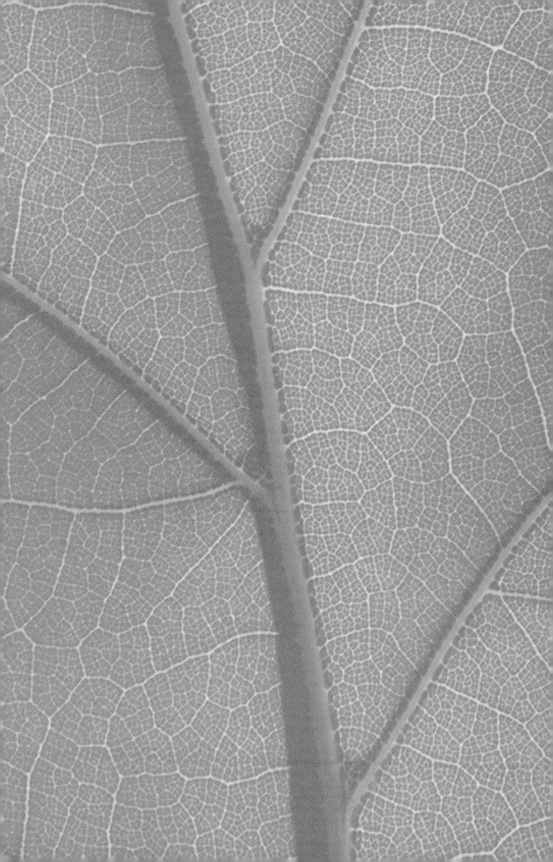

PART FIVE

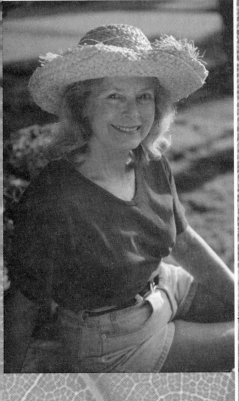

The Musculoskeletal System

CASE STUDY 1

Mrs. DiCenzo

GENDER

Female

AGE

59

SETTING

- Primary Care

ETHNICITY

- Italian American

CULTURAL CONSIDERATIONS

PREEXISTING CONDITIONS

- Myocardial infarction (MI) 17 years ago
- Hypertension (HTN)

COEXISTING CONDITION

COMMUNICATION

DISABILITY

- High risk for disability secondary to progressive nature of disease

SOCIOECONOMIC

SPIRITUAL/RELIGIOUS

PHARMACOLOGIC

- Furosemide (Lasix); atenolol (Tenormin); valsartan (Diovan); methotrexate sodium (Rheumatrex); folic acid (Folvite)

LEGAL

ETHICAL

ALTERNATIVE THERAPY

- Flaxseed; fish oil

PRIORITIZATION

- Client education about disease, treatment, and resources

DELEGATION

- Collaboration with a physical therapist (PT) and occupational therapist (OT)

THE MUSCULOSKELETAL SYSTEM

Level of Difficulty: Easy

Overview: This case requires the nurse to recognize the clinical manifestations of rheumatoid arthritis (RA) and discuss the diagnostic tests to confirm the diagnosis of RA. The nurse educates the client about RA and the medications prescribed as part of her treatment plan. Assistive aids and safety precautions to foster independence and maintain function are discussed. Priority nursing diagnoses and outcome goals for the client are identified.

Client Profile

Mrs. DiCenzo is a 59-year-old female who noticed that in the past three months her left leg, ankle, and toes were slightly swollen and that the rings on her left hand were getting tight. Mrs. DiCenzo's daily medications are furosemide, atenolol, and valsartan. Assuming that the swelling was due to excess fluid, she took an extra dose of furosemide each day for a week. When the swelling did not decrease, Mrs. DiCenzo called to make an appointment with her primary health care provider (HCP).

Case Study

During her assessment by the primary HCP, Mrs. DiCenzo explained that she has been experiencing an aching pain in the joints of her left hand, and noticed she has very little energy at the end of the day. Results of the laboratory tests prescribed by the HCP are erythrocyte sedimentation rate (ESR) elevated, C-reactive protein (CRP) test positive, positive antinuclear antibody (ANA) test, and positive rheumatoid factor (RF). X-rays of her hands show early signs of bone erosion. At a follow-up appointment with the HCP, Mrs. DiCenzo learns that she has RA, and she is prescribed an oral nonsteroidal anti-inflammatory drug (NSAID), methotrexate, and folic acid. The nurse provides informational literature about RA and spends some time educating Mrs. DiCenzo about her diagnosis and newly prescribed medications.

Questions

1. Identify at least five early clinical manifestations of RA.

2. Briefly discuss the incidence of RA and any predisposing risk factors in Mrs. DiCenzo's case.

3. Explain the pathophysiology of RA. Briefly describe the physical changes seen in the joints of a client with RA and potential systemic manifestations of RA.

4. Briefly describe each of the laboratory tests prescribed for Mrs. DiCenzo and the significance of the results: ESR, CRP, ANA, and RF.

5. Briefly describe the indication for each of Mrs. DiCenzo's daily medications: atenolol, valsartan, and furosemide.

Mrs. DiCenzo increased her dosage of furosemide to see if that would decrease the swelling in her left lower extremity and left hand. Explain the rationale for why Mrs. DiCenzo thought increasing this medication would help. What client teaching is appropriate regarding Mrs. DiCenzo's self-treatment decision?

6. Provide client teaching regarding methotrexate sodium. What type of medication is methotrexate sodium? What are the common and serious adverse effects? Explain what laboratory tests will be assessed prior to beginning methotrexate, and how often these tests will be monitored.

7. Briefly explain why folic acid has been prescribed for Mrs. DiCenzo.

Questions (continued)

8. In the future, as the disease progresses, Mrs. DiCenzo may experience a loss of function in completing some of her activities of daily living. When this loss of function occurs, the nurse can help to arrange for Mrs. DiCenzo to have physical and occupational therapy as prescribed by the HCP. What are the goals of this therapy? Describe three assistive devices that foster independence with activities of daily living for the client with RA.

9. The literature the nurse provided includes information about *flaxseed* and *fish oil* as two complementary therapies for RA. Briefly discuss how these dietary supplements are believed to enhance the treatment of RA.

10. Prioritize three nursing diagnoses for Mrs. DiCenzo, and for each diagnosis generate an expected outcome goal.

11. Mrs. DiCenzo is overwhelmed. She states, "I am not even 60 years old yet and I have arthritis. I always thought you got arthritis when you were much older. Is this type of arthritis curable or will I always suffer with this?" How should the nurse respond? Provide Mrs. DiCenzo with information about the later symptoms of RA she may develop and the possibility that her RA could go into remission.

12. Weeks later, Mrs. DiCenzo has returned to the primary HCP for a follow-up visit. During the nursing assessment, Mrs. DiCenzo comments, "One thing that seems to really help reduce the swelling and relieve the pain and stiffness is a heating pad. At night while I am watching television, I wrap my left hand in a heating pad. Provide Mrs. DiCenzo with reminders about the proper way to apply heat to help minimize her risk of injury.

13. Identify a resource where Mrs. DiCenzo can find additional information about RA and support for living with RA.

Questions and Suggested Answers

1. **Identify at least five early clinical manifestations of RA.** Usually symptoms are bilateral and symmetric. Early symptoms indicative of RA include:

- Crepitus (crackling sound or sensation)
- Depression
- Difficulty performing activities of daily living (ADLs)
- Edematous (swelling), erythematous (redness), "boggy" joints (usually in three or more joints and most often in the small joints of the wrists, feet, metacarpophalangeal, and/or proximal interphalangeal joints)
- Fatigue
- Fever
- Generalized aching
- Joint deformity
- Loss of muscle strength
- Loss of mobility or range of motion
- Lymphadenopathy (lymph node enlargement)

- Malaise
- Morning stiffness lasting more than an hour
- Pain and/or tenderness in the joint at rest, with movement, and during the night
- Paresthesias (abnormal sensations such as burning or tingling)
- Positive serum rheumatoid factor test
- Radiographic changes (bone erosion or decalcification) in hand or wrist joints
- Rheumatoid nodules
- Warmth at the joints
- Weight loss

(Marek, 2007; Smeltzer & Bare, 2004).

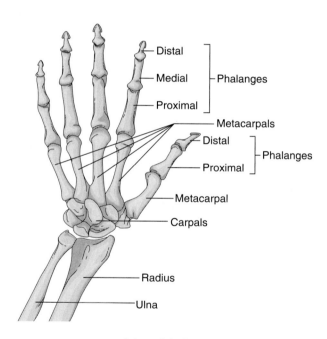

Joints of the hand

2. Briefly discuss the incidence of RA and any predisposing risk factors in Mrs. DiCenzo's case. RA is one of the most common forms of arthritis. A chronic disease, RA affects over 2 million Americans. Women are two to three times more likely than men to have RA. The age of onset in between 20 and 50 years, with women usually diagnosed in later childbearing years. The onset of RA in men is usually later in life. It is uncommon for a male to have symptoms of RA before the age of 45. Native Americans, particularly the Chippewa and Pima, have a higher incidence of RA. Even with attentive management, approximately 10% of clients develop a severe, crippling form of RA. An individual with RA is twice as likely to die as a person of the same age without RA. Almost all individuals with RA will experience pain and a loss of function. Ineffective pain management and loss of function can result in disability and significant financial concerns for clients and their families (Arthritis Foundation, 2005; Marek, 2007; Smeltzer & Bare, 2004). Mrs. DiCenzo's gender and age are predisposing risk factors for RA.

3. Explain the pathophysiology of RA. Briefly describe the physical changes seen in the joints of a client with RA and potential systemic manifestations of RA. RA is a chronic systemic inflammatory disease that primarily affects synovial joints and surrounding soft tissues. Pathologic features characteristic of RA are proliferation of the synovial membrane and erosion of articular cartilage and subchondral bone. Synovial tissue secretes synovial fluid that contains leukocytes, mucin, fat, albumin, and electrolytes. This provides nourishment to the articular cartilage and lubricates the joint. Proliferation of the synovial membrane leads to inflammation, causing edema, vascular congestion, fibrin exudates, and cellular infiltrate to accumulate around the synovial membrane. Articular cartilage covers the ends of articulating bones to reduce joint friction and help distribute weight-bearing forces on the joint. In RA, fibrin develops into an inflammatory exudate (called pannus) that forms at junctions of synovial tissue and articular cartilage and interferes with the nutrition of the cartilage, causing necrosis. This results in the formation of scar tissue. Pannus also invades subchondral bone and supporting ligaments and tendons, causing adhesions between joint surfaces, and a fibrous or bony union (called ankylosis) develops. Ankylosis refers to the immobility and consolidation of a joint due to disease, injury, or a surgical procedure. Affected joints assume the least painful position and then often become permanently fixed in that position. These processes cause destruction of intra-articular and periarticular structures, joint deformity (subluxation or dislocation), and limited joint mobility. The stimulus that triggers the inflammation of the connective tissues throughout the body is unknown. It is believed that RA is an autoimmune process resulting from the interaction of immunoglobulin G with rheumatoid factor, and a genetic predisposition has been identified. Another proposed cause of RA is an altered immune response to an unknown antigen.

RA can also affect other body systems. Systemic manifestations include pulmonary, cardiac, vascular, ophthalmologic, dermatologic, and hematologic effects. Individuals with RA often develop rheumatoid nodules, which are caused by cellular debris that forms near the joints over bony prominences. These rheumatoid nodules can also form in the heart, lungs, and spleen. Manifestations of multisystem involvement include pulmonary fibrosis, pericarditis, aortic valve disease, Raynaud's phenomenon, glaucoma, splenomegaly, brown skin lesions, and anemia (Marek, 2007; Smeltzer & Bare, 2004).

4. Briefly describe each of the laboratory tests prescribed for Mrs. DiCenzo and the significance of the results: ESR, CRP, ANA, and RF. *ESR:* When a tube of well-mixed venous blood is positioned vertically, the red blood cells (also called RBCs or erythrocytes) will tend to fall to the bottom. The ESR measures the rate at which the RBCs fall in one hour. This is a commonly prescribed test to monitor the course of inflammatory disease as well as infection. Elevated levels are seen in clients with conditions that cause increased plasma fibrinogen, increased blood cell size, or increased plasma viscosity. An increased ESR indicates rising inflammation, resulting in the clustering of RBCs, which makes these cells heavier than usual. The ESR of a client with RA is often elevated and the greater the level, the greater the inflammatory activity. The range of 0 to 30 mm/hr is within normal limits for a female over 50 years of age. It is common for a client with RA to have a normal ESR on presentation (up to 40% of clients). The ESR can be helpful in tracking the progression (sometimes called the "sickness index") of a disease such as RA.

CRP: C-reactive protein is an abnormal serum glycoprotein produced by the liver during acute inflammation. This protein appears in the blood in the acute stages of various inflammatory disorders and disappears rapidly when inflammation subsides. C-reactive protein is undetectable in healthy individuals, and, therefore, when detected, it signifies the presence of a current inflammatory process. Normal findings for an adult are less than 6 mg/L. A positive C-reactive protein test is often seen during acute phases of RA. Progressive increases in the amount of C-reactive protein correlate with the amount of inflammatory injury. This test can be used to monitor the therapeutic effect of medications.

ANA: Antinuclear antibodies are antibodies that the body produces against its own DNA and nuclear material in autoimmune disorders that cause tissue damage. Normally, at a 1:20 dilution, no antinuclear antibodies are detected. ANA testing is not diagnostic of all varieties of autoimmune disease, but 30% to 40% of clients with RA have a positive ANA test result. Results are reported as a titer. Higher titers indicate a greater degree of inflammation. If antibodies are present, further testing is prescribed to determine the type of ANA circulating in the blood.

RF: A prolonged exposure to an antigen (an infectious microorganism) can cause normal antibodies to become autoantibodies that attack host tissues. These autoantibodies, called rheumatoid factors, bind with any constituent in the blood capable of stimulating autoimmunity (self-antigens) and the synovial membrane, causing immune complexes to form. In a healthy adult, the rheumatoid factor is usually negative. In clients with RA, rheumatoid factor is positive in 50% to 90% of clients several months after the onset of their disease. Results are reported as a titer (such as 1:80). A higher titer represents greater inflammation. This serum test is valuable in providing early diagnosis of RA and initiating treatment to inhibit the progression of the disease(Chernecky & Berger, 2004; Daniels, 2002; Marek, 2007; Smeltzer & Bare, 2004).

5. Briefly describe the indication for each of Mrs. DiCenzo's daily medications: atenolol, valsartan, and furosemide. Mrs. DiCenzo increased her dosage of furosemide to see if that would decrease the swelling in her left lower extremity and left hand. Explain the rationale for why Mrs. DiCenzo thought increasing this medication would help. What client teaching is appropriate regarding Mrs. DiCenzo's self-treatment decision? *Atenolol* is a beta-adrenergic blocking agent that blocks the stimulation of beta 1 (myocardial)-adrenergic receptors and decreases the blood pressure and heart rate. Used alone or in combination with other antihypertensives, this medication treats hypertension. As an antidysrhythmic, it minimizes the risk of a myocardial infarction.

Valsartan is an angiotensin II receptor blocker. This medication blocks the vasoconstrictor and aldosterone-producing effects of angiotensin II at receptor sites. This action reduces blood pressure and left ventricular hypertrophy. Prescribed alone or in combination with other antihypertensives, valsartan is used to treat hypertension and helps reduce the risk of a stroke.

Furosemide is a loop diuretic that inhibits the reabsorption of sodium and chloride in the proximal and distal tubules and loop of Henle in the kidneys. Furosemide has a slight antihypertensive effect. This medication is used to treat edema and hypertension. Since furosemide leads to diuresis through increased urinary output, Mrs. DiCenzo believed that increasing her urine output would decrease the swelling that she had noted in her left lower extremity and hand. Mrs. DiCenzo's decision to self-treat her symptoms by increasing her dose of furosemide posed a risk of profound diuresis with water and electrolyte depletion, such as sodium, chloride, potassium, and bicarbonate. This fluid and electrolyte depletion can lead to dehydration, hypovolemia, hypokalemia, and thromboembolism. In addition, Mrs. DiCenzo could have experienced weakness, dizziness, or orthostatic (postural) hypotension, placing her at increased risk of injury (Deglin & Vallerand, 2007; Spratto & Woods, 2006). Mrs. DiCenzo should be educated about these risks, instructed to take her medications as prescribed by her HCP, and should increase the dosage and/or frequency only when instructed by her HCP.

6. Provide client teaching regarding methotrexate sodium. What type of medication is methotrexate sodium? What are the common and serious adverse effects? Prior to beginning methotrexate, explain what laboratory tests will be assessed and how often these tests will be monitored. The purpose of medication therapy for the client with RA is to relieve pain, control inflammation, and prevent bone and cartilage destruction. Early aggressive drug therapy is recommended to help prevent irreversible changes in the articular cartilage that often occurs within two years of the onset of RA. The use of NSAIDs and aspirin were traditionally the first line of treatment. However, there is a risk of adverse effects from the COX-2 selective and nonselective NSAIDs, and these medications do not help to prevent long-term damage to the joints. The recommendation is that NSAIDs be used in combination with disease-modifying antirheumatic drugs (DMARDs) or on an as needed basis. The client who is prescribed a DMARD in combination with an NSAID is afforded the benefits of increased functional ability, decreased pain, less joint tenderness and swelling, and lower ESR values than the client using an NSAID alone. Methotrexate sodium is a DMARD that inhibits degradation of folic acid to tetrahydrofolate and thus inhibits the DNA synthesis of inflammatory cells. The X-ray results indicate that Mrs. DiCenzo is already exhibiting signs of bone erosion, and thus her disease appears aggressive. Mrs. DiCenzo should be aware that she might not see the effectiveness of the methotrexate sodium until several weeks or months of therapy. Potential adverse effects of this medication include nausea, diarrhea, and stomatitis (inflammation of the oral mucosa). Serious adverse effects include pneumonitis (inflammation of the lung tissue), bone marrow suppression resulting in anemia, leukopenia or thrombocytopenia, as well as liver and kidney toxicities, and metabolic acidosis. Mrs. DiCenzo will have serum laboratory tests to obtain baseline information about renal function, hepatic toxicity, leukopenia, thrombocytopenia, and anemia, including a complete blood count, uric acid, and liver and renal function studies. These serum tests will be monitored periodically (every four to eight weeks). Mrs. DiCenzo should take her medication as prescribed and notify her HCP if she experiences symptoms of serious adverse effects. Most adverse effects resolve when the medication is discontinued. However, sudden discontinuation of methotrexate sodium is not advised since she may experience a rebound effect. Therefore, careful monitoring of medication effectiveness and adverse effects is advised (Marek, 2007; Smeltzer & Bare, 2004; Spratto & Woods, 2006).

7. Briefly explain why folic acid has been prescribed for Mrs. DiCenzo. Folic acid is necessary for the normal production of RBCs and for the synthesis of nucleoproteins. Folic acid is prescribed in combination with methotrexate sodium to decrease the toxic effects of the methotrexate sodium without decreasing the therapeutic effects (Marek, 2007; Spratto & Woods, 2006).

8. In the future, as the disease progresses, Mrs. DiCenzo may experience a loss of function in completing some of her activities of daily living. When this loss of function occurs, the nurse can help to arrange for Mrs. DiCenzo to have physical and occupational therapy as prescribed by the HCP. What are the goals of this therapy? Describe three assistive devices that foster independence with activities of daily living for the client with RA. Physical therapy (PT) and occupational therapy (OT) are an important part of the treatment plan for a client with RA. In addition to pharmacologic therapy, PT and OT help preserve joint mobility and promote independence. The physical therapist can recommend an exercise program to help maintain mobility and prevent muscle atrophy. The occupational therapist can work with Mrs. DiCenzo and her HCP to prescribe appropriate splints and orthoses to help stabilize or support a joint, protect a body part or joint from external trauma, and mechanically correct a dysfunction, such as foot drop. Assistive devices can aid the client with motor impairments. Utensils with built-up handles or a cuffed handle aid the client who has difficulty closing their hand adequately. A combination knife-fork helps the client who has lost the function of one hand. For the client who is no longer able to bend to reach their feet, long-handled shoehorns and stocking guides maintain their independence in dressing himself or herself. A long-handled reacher provides assistance in reaching or picking up objects out of one's reach. Ambulatory aids often prescribed include a cane, walker, or crutches (Marek, 2007; Smeltzer & Bare, 2004).

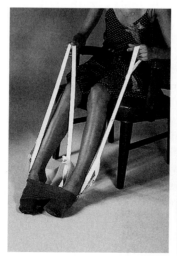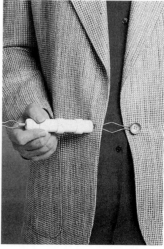

Assistive devices help clients dress independently

9. The literature the nurse provided includes information about *flax-seed* and *fish oil* as two complementary therapies for RA. Briefly discuss how these dietary supplements are believed to enhance the treatment of RA. Flaxseed and fish oil are sources of omega-3 polyunsaturated fatty acids shown to reduce inflammation, which decreases the number of swollen joints, minimizes the duration of morning stiffness, and improves overall function in the client with RA. Flaxseed is derived from the meal or oil of the flax plant. It is available as a pill, flour, or oil. A potential adverse effect to be aware of is diarrhea since flaxseed is also an effective natural laxative. Fish oil may be taken as a dietary supplement or by eating cold-water fish (salmon, tuna, and halibut) two to three times a week. Common adverse effects of fish oil include nausea, diarrhea, and heartburn. Both fish oil and flaxseed can act to slow blood clotting. Mrs. DiCenzo should be aware of the signs and symptoms of bleeding if she takes aspirin or NSAIDs (Arthritis Foundation, 2005; Marek, 2007).

10. Prioritize three nursing diagnoses for Mrs. DiCenzo, and for each diagnosis generate an expected outcome goal. Priority nursing diagnoses and suggested outcome goals for Mrs. DiCenzo include:

- Chronic pain related to (r/t) actual tissue damage and inflammation
  - The client will use the 0 to 10 pain rating scale to identify current level of pain intensity and determine comfort goal by (specify time frame).
  - The client will state that joint pain is decreased to comfort goal level using the 0 to 10 pain rating scale by (specify time frame).
  - The client will verbalize two nonpharmacologic ways to manage her pain at her next follow-up appointment.
  - The client will be able to function at the client's acceptable ability level with minimal interference from pain and adverse effects of medication.
- Fatigue r/t disease state (RA), pain, and emotional stress
  - The client will report reduced fatigue/increased energy after beginning treatment by (specify time frame).
  - The client will state two factors that lead to fatigue and two ways to avoid fatigue at her next follow-up appointment.
- Deficient knowledge (disease, treatment, resources) r/t lack of exposure and unfamiliarity with informational resources
  - The client will demonstrate an understanding of RA, her treatment plan, and symptoms to report to her HCP at the end of her HCP visit.
  - The client will demonstrate an understanding of how to take prescribed medications at the end of her HCP visit.

- ○ The client will explain how she is incorporating her new health regimen into her lifestyle at the next follow-up appointment.
  - ○ The client will demonstrate an ability to cope with RA and remain in control of life.
  - ○ The client will identify at least one resource that can be used for more information and/or support at the end of her HCP visit.
- • Risk for impaired physical mobility r/t pain, musculoskeletal impairment, loss of integrity of bone structures, and joint stiffness
  - ○ The client will maintain active joint range of motion in her left hand and left lower extremity.
  - ○ The client will maintain her acceptable level of function and independence with activities of daily living.

(Ackley & Ladwig, 2006; Marek, 2007; Smeltzer & Bare, 2004)

11. Mrs. DiCenzo is overwhelmed. She states, "I am not even 60 years old yet and I have arthritis. I always thought you got arthritis when you were much older. Is this type of arthritis curable or will I always suffer with this?" How should the nurse respond? Provide Mrs. DiCenzo with information about the later symptoms of RA she may develop and the possibility that her RA could go into remission. As the disease progresses, many joints in the body are affected. The joints most commonly involved are those in the hands, wrists, ankles, elbows, and knees. Later the hips and shoulders may be affected. Bone spurs and osteophytes (an outgrowth of bone) often develop which decrease joint mobility and cause increased pain. Disuse of the affected joints because of pain can lead to muscle atrophy. Twenty percent of individuals with RA will develop rheumatoid nodules, which are caused by cellular debris that forms near the joints over bony prominences (such as the elbow), and are often associated with progressive and destructive disease. Despite these potential complications, disease management and an improved quality of life are realistic goals for the person living with RA and complete remission of symptoms is obtainable by some clients (Marek, 2007).

The course of RA is unpredictable and is marked by periods of exacerbation and remission. The length of time between exacerbations varies with each individual. Physiologic and psychologic stress can bring about an exacerbation of the disease. The diagnostic criteria for remission include the absence of fatigue, no joint pain, joint stiffness that lasts less than 15 minutes, absence of soft tissue swelling, and an ESR less than 30 mm/hr in women and less than 20 mm/hr in men. A client is diagnosed as being in remission if these defining characteristics are present for at least two consecutive months. Remission, however, is unlikely after three years of sustained disease activity (Marek, 2007).

12. Weeks later, Mrs. DiCenzo has returned to the primary HCP for a follow-up visit. During the nursing assessment, Mrs. DiCenzo comments, "One thing that seems to really help reduce the swelling and relieve the pain and stiffness is a heating pad. At night while I am watching television, I wrap my left hand in a heating pad. Provide Mrs. DiCenzo with reminders about the proper way to apply heat to help minimize her risk of injury. Mrs. DiCenzo should avoid placing heat on areas of skin breakdown or redness and should clean her skin of any lotion or ointments before applying the heat to prevent heat intolerance or burning. The heating pad should be applied for 15 to 20 minutes to achieve the maximum effect and then removed to decrease the risk of a burn. If she has a hard time remembering, she can set a timer for 20 minutes as a reminder. She should begin with the temperature on the lowest setting and gradually increase the temperature as she adjusts to the heat. She should use the lowest temperature setting that affords her relief as opposed to always using the highest setting on the heating pad. The heating pad Mrs. DiCenzo is using should have a protective cover or be wrapped in a towel, preventing burns to the skin. If she wraps a towel around the pad, she should secure the towel with tape rather than pins to avoid puncturing the electric wires. She should check her skin every five minutes to assess for redness or evidence of tissue damage. If Mrs. DiCenzo notices decreased sensation in her left hand, she should not apply heat therapy since she risks injury resulting from an inability to detect symptoms of tissue injury or the sensation of burning (Altman, 2004; Marek, 2007).

13. Identify a resource where Mrs. DiCenzo can find additional information about RA and support for living with RA. The client may benefit from involvement in the Arthritis Foundation. Based in Georgia, this foundation publishes *Arthritis Today* magazine and offers a course titled Arthritis Self-Help to assist clients in managing the pain, fatigue, and stress associated with RA. The foundation can provide educational brochures and books, assist with HCP referrals, and connect the client with a local chapter. Information is available on their Web site at www.arthritis.org or by calling 1-800-568-4045. Another network of support is available at www.arthritissupport.com, or by calling the organization at 1-800-366-6056. This Web site community provides current information about treatment options, research news, symptom control advice, and support group listings. The American Chronic Pain Association, located in California, can also offer support and information for clients with chronic pain due to RA. Information is available at www.theacpa.org or by calling 1-800-533-3231 (Arthritis Foundation, 2005; ProHealth, 2006).

References

Ackley, B., & Ladwig, G. (2006). *Nursing diagnosis handbook: A guide to planning care*. St. Louis, MO: Mosby.

Altman, G. (2004). *Delmar's fundamental & advanced nursing skills*. Clifton Park, NY: Thomson Delmar Learning.

Arthritis Foundation. (2005). *Rheumatoid arthritis fact sheet*. Retrieved September 10, 2006 from www.arthritis.org.

Chernecky, C. C., & Berger, B. J. (2004). *Laboratory tests and diagnostic procedures*. Philadelphia, PA: Elsevier.

Daniels, R. (2002). *Delmar's guide to laboratory and diagnostic tests*. Albany, NY: Delmar.

Deglin, J. H., & Vallerand, A. H. (2007). *Davis's drug guide for nurses*. Philadelphia, PA: F. A. Davis.

Marek, J. F. (2007). Osteoarthritis and rheumatoid arthritis. In *Phipps' medical-surgical nursing: Health and illness perspectives* (pp. 1638–1653). St. Louis, MO: Mosby Elsevier.

ProHealth. (2006). *About us*. Retrieved September 10, 2006 from www.arthritissupport.com.

Smeltzer, S., & Bare, B. (2004). Assessment and management of patients with rheumatic disorders. In L. Brunner & D. Suddarth (Eds.), *Textbook of medical-surgical nursing* (pp. 1611, 1621–1623). Philadelphia, PA: Lippincott Williams & Wilkins.

Spratto, G. R., & Woods, A. L. (2006). *PDR nurse's drug handbook*. Clifton Park, NY: Thomson Delmar Learning.

Mrs. Bagnell

GENDER

Female

AGE

36

SETTING

- Hospital

ETHNICITY

- White American

CULTURAL CONSIDERATIONS

PREEXISTING CONDITION

COEXISTING CONDITION

COMMUNICATION

DISABILITY

SOCIOECONOMIC

- Married
- Stay-at-home mother of two daughters (ages 7 and 9 years old)

SPIRITUAL/RELIGIOUS

PHARMACOLOGIC

- Acetaminophen (Tylenol); ibuprofen (Advil, Motrin); doxycycline; hydrocodone bitartrate and acetaminophen (Vicodin)

LEGAL

ETHICAL

ALTERNATIVE THERAPY

PRIORITIZATION

DELEGATION

- Referral to infectious disease specialist
- Referral to physical therapist and occupational therapist as needed

THE MUSCULOSKELETAL SYSTEM

Level of Difficulty: Easy

Overview: The nurse must recognize the characteristic clinical manifestations of Lyme disease and relate an understanding of the serum laboratory tests used to help confirm the diagnosis. Medications prescribed to treat Lyme disease are reviewed. Priority nursing diagnoses for the client are identified, and the potential impact of this disease on the client's quality of life is discussed. The client's family is educated about ways to reduce their risk of exposure to ticks that may be carrying the bacterium that causes Lyme disease.

Client Profile

It is late September in New Haven, Connecticut. **Mrs. Bagnell** is a 36-year-old woman who presents to the emergency department complaining of extreme fatigue, joint pain, and a terrible headache. She is concerned, stating, "About a week ago I noticed a strange mark on my left inner thigh. It was itchy, so I thought it was a mosquito bite. The mark is still there. That part of my leg really hurts. I cannot even wear nylon stockings because anything that rubs against it is very uncomfortable. Also, for the past few days I have felt very sick. I am so tired and ache all over. Do you think I could have Lyme disease?"

Case Study

Mrs. Bagnell's vital signs are blood pressure 108/62, pulse 68, respiratory rate 18, and temperature 99.2°F (37.3°C). Her oxygen saturation is 100% on room air. Further assessment reveals that Mrs. Bagnell has been extremely fatigued for a week. She complains of constant joint pain in her hands, hips, knees, and ankles that is a "7 or 8" out of 10 on a 0 to 10 pain scale. She describes the pain as "throbbing and achy with occasional sharp shooting pains." She states, "I have noticed that even the soles of my feet hurt. I have had such a terrible headache. Basically, I hurt all over." The client has tried acetaminophen and ibuprofen with no relief of her symptoms. Physical assessment reveals that the client has a circular area of erythema migrans on her inner left thigh. The area is approximately three inches in diameter, and the pattern of discoloration resembles a bull's-eye pattern. There is a small red area in the center, surrounded by pallor, and the outer border is red. The area is raised, and the skin is warm to the touch.

Based on Mrs. Bagnell's presenting signs and symptoms and the characteristic erythema migrans rash, the health care provider (HCP) in the emergency department is confident that Mrs. Bagnell has contracted Lyme disease. To help confirm the diagnosis, the HCP requests several serum laboratory tests that include an enzyme-linked immunosorbent assay (ELISA) and Western blot. The HCP prescribes 200 mg of doxycycline by mouth twice daily for four weeks and hydrocodone/acetaminophen by mouth as needed for the client's pain. The HCP refers Mrs. Bagnell to an infectious disease specialist and suggests that she also follow up with her primary HCP as needed. Mrs. Bagnell's laboratory results reveal a positive ELISA that is confirmed by a positive immunoglobulin M (IgM) and immunoglobulin G (IgG) Western blot test.

Questions

1. Why is this condition called Lyme disease?

2. What causes the transmission of Lyme disease, and what is the incubation period? Are there areas in the United States that report a higher incidence of the disease?

3. During which time(s) of the year are individuals at greatest risk of contracting Lyme disease and why?

4. Describe the three stages of Lyme disease. What characteristic clinical manifestations of Lyme disease did Mrs. Bagnell exhibit?

5. Briefly explain why the Western blot test is prescribed to confirm a positive ELISA result.

6. The HCP prescribes doxycycline and hydrocodone/acetaminophen. Provide Mrs. Bagnell with information regarding the most common adverse effects that she should be aware of and ways to minimize these adverse effects.

7. Generate three priority nursing diagnoses that the nurse should consider when creating Mrs. Bagnell's plan of care.

8. Discuss the possible effect of a long-term illness and treatment regimen on Mrs. Bagnell's quality of life.

9. Mrs. Bagnell suspects that she was bitten by a tick while sitting in her backyard. Her husband fears he or the girls will get a tick bite in the yard as well. Identify at least five interventions that the nurse can teach the Bagnells to do to help decrease the family's risk.

10. Briefly discuss the risk that other members of the Bagnell family could become ill with Lyme disease by kissing or being in close contact with Mrs. Bagnell.

Questions and Suggested Answers

1. Why is this condition called Lyme disease? Lyme disease (also called Lyme arthritis) was first identified in Lyme, Connecticut, in 1976 when a group of children developed juvenile rheumatoid arthritis. The Centers for Disease Control and Prevention (CDC) declared Lyme disease a nationally reportable disease in 1991 (Marek, 2007; Zehala, Davis, & Sears, 2007).

2. What causes the transmission of Lyme disease, and what is the incubation period? Are there areas in the United States that report a higher incidence of the disease? Lyme disease is a bacterial infection transmitted by a carrier (called a vector) that transfers an infective agent from one host to another. Blacklegged ticks that reside on mice, squirrels, raccoons, cats, dogs, cows, horses, and deer transmit Lyme disease. The vast majority of Lyme disease cases (95%) are caused by the bite of infected deer ticks. When a young tick feeds on an infected animal, the tick takes the bacterium into its body. If the tick feeds again, it can transmit the bacterium to its new host. Many clients do not remember being bitten because the bite is painless and the deer ticks are very small (3.5 mm to 5.5 mm in length). The bacterium that causes Lyme disease is *Borrelia burgdorferi*, which belongs to a group of bacteria called spirochetes. A spirochete resembles a coiled spring. "A minimum of 24 to 48 hours is necessary for effective transmission of the spirochetes to infect a human" (Marek, 2007, p. 1562). The incubation period usually takes a week to 14 days from the time of exposure to the onset of clinical manifestations. In some clients, however, the incubation period is as brief as three days or as long as 30 days (CDC, 2005; Ignatavicius & Matzko, 2006; Marek, 2007; Zehala, Davis, & Sears, 2007).

The migratory flights of birds contribute to the spread of infected ticks across the country. "The disease has been reported in most European countries, throughout Asia, and in 49 states and the District of Columbia in the United States" (Marek, 2007, p. 1562). More than 85% of the cases of Lyme disease in the United States occur in New England, the mid-Atlantic states including Maryland and Virginia, the upper mid-Western states including Wisconsin and Minnesota, and in northern California. In 2005, there were over 23,000 reported cases of Lyme disease in the United States. The five states with the highest incidence were Delaware (76.6 cases per 100,000 population), Connecticut (51.6 per 100,000), New Jersey (38.6 per 100,000), Massachusetts (36.5 per 100,000), and Pennsylvania (34.5 per 100,000) (CDC, 2006).

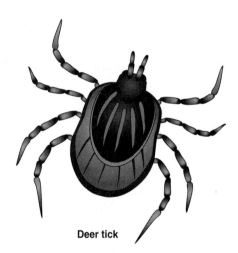

Deer tick

Lyme disease is transmitted with the help of a vector, such as the deer tick. Zehala, A. M., Davis, D., & Sears, R. (2007). Musculoskeletal dysfunction: Nursing management. In Daniels, R., Nicoll, L. H., & Nosek, L. J. (Eds.), *Contemporary medical-surgical nursing (pp. 1966-1969).* St. Louis, MO: Mosby Elsevier.

3. During which time(s) of the year are individuals at greatest risk of contracting Lyme disease and why? Most cases of Lyme disease are diagnosed June through October. Deer ticks are most prevalent during May, June, and

July, when ticks are most active and humans are more likely to participate in outdoor activities. The onset of symptoms is most likely to occur during June, July, and August and least likely from December through March (CDC, 2005; CDC, 2006; Ignatavicius & Matzko, 2006; Marek, 2007).

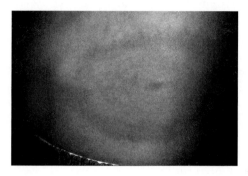

Erythema migrans of Lyme disease. Courtesy of Robert A. Silverman, M.D., Clinical Associate Professor, Department of Pediatrics, Georgetown University

4. Describe the three stages of Lyme disease. What characteristic clinical manifestations of Lyme disease did Mrs. Bagnell exhibit? Lyme disease is a form of rheumatic joint disease. For some clients, the first and only clinical manifestation they exhibit is arthritis. The disease is also considered a connective tissue disorder since the skin, joints, nervous system, and heart are also involved. In the early (stage I or localized) stage of Lyme disease, the client often complains of flulike symptoms, including fever, headache, fatigue, and lethargy. The client has an erythema migrans rash that has a bull's-eye appearance (the first sign of infection in 70% to 80% of cases), pain and stiffness of their joints (arthralgia) and muscles (myalgia), and may have lymphadenopathy (lymph node enlargement). The clinical manifestations of stage I of this systemic inflammatory disease begin three to 32 days after an infected deer tick has bitten the client. The early disseminated stage of the disease (stage II) occurs two to 12 weeks after the tick bite. Clients in this stage may experience carditis (inflammation of the heart), dysrhythmias, pericarditis (inflammation of the pericardium), palpations, dizziness, shortness of breath, and generalized lymphadenopathy. Since *B. burgdorferi* crosses the blood-brain barrier, the client with Lyme disease will often have central nervous system disorders such as meningitis, encephalitis, facial paralysis (usually unilateral), and peripheral neuropathy. If not treated, Lyme disease can progress to chronic complications. Approximately 60% of clients with untreated infection have intermittent bouts of arthritis with severe joint pain and swelling. The large joints, especially the knees, are most often affected (CDC, 2005). Manifestations of this chronic stage III include chronic fatigue, arthritis, lack of muscular coordination (called ataxia), spastic paresis (also referred to as intermittent incomplete paralysis), and arthralgia (joint pain). Lyme encephalitis, an inability to think clearly, difficulty concentrating, and memory loss can also occur. Rare, but serious long-term complications of Lyme disease include ocular changes such as conjunctival erythema, retinal hemorrhage, inflammation of the cornea (keratitis), and edema of the optic disc (papilledema). Stage III occurs weeks, months, or years after being infected by a tick bite (CDC, 2005; Ignatavicius & Matzko, 2006; MacDonald, 2005; Marek, 2007; Zehala, Davis, & Sears, 2007).

The characteristic manifestations that Mrs. Bagnell exhibited include an erythema migrans rash with a "bull's-eye" appearance on her left thigh, a severe headache, joint pain in several joints, fatigue, and a low-grade fever.

5. Briefly explain why the Western blot test is prescribed to confirm a positive ELISA result. An ELISA test is designed to be very "sensitive," meaning that almost every client with Lyme disease and some individuals who do not have Lyme disease will test positive (reactive). False-positive ELISA results can occur in 40% to 60% of cases. Therefore, if the ELISA is positive (reactive) or indeterminate (equivocal), a Western blot test should be conducted to confirm the results. A Western blot test is designed to be "specific," meaning that it will be positive only if a client is truly infected with the *B. burgdorferi* bacteria. If the Western blot result is negative, the client's ELISA was a false positive. If the Western blot is positive, as in Mrs. Bagnell's case, it confirms the diagnosis of Lyme disease (CDC, 2005; Daniels, 2002).

6. The HCP prescribes doxycycline and hydrocodone/acetaminophen. Provide Mrs. Bagnell with information regarding the most common adverse effects that she should be aware of and ways to minimize these adverse effects. Common adverse effects of the antibiotic doxycycline include dizziness, diarrhea, nausea, and vomiting. Mrs. Bagnell should avoid driving or any activities that require alertness until her reaction to the medication is known. The client may experience a heightened reactivity of her skin to sunlight (photosensitivity) and should avoid direct exposure to sunlight whenever possible. When in the sun, she should wear sunscreen and protective clothing. Many clients experience gastric reflux and an upset stomach. Taking doxycycline with food and a full glass of water or milk, and remaining upright for at least 45 minutes afterward, can help prevent gastric reflux and esophageal ulceration (Deglin & Vallerand, 2007; Spratto & Woods, 2006).

Taking the narcotic hydrocodone/acetaminophen may cause drowsiness, confusion, sedation, constipation, respiratory depression, and hypotension.

As with the doxycycline, the nurse should educate Mrs. Bagnell about the importance of avoiding driving a vehicle and activities requiring her to be alert. Increasing her fluid intake and bulk in her diet can help prevent constipation. She should notify her HCP if she has a change in her bowel pattern. The HCP can suggest an over-the-counter laxative or prescribe a stimulant laxative to minimize the constipating effects while she is taking this narcotic. She should rise slowly from a lying or sitting position to prevent orthostatic hypotension and report any excessive sedation or difficulty breathing to her HCP immediately. The nurse should instruct Mrs. Bagnell to avoid the use of alcohol while taking this narcotic analgesic to prevent increased risk of sedation and central nervous system depression (Deglin & Vallerand, 2007; Spratto & Woods, 2006).

7. Generate three priority nursing diagnoses that the nurse should consider when creating Mrs. Bagnell's plan of care. Priority nursing diagnoses to consider when creating Mrs. Bagnell's plan of care include:

- Acute pain related to (r/t) inflammation of the joints, urticaria, and rash
- Deficient knowledge r/t lack of information concerning disease, prevention, and treatment
- Fatigue r/t increased energy requirements
- Activity intolerance r/t fatigue and weakness
- Anxiety r/t unknown progression of disease
- Risk for decreased cardiac output r/t dysrhythmia
- Risk for infection r/t long-term antibiotic use
- Risk for powerlessness r/t possible chronic condition
- Risk for disturbed body image r/t facial paralysis
- Risk for impaired role performance r/t fatigue, chronic pain, and memory and concentration difficulties
- Risk for self-care deficit (bathing/hygiene, dressing/grooming) r/t fatigue and chronic pain

(Ackley & Ladwig, 2006; Zehala, Davis, & Sears, 2007).

8. Discuss the possible effect of a long-term illness and treatment regimen on Mrs. Bagnell's quality of life. Most clients who are diagnosed in the early stage of Lyme disease and treated with the proper antibiotic recover quickly and completely. If Lyme disease is not treated in the early stages or if the client does not respond to antibiotics, the client can develop chronic complications. Once Mrs. Bagnell has completed her month-long prescription of dozycycline, her clinical manifestations may not have resolved. A second round of antibiotic therapy will be prescribed. It is possible, however, that despite pharmacological therapy, she will continue to be fatigued, have aching joints, and suffer with frequent headaches. The extreme fatigue may result in the need for frequent naps and a lack of energy to complete her daily tasks and fulfill her role as wife and mother of two children. Permanent damage to the nervous system can leave the client with memory difficulties and a decreased ability to concentrate for years after the initial infection. It can be a long-term illness requiring months to years of treatment. Clients who continue to have joint pain and musculoskeletal symptoms that result in impaired mobility, activity intolerance, or a decreased ability to complete their activities of daily living may be referred to a physical and/or occupational therapist. Careful monitoring by an HCP and the support of family and friends is essential for maximizing the client's ability to maintain their highest degree of function and quality of life (CDC, 2005; Ignatavicius & Matzko, 2006; MacDonald, 2005; Marek, 2007).

9. Mrs. Bagnell suspects that she was bitten by a tick while sitting in her backyard. Her husband fears he or the girls will get a tick bite in the yard as well. Identify at least five interventions that the nurse can teach the Bagnells to do to help decrease the family's risk. Interventions to help prevent Lyme disease include:

- Avoid heavily wooded areas or areas with thick underbrush. Do not sit directly on the ground.
- Bathe immediately after spending time in an area that may be infested with ticks.
- Inspect your/each other's body (especially arms and legs), hairline, and clothes for ticks (ticks are the size of the head of a pin).
- Pets should wear tick collars and be kept off furniture since they can carry ticks into the house.
- Place wood chips or gravel between wooded areas and the lawn to prevent the migration of ticks into the yard.
- Prune trees, clear brush and tall grasses, remove leaf litter, and mow the lawn frequently since ticks are susceptible to dehydration. Ticks die quickly in dry, sunny environments, and landscaping can reduce humidity.
- Remove any ticks with tweezers or fingers by gently pulling the tick straight out of the skin. Dispose of ticks down the toilet. Squeezing or burning a tick is not advised, since doing so can spread the infection. Disinfect the tweezers. The client may choose to save the tick in a jar and have it tested for Lyme disease by the health department or a local veterinarian.
- Remove bird feeders and birdbaths from the yard since these attract animals that may carry ticks.
- Spray the yard with a pesticide designed to kill ticks (called an acaricide). A single application at the end of May or beginning of June can reduce tick populations by 68% to 100%.

- Use insect repellent containing diethyl toluamide (DEET) on skin and clothes when spending time in the yard or in other areas where ticks may be found. Be sure to use repellent that is safe for children.
- A vaccine for Lyme disease was introduced in 1998. However, the vaccine was withdrawn from the market in 2002. The vaccine manufacturer cited insufficient consumer demand as the reason for discontinuing production of the vaccine. Clients who received the vaccine are no longer protected because the vaccine's effectiveness diminishes over time.
- Wash the tick site thoroughly with warm water and soap and apply an antiseptic. Wash hands and clothes thoroughly.
  - Wear a hat or cap.
  - Wear closed shoes.
  - Wear light-colored clothing so that ticks can be spotted more easily.
  - Wear long-sleeved shirts and long pants. Tuck shirts into pants and pants into socks.
  - Woodpiles should be kept away from the house.

(CDC, 2005; Ignatavicius & Matzko, 2006; Marek, 2007)

10. Briefly discuss the risk that other members of the Bagnell family could become ill with Lyme disease by kissing or being in close contact with Mrs. Bagnell. There is no evidence of any risk that others could contract Lyme disease by being in contact with Mrs. Bagnell. The disease is not transmitted from person-to-person through touching, kissing, sexual intercourse, or any other means of contact with an infected client (CDC, 2005).

References

Ackley, B., & Ladwig, G. (2006). *Nursing diagnosis handbook: A guide to planning care*. St. Louis, MO: Mosby.

Centers for Disease Control and Prevention (CDC). (2005). *Learn about Lyme disease.* Retrieved February 8, 2007, from www.cdc.gov.

Centers for Disease Control and Prevention (CDC). (2006). *Reported Lyme disease cases by state, 1993–2005.* Retrieved February 8, 2007, from www.cdc.gov.

Daniels, R. (2002). *Delmar's guide to laboratory and diagnostic tests* (pp. 500–501). Clifton Park, NY: Thomson Delmar Learning.

Deglin, J. H., & Vallerand, A. H. (2005). *Davis's drug guide for nurses (9th ed.)* (pp. 604–606, 1122–1125). Philadelphia, PA: F.A. Davis Company.

Ignatavicius, D. D., & Matzko, C. K. (2006). Interventions for clients with connective tissue disease and other types of arthritis. In D. Ignatavicius & L. Workman (Eds.), *Medical-surgical nursing: Critical thinking for collaborative care* (p. 418). St. Louis, MO: Elsevier.

MacDonald, P. A. (2005). Management of clients with rheumatic disorders. In J. M. Black & J. H. Hawk (Eds.), *Medical-surgical nursing: Clinical management for positive outcomes* (p. 2372). St. Louis, MO: Elsevier.

Marek, J. F. (2007). Degenerative disorders. In F. Monahan, J. Sands, M. Neighbors, J. Marek, & C. Green (Eds.), *Phipps' Medical-surgical nursing: Health and illness perspectives* (pp. 1562–1563). St. Louis, MO: Mosby Elsevier.

Spratto, G. R., & Woods, A. L. (2006). *PDR nurse's drug handbook* (pp. 456–458, 671–672). Clifton Park, NY: Thomson Delmar Learning.

Zehala, A. M., Davis, D., & Sears, R. (2007). Musculoskeletal dysfunction: Nursing management. In R. Daniels, L. H. Nicoll, & L. J. Nosek (Eds.), *Contemporary medical-surgical nursing* (pp. 1966–1969). St. Louis, MO: Mosby Elsevier.

CASE STUDY 3

Mr. Rodriquez

GENDER

Male

AGE

23

SETTING

- Home

ETHNICITY

- Hispanic

CULTURAL CONSIDERATIONS

- Injury resulting from an act of violence

PREEXISTING CONDITION

COEXISTING CONDITION

- Sacral pressure ulcer

COMMUNICATION

DISABILITY

- Spinal cord injury
- Unemployed

SOCIOECONOMIC

- Lives with his family in a predominantly Hispanic urban community
- Has a girlfriend
- No health insurance

SPIRITUAL/RELIGIOUS

PHARMACOLOGIC

LEGAL

ETHICAL

ALTERNATIVE THERAPY

PRIORITIZATION

DELEGATION

MODERATE

THE MUSCULOSKELETAL SYSTEM

Level of Difficulty: Moderate

Overview: The client in this case sustained a spinal cord injury (SCI) as a result of a gunshot wound. His quality of life is affected by the long-term physical, psychological, and financial sequelae of this devastating injury. The most common causes of SCI in specific client populations are identified. Factors that contribute to the development and prevention of pressure ulcers are reviewed. This case challenges the nurse to consider how the client's SCI has affected his relationship with his girlfriend, his family, and his future. Priority nursing diagnoses to address the client's physical and psychological concerns are identified. The potential for caregiver role strain is acknowledged.

Client Profile

Less than two years ago, **Mr. Rodriquez** was the victim of a drive-by shooting. Walking home from work late in the evening, Mr. Rodriquez was mistaken for another man and was shot from behind. The bullet caused a penetrating SCI at the eleventh thoracic (T11) vertebra, leaving the client with a complete SCI.

Case Study

Mr. Rodriquez is independent with most of his activities of daily living and can transfer from bed to wheelchair and from wheelchair to chair. He performs scheduled straight catheterizations throughout the day, but has occasional episodes of incontinence, particularly at night. He lives in his home with his parents and younger brother, who assist with his care as needed. The client recently developed a pressure ulcer. He has a 3.5 cm by 4 cm area of partial-thickness skin loss involving the epidermis and dermis that looks like an abrasion on his sacrum.

The client is no longer employed. Since losing his health insurance coverage, his immediate and extended family (grandparents, aunts, and uncles) have been paying for his medical expenses. A fund-raising event coordinated by the client's girlfriend also provided initial monies to help pay for a wheelchair and other safety equipment for the home. The client's parents have taken a second mortgage on their home to pay his medical bills. Mr. Rodriquez's girlfriend has been supportive since his injury. Lately, however, she has been visiting less often. She explains to the client's mother, "It is getting harder to visit every day. I can't stand to see him so depressed and I think by visiting, I only make things worse. Before the accident, we talked about getting married. Now he thinks I should find someone else. He tells me I deserve better—a whole man."

Questions

1. Briefly discuss the incidence of SCI in the United States, and Mr. Rodriquez's risk of sustaining a SCI according to his age, gender, and ethnicity.

2. Explain the loss of function caused by an injury at the T11 vertebra. Does Mr. Rodriquez have tetraplegia (also called quadriplegia) or paraplegia?

3. Discuss the factors that contribute to the development of a pressure ulcer, and define the stages of a pressure ulcer. What stage is Mr. Rodriquez's pressure ulcer?

4. Identify three ways the client and client's family can help the pressure ulcer heal and prevent the development of other pressure ulcers.

5. Identify at least five priority nursing diagnoses that address the physiologic issues of concern in Mr. Rodriquez's care.

Questions (continued)

6. Briefly discuss spasticity, a common complication of SCI. What intervention(s) might be included in the client's plan of care to help manage spasticity?

7. To help reduce his risk for impaired airway clearance, instruct Mr. Rodriquez in the proper technique for using an incentive spirometer (IS).

8. Mr. Rodriquez has expressed to his girlfriend that he feels that he is less of a man. Discuss the client's struggle to adapt to role changes and sexuality concerns.

9. Identify at least three priority nursing diagnoses that address the psychological issues of concern in Mr. Rodriquez's care.

10. Briefly discuss the factors that may contribute to caregiver role strain. Identify at least two priority nursing diagnoses that address the potential issues of caregiver role strain facing Mr. Rodriquez's family.

11. Identify at least one formal organization that serves as a resource to provide support to clients living with an SCI and the families that care for them.

Questions and Suggested Answers

1. Briefly discuss the incidence of SCI in the United States and Mr. Rodriquez's risk of sustaining a SCI according to his age, gender, and ethnicity. In the United States, there are approximately 11,000 new cases of SCI each year. The most common causes of SCI are motor vehicle accidents, followed by falls, then acts of violence (primarily gunshot wounds), and lastly sports-related injuries. More than half of all SCIs affect individuals 16 to 30 years old. The majority (approximately 80%) of SCIs occur in men. Since the year 2000, the majority of individuals with an SCI have been Caucasian (63%). Black Americans were injured in 22.7% of cases, and 11.8% were Hispanic. Hispanic youth are at an increased risk for injuries resulting from violence. The National Center for Injury Prevention and Control (NCIPC) suggests that this increased risk is due in part to the fact that "a greater percentage of Hispanic Americans have lower education levels and higher poverty levels" (Centers for Disease Control and Prevention, 2002). Also proposed as contributing factors are that the Hispanic community is more likely to face family disruption and a lack of intergenerational ties in families and communities. These factors have been shown to increase the risk of violent behavior and thus injuries sustained in violent acts (Mahanes & Sands, 2007; National Center for Injury Prevention and Control, 2006; National Spinal Cord Injury Statistical Center, 2006).

2. Explain the loss of function caused by an injury at the T11 vertebra. Does Mr. Rodriquez have tetraplegia (also called quadriplegia) or paraplegia? Mr. Rodriquez has suffered a complete SCI. A complete SCI results in the total loss of sensory and voluntary function below the level of injury (T11). A client with an injury to the thoracic, lumbar, or sacral segments of the spinal cord is described as having paraplegia. These clients have lost the function of their legs, bladder, bowel, and reproductive organs.

An SCI above the level of T12 affects upper motor neuron control. This results in the loss of one's voluntary control of urination. Following the initial period of spinal shock, spinal reflex activity resumes. However, a spastic bladder develops, and the client is unable to sense bladder fullness or the urge to void. The client experiences spontaneous voiding, often with incomplete emptying of the bladder.

Voluntary control of the anal sphincter is also lost because the ascending impulses to the brain are blocked. The client no longer feels rectal fullness or the urge to defecate, resulting in constipation and possibly bowel incontinence. Bladder and bowel retraining programs can assist the client in achieving control over the elimination of urine and stool.

Sexual function is impaired in the client who has suffered damage of the upper motor neurons. Men have difficulty establishing an erection, but may be able to have an erection in response to direct stimulation of the genitalia (called reflexogenic erection). The ability to ejaculate is usually not present.

Mr. Rodriquez is also at risk for impaired respiratory function since the abdominal muscles, which play a role in ventilation, are innervated from the spinal cord at the level of T6 to T12. The loss of abdominal muscle function and strength can cause the client to have difficulty taking deep breaths. This presents the risk of impaired airway clearance and the progressive accumulation of secretions, as well as possible atelectasis (collapse of alveolar sacs).

Mr. Rodriquez has paraplegia. A client with tetraplegia (formerly referred to as quadriplegia) has sustained an injury of the cervical spinal cord that leaves the client with a loss of function in the arms, legs, trunk, bowel, bladder, and reproductive organs (Hausman, 2006; Mahanes & Sands, 2007).

3. Discuss the factors that contribute to the development of a pressure ulcer and define the stages of a pressure ulcer. What stage is Mr. Rodriquez's pressure ulcer? Pressure ulcers, also called decubitis ulcers or bedsores, are localized areas of impaired skin integrity "that tend to develop when soft tissue is compressed between a bony prominence and an external surface for a prolonged period of time" (Delaune & Ladner, 2006, p. 1228). Immobility and diminished sensation, as in the client with an SCI, are the primary factors that contribute to the development of a pressure ulcer. Shearing force, friction, and moisture also play a role in impaired skin integrity. When the client is moved or repositioned in bed, a shearing force is exerted against his skin. As well, if the client is positioned in an upright position in bed and he slides down, the outer layer of skin and subcutaneous tissue will adhere to the surface of the bed and the deeper layers of

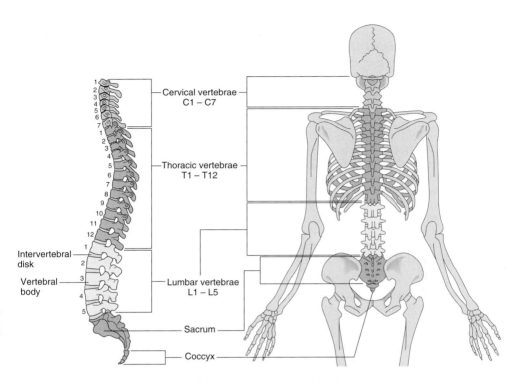

1
2
3
4
5
6
7
1
2
3
4
5
6
7
8
9
10
11
12
1
2
3
4
5

Cervical vertebrae
C1 – C7

Thoracic vertebrae
T1 – T12

Intervertebral disk

Vertebral body

Lumbar vertebrae
L1 – L5

Sacrum

Coccyx

Lateral and posterior views of the spinal column

tissue will move in the direction of the body's movement. This shearing (common in the sacral area) causes stretching and tearing of blood vessels, reduces blood flow to the area, and can lead to tissue necrosis. Friction is another factor that contributes to the development of a pressure ulcer. When a client moves, or is pulled up in the bed, the skin rubs against the sheets and creates friction. This friction damages and/or removes the superficial layer of skin and increases the risk of skin breakdown. The risk is further increased in clients with urinary or bowel incontinence. Moisture from urinary incontinence exposes the skin to irritating excretions that soften the skin tissue and lead to skin breakdown and potential infection. Pressure ulcers are described according to four stages of tissue destruction. The clinical manifestations of each stage are:

Stage 1: This is a pressure-related change of intact skin. There is persistent, nonblanchable erythema. Discoloration of the skin, edema, induration, and warmth may also be noted.

Stage 2: There is partial-thickness skin loss involving the epidermis or dermis, or both. A stage 2 ulcer is superficial and often appears as an abrasion, blister, or shallow crater.

Stage 3: This is a full-thickness loss of skin that involves damage or necrosis of the subcutaneous tissue. The damage may extend down to (but not through) the underlying fascia. A stage 3 ulcer is often a deep crater that may or may not involve undermining of the adjacent tissue.

Stage 4: These ulcers manifest as extensive, full-thickness tissue necrosis and destruction. There is often damage to the muscle, bone, and supporting structures (such as the tendon or joint capsule). Undermining, tunneling, and sinus tracks are often noted in these wounds.

(Delaune & Ladner, 2006)

Mr. Rodriquez has a stage 2 pressure ulcer on his sacrum.

4. Identify three ways the client and client's family can help the pressure ulcer heal and prevent the development of other pressure ulcers. Every day the family should inspect Mr. Rodriquez's skin for manifestations of a pressure ulcer. Early detection of areas of increased pressure and initiation of interventions is essential for maintaining the client's skin integrity. To help promote healing of the client's pressure ulcer and to prevent the development of others, his family can encourage proper dietary intake, provide appropriate hygiene, limit the skin's exposure to moisture, and change the client's position frequently to decrease pressure over bony prominences.

Proper dietary intake

The client's diet should include foods high in protein with adequate vitamins and minerals, such as meats, poultry, fish, eggs, and soy. The client should drink liberal amounts of fluid each day, while complying with the guidelines of a bladder or bowel program if prescribed.

Appropriate hygiene/Limit exposure to moisture

The client's skin should be washed with a mild soap and warm water. The skin should be dried thoroughly after cleansing and care should be taken to dry any moisture in skin folds and creases. To protect the skin from chemical exposure due to incontinence, a protective skin barrier cream should be applied to the client's skin after bathing. Since the client has occasional incontinence, particularly at night, perhaps setting an alarm clock would remind a family member to check to see if Mr. Rodriquez's clothing or linens need to be changed and to clean his skin and perineum. Pads and undergarments can be used to prevent soiling of linens. However, pads and undergarments that trap moisture next to the skin overnight should be avoided.

Change position frequently/Decrease pressure over bony prominences

The client should change position at least every two hours. Family members should assist one another in changing Mr. Rodriquez's position to limit the risk of shearing force and friction when pulling him up in the bed or across the sheets to position him on his side. Care should be taken to distribute his body weight evenly in the bed and while seated in a chair. Mr. Rodriquez should shift his weight every 15 to 20 minutes (with assistance as needed). Pressure reduction devices such as foam and air mattresses, gel pads, and elbow and heel protectors are effective in decreasing pressure over the bony prominences of the client's spine, ischial tuberosities, head, shoulders, elbows, and heels. The client's health care provider (HCP) may also prescribe a protective dressing such as a DuoDERM (Delaune & Ladner, 2006; Mahanes & Sands, 2007).

5. Identify at least five priority nursing diagnoses that address the physiologic issues of concern in Mr. Rodriquez's care. Priority nursing diagnoses for Mr. Rodriquez include:

- Impaired physical mobility related to (r/t) neuromuscular impairment
- Impaired skin integrity (coccyx) r/t immobility and paralysis
- Impaired urinary elimination r/t neuromuscular dysfunction
- Self-care deficit r/t neuromuscular impairment
- Risk for constipation r/t neurological disorder and immobility and adverse effect of medication(s)
- Risk for bowel incontinence r/t neurological disorder
- Sexual dysfunction r/t altered body function
- Risk for ineffective airway clearance r/t neuromuscular dysfunction
- Risk for disuse syndrome r/t paralysis
- Risk for injury (pulmonary complications; deep vein thrombosis; infection) r/t paralysis and immobilization
- Risk for infection r/t chronic disease and stasis of body fluids

(Ackley & Ladwig, 2006; Mahanes & Sands, 2007).

6. Briefly discuss spasticity, a common complication of SCI. What intervention(s) might be included in the client's plan of care to help manage spasticity? When the period of spinal shock resolves and spinal activity returns, muscle spasticity poses a serious concern for clients. This "heightened muscle responsiveness adds resting tone to flaccid muscles" (Mahanes & Sands, 2007, p. 1469). Most clients will experience the peak of their spasticity within the first year following their injury, and the condition will stabilize within two years. While this increased muscle tension helps minimize the effects of muscle wasting and makes it easier to assist the client with movement, it poses the risk of contracture and creates safety concerns. Clients may experience both clonic (intermittent) and tonic (sustained) muscle spasms. Clients may find that clonic spasms can assist in self-propelling them out of bed or to change position. However, a tonic episode can leave them in one position for extended periods. Passive range of motion exercises done daily and frequently (fours times a day) can help decrease muscle stiffness and decrease spasticity. When exercise and positioning are not effective in decreasing the adverse effects of spasticity, medications such as baclofen (Lioresal) and tizanidine hydrochloride (Zanaflex), may be prescribed (Mahanes & Sands, 2007).

7. To help reduce his risk for impaired airway clearance, instruct Mr. Rodriquez in the proper technique for using an IS. An IS is a deep-breathing exerciser that increases lung expansion, keeps alveoli open, helps remove mucous secretions, and strengthens respiratory muscles. Mr. Rodriquez should hold the IS upright. The steps for using the IS correctly include:

1. Take a normal breath and exhale.
2. Seal his lips around the IS mouthpiece.
3. Take a slow, deep breath to elevate the ball or plastic bar within the plastic chamber/tube.
4. Hold his inspiration for at least three seconds.
5. Simultaneously, he should measure the amount of inspired air volume using the calibrated plastic tube.
6. Remove the mouthpiece and exhale normally.
7. Take several normal breaths.
8. Repeat these steps four to five times.
9. Mr. Rodriquez should cough after using the IS to facilitate the removal of secretions.

The recommendation is that the client use his IS every hour while awake.

(Johnson & Altman, 2004)

8. Mr. Rodriquez has expressed to his girlfriend that he feels that he is less of a man. Discuss the client's struggle to adapt to role changes and sexuality concerns. Clients with an SCI face significant physical and emotional challenges that affect their quality of life, body image, role performance, and self-concept. The client is facing an acute and drastic change in his identity from that of a young, healthy, self-sufficient man, to that of a man in need of other's care and with significant physical limitations. Prior to his SCI, Mr. Rodriquez and his girlfriend were planning a life together. It is likely that their plans included Mr. Rodriquez's intentions to provide for the couple financially and a desire to convey a sense of strength and protection for his future wife. They anticipated a healthy sexual relationship and likely looked forward to having children. Mr. Rodriquez's injury threatens these desires and dreams. Statistics show that the likelihood of getting married after an SCI is reduced (NSCISC, 2006). The client is not currently able to contribute to the couple's financial stability and is physically unable to offer his girlfriend protection, participate in sexual intercourse; and starting a family appears impossible. Alternatives do exist that could allow many of their plans to be realized. The couple could consider alternatives such as penile implants, in vitro fertilization, and adoption. Mr. Rodriquez could find employment, perhaps working from home. Many clients with paraplegia are employed within 10 years of their injury (Hausman, 2006). Many aspects of the life that Mr. Rodriquez knew prior to his accident have been lost. He will need the support and understanding of his family, girlfriend, and friends to work toward coping and adapting to these changes. A peer support group of fellow SCI clients and/or work with a counselor can also offer support and assist Mr. Rodriquez in validating his feelings, developing coping strategies, and setting goals for the future. Many support groups are available online and can be accessed from a home computer if transportation is a concern.

9. Identify at least three priority nursing diagnoses that address the psychological issues of concern in Mr. Rodriquez's care. Nursing diagnoses that address the psychological concerns in Mr. Rodriquez's case include:

- Powerlessness r/t loss of function
- Disturbed body image r/t injury and change in body function
- Dysfunctional grieving r/t loss of usual body function
- Ineffective coping r/t situational crisis, inadequate opportunity to prepare for stressor, inadequate level of confidence in ability to cope, and uncertainty
- Ineffective sexual patterns r/t altered body function or structure, knowledge deficit about alternative responses to health-related transitions, and lack of privacy
- Fear r/t powerlessness over loss of body function
- Risk for impaired social interaction r/t limited physical mobility and self-concept disturbance
- Risk for loneliness r/t physical immobility
- Risk for chronic sorrow r/t immobility and change in body function

(Ackley & Ladwig, 2006).

10. Briefly discuss the factors that may contribute to caregiver role strain. Identify at least two priority nursing diagnoses that address the potential issues of caregiver role strain facing Mr. Rodriquez's family. There are many stressors inherent in the role of caregiver. The caregiver faces physical, emotional, and financial strains. Often caregivers maintain full-time employment and spend the remaining hours of the day caring for their loved one. Family members may create a schedule of "shifts" during which each is responsible for the client's care. Family members are often sleep deprived and physically exhausted. The emotional strain is immeasurable as they struggle to support the physical and emotional needs of their loved one while struggling with their own issues of fear, powerlessness, and uncertainty. The cost of equipment, supplies, medications, personal care, rehabilitation services, and HCP visits can be staggering. As the client develops complications, such as a pressure ulcer, the cost of supplies, additional medications, and need for follow-up HCP care escalates the expense. Although estimated costs vary greatly according to the severity of injury and individual needs, the average annual cost of health care and living expenses for the client with paraplegia is over $270,900 for the first year and over $27,500 for each year thereafter (NSCISC, 2006). Some clients are fortunate to have health insurance coverage for rehabilitation and care. Others, like Mr. Rodriquez, may have insufficient coverage or no coverage at all. If family members draw from their financial resources to supplement care, as the Rodriquez family has done, future savings and retirement resources are depleted, creating an ongoing struggle to sustain the needs of the client as well as those of the family (NCIPC, 2006).

Suggested nursing diagnoses to address the Rodriquez family's potential for caregiver role strain include:

- Interrupted family processes r/t shift in health status of family member, family roles shift, and modification in family finances
- Compromised family coping r/t role changes and prolonged disability that exhausts supportive capacity of significant people
- Parental role conflict r/t home care of child with special needs and interruptions of family life as a result of home care regimens
- Risk for caregiver role strain r/t duration of care giving required and situational stressors (major life event and economic vulnerability)
- Risk for impaired home maintenance r/t change in health status, insufficient family planning for finances, and deficient knowledge
- Risk for fatigue r/t stress, anxiety, and sleep deprivation

(Ackley & Ladwig, 2006).

11. Identify at least one formal organization that serves as a resource to provide support to clients living with an SCI and the families that care for them. Example of resources to provide support for those living with a SCI or those caring for someone with an SCI include the National Spinal Cord

Injury Association, National Rehabilitation Information Center, and the Christopher Reeve Foundation.

References

Ackley, B., & Ladwig, G. (2006). *Nursing diagnosis handbook: A guide to planning care*. St. Louis, MO: Mosby.

Centers for Disease Control and Prevention (CDC). (2002). *CDC Fact Book 2001–2002: Different people, different injuries.* Retrieved February 3, 2007, from www.cdc.gov.

Delaune, S. C., & Ladner, P. K. (2006). Skin integrity and wound healing. In *Fundamentals of nursing: Standards & practice* (pp. 1228–1230). Clifton Park, NY: Thomson Delmar Learning.

Hausman, K. A. (2006). Interventions for clients with problems of the central nervous system. In D. Ignatavicius & L. Workman (Eds.), *Medical-surgical nursing: Critical thinking for collaborative care* (pp. 983–995). St. Louis, MO: Elsevier.

Johnson, K., & Altman, G. (2004). Postoperative exercise instruction. In G. Altman (Ed.), *Delmar's fundamental & advanced nursing skills* (pp. 522–523). Clifton Park, NY: Thomson Learning.

Mahanes, D., & Sands, J. K. (2007). Spinal cord and peripheral nerve problems. In F. Monahan, J. Sands, M. Neighbors, J. Marek, & C. Green (Eds.), *Phipps' Medical-surgical nursing: Health and illness perspectives* (pp. 1459–1482). St. Louis, MO: Mosby Elsevier.

National Center for Injury Prevention and Control (NCIPC). (2006). *Spinal cord injury (SCI): Fact sheet.* Retrieved February 3, 2007, from www.cdc.gov/ncipc.

National Spinal Cord Injury Statistical Center (NSCISC). (2006). *Spinal cord injury: Facts and figures at a glance, June 2006.* Retrieved February 3, 2007, from www. spinalcord.uab.edu.

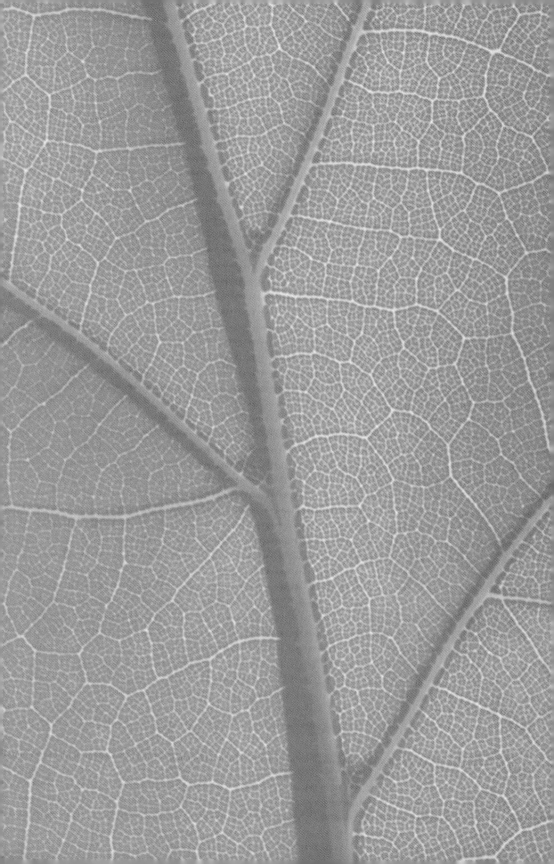

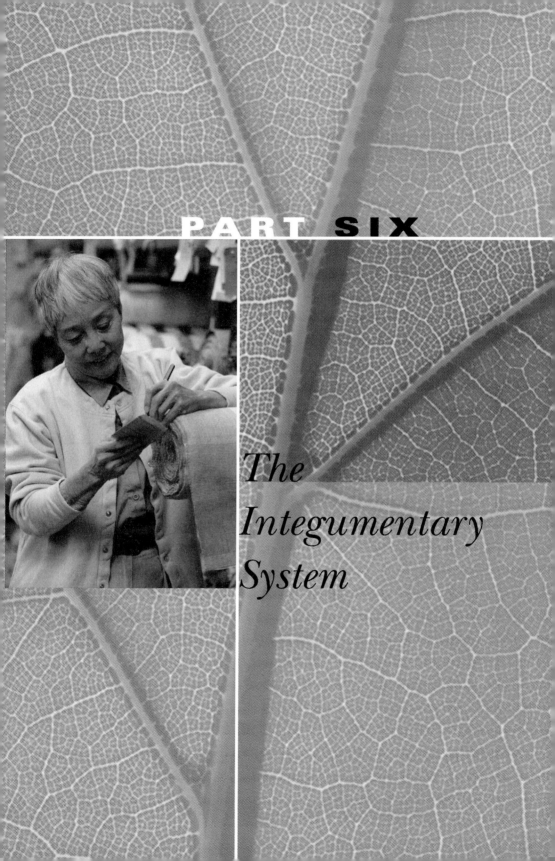

PART SIX

The Integumentary System

CASE STUDY 1

Mr. Shannon

GENDER

Male

AGE

80

SETTING

- Hospital

ETHNICITY

- Irish American

CULTURAL CONSIDERATIONS

PREEXISTING CONDITIONS

- Diabetes mellitus type 2, hyperlipidemia, hypertension (HTN), coronary artery disease (CAD), pneumococcal vaccine (Pneumovax) six years ago, influenza vaccine (Fluzone) six months ago

COEXISTING CONDITION

COMMUNICATION

DISABILITY

SOCIOECONOMIC

- Married, retired, recently returned from spending the winter in Florida

SPIRITUAL/RELIGIOUS

PHARMACOLOGIC

- Levofloxacin (Levaquin); tramadol hydrochloride (Ultram); glipizide (Glucotrol); insulin aspart (NovoLog); clopidogrel bisulfate (Plavix); amlodipine (Norvasc)

LEGAL

ETHICAL

ALTERNATIVE THERAPY

PRIORITIZATION

DELEGATION

- Delegation of a prescribed client treatment to a certified nursing assistant

THE INTEGUMENTARY SYSTEM

Level of Difficulty: Easy

Overview: The client in this case presents with left foot cellulitis. The impact of the client's history of diabetes mellitus is considered when planning the treatment regimen. The rationales for medications prescribed for the client are discussed. The nurse provides client teaching to reinforce the importance of proper foot care. Nursing diagnoses appropriate for this client are prioritized. Safety considerations when implementing warm compress therapy are discussed.

Client Profile

Mr. Shannon is an 80-year-old man who presents to the emergency department with complaints of pain in his left foot. The pain is worse with weight bearing on the foot when walking. He states, "I just don't feel well. I was fine when I came back home from Florida last week. My foot had a slight ache, but I was not concerned. Then this week I noticed the pain in my foot becoming worse and I feel sick. It feels like I have the flu."

Case Study

Mr. Shannon's vital signs are blood pressure 132/70, pulse 94, respiratory rate 20, and temperature 101.4°F (38.6°C). His blood glucose is 200 mg/dL. Further assessment reveals a small laceration on the bottom of Mr. Shannon's foot. When asked about the laceration, Mr. Shannon recalls, "I do remember cutting the bottom of my foot on a seashell while walking along the beach. It was just a tiny cut. I didn't think much of it." The area of skin surrounding the cut has become reddened and warm. His foot and ankle are swollen, and the diffuse redness is beginning to spread up to his left ankle. Mr. Shannon is noted to have an unsteady gait. He is diagnosed with cellulitis of the left foot. Intravenous (IV) levofloxacin and tramadol hydrochloride by mouth (per os, PO) are prescribed. The health care provider (HCP) prescribes that the client's left foot be elevated and a warm aquathermia pad applied every two hours. Mr. Shannon takes glipizide PO twice daily before meals. In addition the HCP prescribes sliding scale subcutaneous (SC) NovoLog insulin while the client is hospitalized.

Questions

1. Mr. Shannon asks, "What is cellulitis and how did this happen?" Explain cellulitis, the characteristic clinical manifestations with which Mr. Shannon presented, and what likely caused Mr. Shannon to develop cellulitis.

2. In priority order, identify at least three nursing diagnoses appropriate for Mr. Shannon's diagnosis of cellulitis.

3. Discuss the difference between type 1 and type 2 diabetes mellitus.

4. The nurse wishes to provide Mr. Shannon with teaching about diabetic foot care. Highlight five principles of good foot care that the nurse will discuss.

5. Mr. Shannon takes glipizide twice daily before meals. His breakfast tray arrives at 0830 each morning. When should he take his morning dose of glipizide, and when should the nurse anticipate the onset of glipizide's effect?

6. Discuss the rationale for prescribing sliding scale NovoLog insulin for Mr. Shannon.

Questions (continued)

7. Mr. Shannon takes clopidogrel bisulfate and amlodipine. Briefly explain the action of both medications, and why each is prescribed as part of his daily medication regimen.

8. Discuss the steps the nurse will follow to implement the HCP's request that a warm aquathermia pad be applied to Mr. Shannon's left foot and ankle every two hours. Is it appropriate for the nurse to delegate the implementation of this therapy to a certified nursing assistant (CNA)?

9. Mr. Shannon received a pneumococcal vaccine six years ago and an influenza vaccine prior to leaving for Florida six months ago. Should Mr. Shannon be offered either vaccine prior to his discharge from the hospital? Explain your answer.

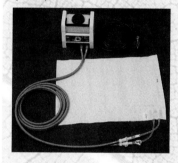

Aquathermal Heating Unit

Questions and Suggested Answers

1. Mr. Shannon asks, "What is cellulitis and how did this happen?" Explain cellulitis, the characteristic clinical manifestations with which Mr. Shannon presented, and what likely caused Mr. Shannon to develop cellulitis. Cellulitis is an infection of the subcutaneous tissue. It is the most common cause of limb swelling and may occur as an isolated event or a series of recurrent infections. Cellulitis occurs when there is a loss of skin integrity creating a portal of entry for bacteria. The bacteria release toxins into the subcutaneous tissue causing an infection. Characteristic clinical manifestations of cellulitis noted in Mr. Shannon's case include an acute onset of swelling, pain, and localized diffuse erythema. The area is warm on palpation, and the client has a fever and slight tachycardia. Mr. Shannon most likely developed cellulitis because of the laceration on the bottom of his foot from the seashell. Untreated, this wound created a portal of entry for bacteria and became infected (Nicol & Black, 2005; Smeltzer & Bare, 2004).

2. In priority order, identify at least three nursing diagnoses appropriate for Mr. Shannon's diagnosis of cellulitis.

1. Impaired skin integrity related to (r/t) inflammatory process and infection damaging skin/tissues
2. Risk for falls r/t older than 65 years of age, presence of acute illness, unsteady gait, antihypertensive agents, and unfamiliar environment
3. Acute pain r/t edema and inflammatory changes in tissues secondary to infection
4. Hyperthermia r/t infectious process
5. Ineffective health maintenance r/t lack of knowledge regarding care of diabetic condition and prevention of further incidence of infection
6. Deficient knowledge (diabetes, foot care) r/t unfamiliarity with information resources
7. Risk for injury (physical) r/t use of warm compress and unsteady gait
8. Risk for disturbed sensory perception r/t ineffective tissue perfusion

(Ackley & Ladwig, 2006)

3. Discuss the difference between type 1 and type 2 diabetes mellitus. Type 1 diabetes mellitus was previously referred to as insulin-dependent diabetes mellitus (IDDM) or juvenile diabetes. A destruction or genetic lack of development of pancreatic beta cells causes clients with type 1 diabetes mellitus to have either relatively low insulin production or insulin resistance or both. As a result, type 1 diabetics depend on exogenous insulin (injected subcutaneously) for their survival. Type 1 diabetes mellitus is usually diagnosed before the age of 30, and affects 10% of all individuals who have diabetes. Males and females are affected equally, with an increased incidence in African Americans, Native Americans, Hispanic Americans, and Asian Americans.

Type 2 diabetes mellitus was formerly known as non–insulin-dependent diabetes (NIDDM) or adult onset diabetes mellitus. The more common form of diabetes, type 2 affects 90% to 95% of the diabetic population and is often diagnosed after the age of 40. The primary defect in type 2 diabetes mellitus is thought to be an impaired liver and muscle sensitivity to insulin or impaired insulin secretion. Most type 2 diabetics manage their blood glucose levels with oral hypoglycemic medication. Some individuals, however, require insulin administration when oral medication alone becomes inadequate in controlling blood glucose levels. Populations that are at greater risk for type 2 diabetes mellitus include African Americans,

Hispanic Americans, Native Americans, obese individuals, and older adults (Fain, 2005).

4. The nurse wishes to provide Mr. Shannon with teaching about diabetic foot care. Highlight five principles of good foot care that the nurse will discuss. Critical elements of any educational plan are an assessment of the client's current knowledge of the topic and the client's readiness to learn. The nurse might choose to collaborate with a diabetic educator to develop the teaching plan. As may have been the situation in Mr. Shannon's case, decreased circulation and sensation (neuropathy) of the lower extremities can result in undetected foot wounds. Mr. Shannon, perhaps with his wife's assistance, should assess his feet daily with an understanding of five principles of proper foot care, which include inspection and palpation, hygiene, protection, and circulation.

Inspection and palpation

The feet should be inspected for dry, rough skin, fissures (a narrow slit), areas of discoloration, blisters, lesions, calluses, and changes in the toenails (discoloration or thickening). The client should be taught to note the color and temperature of the skin as well as any changes in hair distribution, especially decreased or absent hair growth. The extremities should be assessed for wounds, swelling, or signs of infection. It is likely that Mr. Shannon will have difficulty visualizing the bottom of his feet and his heels. Mrs. Shannon can be of assistance to him by inspecting these skin surfaces for wounds or signs of infection. Mr. Shannon should inform his HCP if any changes are noted, and see his HCP as soon as possible to assess any wounds or signs of infection.

Hygiene

Proper hygiene is encouraged. Mr. Shannon should wash his feet with a mild soap and warm water with careful attention paid to cleaning between the toes. The client (or his wife) should check the temperature of the bath (or shower) water with the hand to be sure that the water is not too hot. After bathing, he should dry his feet thoroughly and apply lotion. The lotion should not be applied between the toes however since this creates a moist environment that increases his chance of infection. Toenails should be kept trimmed, and it is recommended that toenails be cared for by a podiatrist to prevent cuts that may lead to infection.

Protection

In an effort to decrease the likelihood of wounds and infection, the feet should be protected. Properly fitting shoes and shoes appropriate for the weather are important safety measures. He should shake out his shoes before putting them on. Wearing clean cotton socks is recommended. Mr. Shannon should not walk barefoot, even at home.

Circulation

Good nutrition and adequate fluid intake are important for healthy peripheral circulation. Conversely, restrictive socks or clothing, crossed legs, and smoking all contribute to impaired vascular circulation and should be avoided. To help increase circulation to the extremities, clients should be taught to do range of motion exercises and keep their legs elevated whenever possible.

(Doughty, 2004; Fain, 2005)

5. Mr. Shannon takes glipizide twice daily before meals. His breakfast tray arrives at 0830 each morning. When should he take his morning dose of glipizide, and when should the nurse anticipate the onset of glipizide's effect? Glipizide is an oral antidiabetic medication that should be taken 30 minutes before eating a meal. Therefore, Mr. Shannon should take his glipizide at 0800. The nurse anticipates that the glipizide will take effect in one to three hours, therefore, between approximately 0900 and 1100 (Spratto & Woods, 2006).

6. Discuss the rationale for prescribing sliding scale NovoLog insulin for Mr. Shannon. Illness places the body under stress. In response to physiologic stress, the body releases hormones to fight the illness. These hormones can elevate blood glucose levels and impair the effects of insulin causing hyperglycemia. Extreme hyperglycemia that goes untreated may lead to diabetic ketoacidosis (DKA) and coma in the type 1 diabetic and hyperosmolar hyperglycemic nonketotic (HHNK) coma in the type 2 diabetic. In addition, abnormal serum glucose levels are a potential adverse effect of the prescribed antibiotic levofloxacin. While Mr. Shannon's body is recovering from cellulitis, he will require serum glucose monitoring four times per day. Clients who take oral agents may need to administer insulin during episodes of illness to help maintain their serum glucose level within normal limits. Episodic elevated serum glucose levels are most effectively treated with short-acting insulin such as NovoLog using a sliding scale to determine the appropriate dosage (American Diabetes Association, 2005; Fain, 2005; Spratto & Woods, 2006).

7. Mr. Shannon takes clopidogrel bisulfate and amlodipine. Briefly explain the action of both medications, and why each is prescribed as part of his

daily medication regimen. *Clopidogrel bisulfate* inhibits platelet aggregation to help reduce atherosclerotic events such as myocardial infarction and stroke in high-risk clients. Mr. Shannon is considered high risk because of his history of hyperlipidemia, hypertension, and coronary artery disease (Spratto & Woods, 2006).

Amlodipine is a calcium channel blocker used alone or with other agents to manage Mr. Shannon's hypertension. This antihypertensive medication works by "inhibiting the transport of calcium into myocardial and vascular smooth muscle cells, resulting in inhibition of excitation-contraction coupling and subsequent contraction" (Deglin & Vallerand, 2007, p. 128). The resulting systemic vasodilation decreases blood pressure (Spratto & Woods, 2006).

8. Discuss the steps the nurse will follow to implement the HCP's request that a warm aquathermia pad be applied to Mr. Shannon's left foot and ankle every two hours. Is it appropriate for the nurse to delegate the implementation of this therapy to a CNA? Clients with sensory and circulatory deficits, such as those with diabetes mellitus, are at increased risk for burns from a warm compress. Aquathermia pads are rubber heating pads through which water circulates. Tubing connects the pad to a water reservoir unit. This heating device is also called an aqua pad, k-pad, t-pump, or hydroculator. The nurse should follow the appropriate steps and precautions when implementing the HCP's prescription for warm compress therapy using an aquathermia pad.

1. Assessment

Prior to initiating warm compress therapy, the nurse should assess the skin integrity and circulation of the area to be treated. Skin breakdown, erythema, swelling, or scar tissue should be evaluated before heat is applied. Therapy should be held and the HCP notified if the area has scar tissue or appears blistered or burned. Adequate circulation, evaluated by assessing peripheral pulses, skin color and temperature, and results of vascular studies, is necessary for effective heat therapy and prevention of tissue and vessel damage. The nurse should document circulation, condition of the skin, and the client's pain level prior to the therapy. Also important is an assessment of the client's ability to sense a change in temperature or comfort level. The client's safety is at greater risk if they are unable to sense pain or burning, and/or if their level of sedation, agitation, or confusion prevents them from being able to report such sensations. If this is the case, the client should not be left alone during heat therapy.

2. Clean the area

Lotion, creams, or ointments on the skin can retain heat and increase the risk of heat intolerance and burning. If such a product has been applied to the skin, it should be cleansed from the area prior to applying the aqua-thermia pad.

3. Client education

The client should be educated about the purpose and desired outcome of the heat therapy, as well as the importance of reporting any increase in pain or sensation of burning. The aquathermia device used should have a temperature gauge to be set such that the temperature of the compress remains lukewarm. The client should be instructed not to change the temperature setting of the device. The client's understanding that the pad should not remain in place for longer than 20 to 30 minutes fosters safe implementation of heat therapy.

4. Initiate therapy

The nurse should wash his/her hands and set up the aquathermia pad equipment according to the manufacturer's instructions. The integrity of the pad, heating device, temperature gauge, and electrical cord should be ensured and a new device obtained if the nurse notes a leak, broken gauge, or frayed cord. The pad should be covered with a protective cover (not a bath towel) if not supplied by the manufacturer. Tape, not pins, should be used to secure the cover. The temperature of the heating device should be set to low and the pad applied to the area. The nurse should set a timer or note the time when the pad is applied to be reminded to remove the heat after 20 to 30 minutes. The temperature may be increased to 105°F (40.5°C) after the client adjusts to the heat. The highest temperature gauge setting is avoided, to decrease the risk of injury.

5. Discontinue therapy

After 20 to 30 minutes maximum, the pad should be removed and the aquathermia device turned off.

6. Evaluation

The nurse should evaluate the client's response to the treatment. In the minutes immediately following removal of the heated pad, the skin may appear red. This expected color change should resolve 15 to 20 minutes after discontinuing therapy.

7. Documentation

A nursing note includes the date, time, and purpose of treatment, prepro-cedure education and client understanding, assessment and condition of the skin prior to the application of heat, type of equipment used, duration of heat therapy, evaluation of the effectiveness of the treatment, condition of the skin after therapy, and client's tolerance of heat therapy.

Yes. It is appropriate for the nurse to delegate the implementation of this therapy to properly trained ancillary personnel such as a CNA. It remains the nurse's responsibility, however, to assess the client prior to and following the therapy and to evaluate the effectiveness of the therapy as part of the nursing documentation.

(Altman, 2004; Smeltzer & Bare, 2004)

9. Mr. Shannon received a pneumococcal vaccine six years ago and an influenza vaccine prior to leaving for Florida six months ago. Should Mr. Shannon be offered either vaccine prior to his discharge from the hospital? Explain your answer. Yes. Mr. Shannon should be offered the pneumococcal vaccine. This vaccine is recommended for all adults over the age of 65 years, especially for those with a chronic illness. Adults should have a booster after six years. Mr. Shannon does not need the influenza vaccine since this is an annual vaccine (Deglin & Vallerand, 2007).

References

Ackley, B., & Ladwig, G. (2006). *Nursing diagnosis handbook: A guide to planning care*. St. Louis, MO: Mosby.

Altman, G.B. (2004). *Delmar's physical assessment skills* (pp. 310–317). Clifton Park, NY: Thomson Learning.

American Diabetes Association (2005). *Using the diabetes food pyramid*. Retrieved November 1, 2005, from www.diabetes.org.

Deglin, J. H., & Vallerand, A. H. (2007). *Davis's drug guide for nurses*. Philadelphia, PA: F. A. Davis.

Doughty, D. B. (2004). Skin integrity and wound healing. In R. Daniels (Ed.), *Nursing fundamentals: Caring & clinical decision making* (p. 1078). Clifton Park, NY: Delmar Learning.

Fain, J. A. (2005). Management of clients with diabetes mellitus. In J. M. Black & J. H. Hawks (Eds.), *Medical-surgical nursing: Clinical management for positive outcomes* (pp. 1243–1288). St. Louis, MO: Elsevier.

Nicol, N. H., & Black, J. M. (2005). Management of clients with integumentary disorders. In J. M. Black & J. H. Hawks (Eds.), *Medical-surgical nursing: Clinical management for positive outcomes* (p. 1418). St. Louis, MO: Elsevier.

Smeltzer, S., & Bare, B. (2004). Assessment and management of patients with vascular disorders and problems of peripheral circulation. In *Brunner & Suddarth's textbook of medical-surgical nursing* (pp. 850–851). Philadelphia, PA: Lippincott, Williams & Wilkins.

Spratto, G. R., & Woods, A. L. (2006). *PDR nurse's drug handbook*. Clifton Park, NY: Thomson Delmar Learning.

CASE STUDY 2

Ms. Champlin

GENDER

Female

AGE

52

SETTING

- Hospital

ETHNICITY

- White American

CULTURAL CONSIDERATIONS

PREEXISTING CONDITIONS

- Depression
- Completed tetanus vaccination series as a child
- Most recent tetanus toxoid booster was 15 years ago

COEXISTING CONDITION

COMMUNICATION

DISABILITY

- Risk of contracture

SOCIOECONOMIC

SPIRITUAL/RELIGIOUS

PHARMACOLOGIC

- Morphine sulfate; tetanus toxoid (human tetanus immunoglobulin, TIG)

LEGAL

ETHICAL

ALTERNATIVE THERAPY

- Topical creams to minimize scarring

PRIORITIZATION

- First aid management of a burn injury

DELEGATION

THE INTEGUMENTARY SYSTEM

Level of Difficulty: Difficult

Overview: This case requires the nurse to recognize the emergent needs of a burn victim and potential complications of recovery. The different types of burn injuries and characteristics of first-, second-, third-, and fourth-degree burns are reviewed. Appropriate interventions for the client during the emergent, acute, and rehabilitative phase of burn care are discussed. Priority nursing diagnoses for the client who has suffered a burn injury are reviewed. The psychological impact of a burn injury is acknowledged.

DIFFICULT

Client Profile

Ms. Champlin is a 52-year-old woman who was cooking New England clam cakes in a skillet filled with hot oil. While dropping the dough into the skillet, oil splattered onto the gas stove catching on fire and filling the skillet with flames. In a panic, Ms. Champlin grabbed the handle of the burning skillet to remove it from the stove, spilling the hot oil all over her right arm and hand. The oil also splashed onto the right side of her face and neck, and across her chest, burning her skin through her T-shirt. She is transported to the emergency department by emergency medical technicians (EMTs).

Case Study

Upon arrival at the hospital, she is alert and oriented, without signs or symptoms of respiratory distress. She is screaming in pain. Ms. Champlin's vital signs are blood pressure 130/60, pulse 94, respiratory rate 22, and temperature 97°F (36.1°C). Her oxygen saturation is 99% on 2 liters of oxygen. She has suffered superficial and superficial partial-thickness burns on her face, neck, and chest, and deep partial-thickness burns over her right arm and hand. The right side of her face and neck and her chest are red with several blisters noted. Her right arm and hand are swollen and have sloughing skin with a mottled appearance of cherry red, tan, and pale areas. The health care provider (HCP) does not observe any discoloration of soot around Ms. Champlin's nose or mouth, singed nasal hair, or burned eyebrows. Acute care in the emergency department includes oxygen, intravenous (IV) fluids, the insertion of an indwelling urinary catheter, nasogastric tube attached to low wall suction, and the administration of IV morphine sulfate and tetanus toxoid. Ms. Champlin is transferred to a burn unit for continued care.

Questions

1. Describe each of the five types of burn injury and provide examples of each. Which type of burn has Ms. Champlin sustained?

2. Describe the appropriate first aid interventions the EMTs will initiate while en route to the hospital.

3. Using the "Rule of Nines," estimate the extent of the client's burn injury.

4. Why did the HCP assess Ms. Champlin for discoloration around her nose and mouth, singed nasal hair, and burned eyebrows? What other related manifestations should be assessed to determine if there is need for concern?

5. In the emergency department, treatment of the client included the insertion of an indwelling urinary catheter, insertion of a nasogastric (NG) tube, and administration of tetanus toxoid. Provide a brief rationale for each of these interventions.

Questions (continued)

6. Briefly describe the skin depth and manifestations that define each degree of burn injury (first-, second-, third-, and fourth-degree). What degree(s) of burn injury does Ms. Champlin have?

7. Ms. Champlin cries to the nurse, "It seems as if my arm is getting bigger by the minute! Can't you do something?" Help the nurse explain to the client what is causing the edema and the expected progression and resolution of the swelling.

8. Ms. Champlin weighs 180 lbs. Using the Parkland Formula below, estimate the IV fluid replacement needs of this client in the first 24 hours following her injury.

Parkland Formula: 2 to 4 mL of solution
  × body weight (in kilograms)
  × percent burn

9. Help the nurse identify five priority nursing diagnoses for Ms. Champlin's plan of care during the acute phase of her treatment.

10. The HCP is concerned that Ms. Champlin may develop a contracture of her right arm because of the burn injury over her right elbow. Discuss what a contracture is and why this client is at increased risk of developing one.

11. The HCP caring for Ms. Champlin tells her that it may become necessary to apply a skin graft to the deep partial thickness area over her elbow to speed healing and minimize the risk of contracture. Skin grafts are obtained from various sources. Briefly explain these four types of grafts: autograft, allograft, heterograft, synthetic skin substitute graft. Is there any benefit(s) to selecting one type of graft over another? If so, explain.

12. Briefly discuss why environmental temperature control is an important intervention while caring for the client with a burn injury. At what temperature should the nurse maintain the client's room?

13. Ms. Champlin has asked the nurses that no visitors be allowed in to see her. Briefly discuss Ms. Champlin's psychological reaction to her burn. How should the nurse respond?

14. Ms. Champlin is being discharged. She will wear a custom molded hand and arm splint at home. Briefly describe the teaching points the nurse should address regarding limb assessment and proper use of the splint.

15. Ms. Champlin asks the nurse, "I have heard there is a cream you can apply to decrease scarring." What types of cream might Ms. Champlin be referencing?

Questions and Suggested Answers

1. Describe each of the five types of burn injury and provide examples of each. Which type of burn has Ms. Champlin sustained? A burn injury is caused by (1) a thermal source such as a flame, scalding, or direct contact with a hot surface; (2) chemicals; (3) inhalation; (4) electric currents; or (5) radiation.

Thermal burns are the leading type of tissue and inhalation burn injuries in the United States. Individuals suffer thermal burns from house fires, contact with hot substances or objects (such as food, a stove, or an iron), scalding from hot fluid or steam, and ignited gasoline or propane. The injury is often a combined partial- and full-thickness burn, and confined to the area of skin that is in direct contact with the thermal source.

Chemical burns are the second leading type of burn injury in the United States. These injuries are caused by direct contact with, splashing of, or inhalation of fumes from chemical solutions used in the industrial (e.g., hydrochloric acid, petroleum products, and gasoline), military (e.g., white phosphorus, sulfur mustard), or agricultural (e.g., lime or lye) industries. In the home, cleaning products (e.g., drain cleaner and bleach) and disinfectants are common sources of injury. The severity of the injury is dependent on the type of chemical exposure.

When an individual inhales smoke, hot air, or toxins, an *inhalation burn* injury can result. Visible burns on the skin of the face often mask the clinical manifestations of an inhalation injury, which include singed nasal hair, soot around the mouth and nose, and respiratory distress. Failure to assess for these signs and symptoms increases the risk of fatality from an undiagnosed inhalation burn.

Low-voltage electrical currents often cause mild *electrical burns*, whereas contact with a high-voltage electrical current can produce a severe and potentially fatal burn injury. The extent of the injury is affected by several situational factors. "The amount of current (low voltage, high voltage, or high tension), type of current (direct or alternating), path of current (e.g., hand to toe), length of contact, and extenuating events (in contact with water or resulting in a fall) are factors that determine the extent or lethality of an electrical injury" (Green, 2007, p. 1911). Electrical burn injuries are particularly threatening since the electrical insult disrupts the body's electrical activity and can cause asystole and apnea.

Radiation burns can be quite serious. Skin exposure to the ultraviolet radiation of the sun or artificial tanning beds, industrial radiation, and therapeutic radiation are the most common sources of radiation burn injury. The length of exposure, strength of radiation, amount of body surface exposed, and distance from the source are factors that affect the severity of the burn injury. Clinical manifestations may not emerge until days or weeks after exposure and include localized erythema, blistering, and ulceration. Some individuals develop acute radiation syndrome, an illness caused by radiation to the entire body. Those with acute radiation syndrome present with nausea, vomiting, anorexia, fatigue, fever, diarrhea, and/or respiratory distress. (Green, 2007)

Ms. Champlin has sustained a thermal burn.

2. Describe the appropriate first aid interventions the EMTs will initiate while en route to the hospital. EMTs will remove any clothing (except clothing adhered to the burned area), jewelry, or debris to stop the burn process. EMTs will conduct an initial assessment of airway, breathing, and circulation. An airway is established as needed. Oxygen will be administered.

If the client is alert and able to respond, a medical history, list of medications taken, and allergies will be obtained. Dressings dampened with sterile saline or water are applied to the injured areas of skin to provide immediate cooling, prevent evaporation of body fluid, reduce edema, and ease pain. Ice is not recommended since this will cause local vasoconstriction, deepening tissue injury, and increases the client's risk of hypothermia. The client is covered with a dry blanket to prevent the loss of body heat through evaporation. An IV line is obtained and lactated Ringer's solution administered. The EMTs will notify the emergency department (ED) of their anticipated arrival, allowing the ED staff to prepare for the client's arrival and treatment needs (Green, 2007; National Library for Health, 2006).

3. Using the "Rule of Nines," estimate the extent of the client's burn injury. Used to estimate the percentage of total body surface area (TBSA) that is burned, the "Rule of Nines" divides the body into areas equal to multiples of 9%. In the adult, the back of the head and the face are each equal to 4.5%, the chest and back are each 18%, each aspect of the arm is 4.5%, the front and back of each leg are each 9%, and the genitalia and perineal area are 1%. Ms. Champlin has burns on the right side of her face and neck (2.25%), across her chest (18%), and on the anterior (4.5%) and posterior (4.5%) aspect of her right arm and hand. Using the "Rules of Nines," an estimated 29.25% of the client's TBSA has been burned (Green, 2007; National Library for Health, 2006).

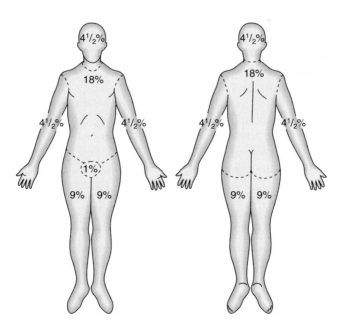

The Rule of Nines is used to estimate the percentage of body surface area burned

4. Why did the HCP assess Ms. Champlin for discoloration around her nose and mouth, singed nasal hair, and burned eyebrows? What other related manifestations should be assessed to determine if there is need for concern? The HCP was assessing Ms. Champlin for signs of an inhalation burn. An inhalation burn results when the client inhales smoke, hot air, or flames. Smoke inhalation can cause bronchospasm as well as pulmonary and laryngeal edema. The HCP should suspect potential airway problems if there is discoloration from soot around the nose and mouth, singed nasal hair, and/or burned eyebrows. Other clinical manifestations of an inhalation burn include a severe or brassy cough, wheezing, stridor, hoarseness, carbon-containing sputum, lacrimation (tearing eyes), and confusion. It is important to rule out the possibility of an inhalation burn injury since burn fatalities often are attributed to inhalation injuries that are masked by the more obvious external burns (Green, 2007; National Library for Health, 2006).

5. In the ED, treatment of the client included the insertion of an indwelling urinary catheter, insertion of an NG tube, and administration of tetanus toxoid. Provide a brief rationale for each of these interventions. A *urinary catheter* is inserted to monitor hourly urine output. The client's output is used to evaluate the adequacy of fluid resuscitation (replacement).

Clients with burns that extend to more than 20% of their TSBA are at risk of nausea, vomiting, aspiration, and the development of a paralytic gastric ileus (obstruction). An *NG tube* is inserted and attached to wall suction to empty gastric contents and prevent gastric distention.

Tetanus is a potentially fatal bacterial infection characterized by muscle rigidity and spasm, trismus (lock jaw), difficulty swallowing, and convulsions. Tetanus bacteria (*Clostridium tetani*) enter the body through breaks in the skin or mucous membranes and thrive in anaerobic (low oxygen) conditions. The deeper and more narrow the wound, the greater the possibility of developing tetanus. Contracting tetanus is a concern for clients with burn injuries because of their high risk of wound infection. *Tetanus toxoid* is prescribed for tetanus prophylaxis in the client who has received the tetanus toxoid immunization in their lifetime but has not been given a booster dose within the past five years (CDC, 2006).

6. Briefly describe the skin depth and manifestations that define each degree of burn injury (first-, second-, third-, and fourth-degree). What degree(s) of burn injury does Ms. Champlin have? The severity of a burn is classified according to the depth of the layers of skin involved. The depth of a burn will depend on the temperature of the agent and the length of time the agent is in contact with the skin. A *first-degree* burn is a superficial burn with nonblistering damage to the epidermis.

Manifestations of a first-degree burn are blanchable erythema, swelling, edema, and pain at the site. Regeneration of the epidermis usually heals the skin in approximately seven days with minimal scarring. A *second-degree* burn is a superficial partial-thickness or deep partial-thickness injury that causes skin damage to the epidermis and dermis. The area of injury often takes on a mottled appearance of pink, red, tan, and pale areas. The site is very painful, moist, and swollen, often developing blisters that increase in size. In first- and second-degree burns, hair follicles, sweat glands, and nerve endings remain intact. The healing of injuries with minimal involvement of the dermis takes approximately two weeks, and scarring is often minimal. Greater involvement of the dermal layer extends the healing time to several months, and scar tissue often develops. *Third- and fourth-degree* burns involve full-thickness damage to the epidermis, dermis, and subcutaneous layers. It is possible that a full-thickness (fourth-degree) burn extends to the muscle and bone below. The skin will appear leathery (eschar) and is white, red, black, tan, or brown. There is no blanching when fingertip pressure is applied. Hair follicles, sweat glands, and nerve endings are destroyed at the site of the injury, thus the injury is painless. However, the individual often experiences a pain sensation from the surrounding area of skin, which has often suffered first- and second-degree burns. Since the epidermis and dermis are destroyed in third- and fourth-degree burns, the recovery is long and necessitates skin grafting to speed healing and minimize scarring. A client will often have varying degrees of burn injuries (Ehrlich & Schroeder, 2005; Green, 2007; Rizzo, 2006; Zator Estes, 2006).

Ms. Champlin has first- and second-degree burns. She has superficial (first-degree) and superficial partial-thickness (second-degree) burns on her face, neck and chest, and deep partial- thickness (second-degree) burns over her right arm and hand. She arrived in the emergency department screaming in pain, which is a symptom indicative of first- and second-degree burns.

7. Ms. Champlin cries to the nurse, "It seems as if my arm is getting bigger by the minute! Can't you do something?" Help the nurse explain to the client what is causing the edema and the expected progression and resolution of the swelling. The swelling (edema) is caused by the body's inflammatory response to the injury and the release of certain body chemicals (vasoactive mediators) that cause the blood vessels to dilate (vasodilation) and fluid to shift. Fluid moves from within the blood vessels (intravascular) to the surrounding tissues (interstitial space). These natural reactions by the body when it has been injured result in rapid swelling of the area that has been burned. The swelling will continue for the next eight to 24 hours but should begin to subside in approximately 72 hours (Green, 2007).

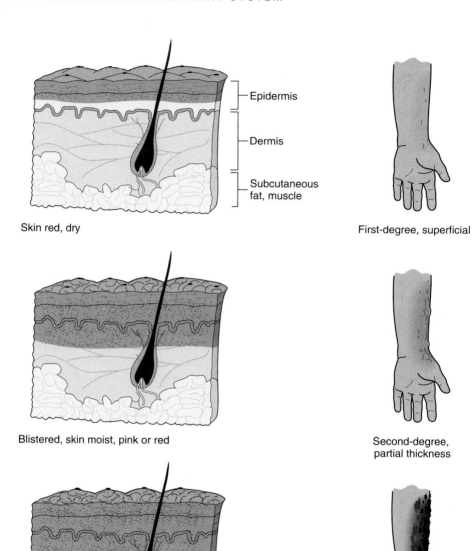

Skin red, dry

Epidermis

Dermis

Subcutaneous fat, muscle

First-degree, superficial

Blistered, skin moist, pink or red

Second-degree, partial thickness

Charring, skin black, brown, red

Third-degree, full thickness

The degree of a burn is determined by the layers of skin involved

8. Ms. Champlin weighs 180 lbs. Using the Parkland Formula below, estimate the IV fluid replacement needs of this client in the first 24 hours following her injury.

Parkland formula:

2 to 4 mL of solution × body weight (in kilograms) × percent burn

Ms. Champlin weighs 180 lbs, or 81.8 kg (1 kg = 2.2 lb). She has suffered burns to approximately 29% of her TBSA. Using the Parkland formula,

$$2 \text{ mL} \times 81.8 \text{ kg} \times 29\% = 4{,}744.4 \text{ mL}$$

and

$$4 \text{ mL} \times 81.8 \text{ kg} \times 29\% = 9{,}488.8 \text{ mL}$$

Therefore, the client should receive 4744 mL to 9489 mL of IV lactated Ringers in the first 24 hours following her injury. It is recommended that 50% of the calculated volume of fluid be administered in the first eight hours following the injury (not from the time care is initiated) and the remaining half delivered over the next 16 hours. Therefore, if the HCP requested that the client receive 9000 mL, for example, the client should be given 4500 mL over the first eight hours (or 563 mL/hour) and 4500 mL over the next 16 hours (or 281 mL/hour). Despite the calculation and recommended rate of infusion, the nurse must assess the client's physiologic response and collaborate with the HCP to individualize the fluid rate to meet the specific needs of the client and prevent inadequate hydration or overhydration (Green, 2007).

9. Help the nurse identify five priority nursing diagnoses for Ms. Champlin's plan of care during the acute phase of her treatment. Suggested nursing diagnoses for Ms. Champlin's plan of care in priority order include:

- Acute pain related to (r/t) burn injury and treatment
- Impaired skin integrity (25% of TBSA) r/t burn injury
- Risk for infection r/t impaired skin integrity and altered immune response
- Imbalanced nutrition: Less than body requirements r/t increased metabolic needs, protein, and fluid loss
- Risk for deficient fluid volume r/t increased insensible loss and evaporation from skin surface and fluid shift
- Risk for hypothermia r/t impaired skin integrity
- Risk for ineffective peripheral tissue perfusion (right arm) r/t circumferential burn and impaired arterial/venous circulation
- Risk for peripheral neurovascular dysfunction r/t eschar formation with circumferential burn

- Risk for impaired physical mobility (right arm) r/t pain and contracture formation
- Disturbed body image r/t altered physical appearance
- Fear r/t pain from treatments and possible permanent disfigurement
- Risk for posttrauma syndrome r/t life-threatening event

(Ackley & Ladwig, 2006; Green, 2007)

10. The HCP is concerned that Ms. Champlin may develop a contracture of her right arm because of the burn injury over her right elbow. Discuss what a contracture is and why this client is at increased risk of developing one. A circumferential, or encircling, burn on a limb can cause a constrictive contraction of the skin. A contracture is an abnormal shortening of tissue that renders the tissue resistant to stretching and limits joint mobility. In addition to the constrictive contraction of burned skin, a client with a serious burn injury may assume a position that provides the most comfort while healing and resist frequent changes in position to avoid pain. When a joint is allowed to remain in an immobile position for too long, the muscle fibers will stretch or shorten to accommodate the position and eventually lose the ability to contract or relax normally. Contractures can lead to significant loss of function and permanent disability. Active and passive range of motion exercises help to prevent a contracture (Green, 2007).

11. The HCP caring for Ms. Champlin tells her that it may become necessary to apply a skin graft to the deep partial thickness area over her elbow to speed healing and minimize the risk of contracture. Skin grafts are obtained from various sources. Briefly explain these four types of grafts: autograft, allograft, heterograft, synthetic skin substitute graft. Is there any benefit(s) to selecting one type of graft over another? If so, explain. An *autograft* is a skin graft that is obtained from an area of the client's own body, usually the thigh. An *allograft* (or homograft) is a cryopreserved skin graft that has been harvested from a deceased donor within six to 24 hours after the donor's death, or may come from a live donor other than the client. A *heterograft* (also called a xenograft) is a skin graft that comes from another species, such as a pig. Synthetic skin substitutes are fabricated forms of dermal replacement. Products such as Integra, AlloDerm, and Epicel are examples of products available in the United States and Canada. These synthetic products, as well as an autograft, are permanent grafts, whereas the others are used to provide temporary coverage of the injured area to prevent fluid and electrolyte loss and promote healing until a more permanent option is available. As the wound heals, the temporary graft is gradually rejected and removed from the healed skin. An autograft is the preferred method of treatment. Allografts and heterografts are more cost-effective than skin substitutes. Allografts, however, do pose a risk of blood-borne disease transmission (Green, 2007).

12. Briefly discuss why environmental temperature control is an important intervention while caring for the client with a burn injury. At what temperature should the nurse maintain the client's room? Impaired skin integrity causes altered thermoregulation, which can result in hypothermia. Environmental temperature control is an important intervention when caring for the client who has suffered a burn injury. The nurse should monitor the environmental temperature in the client's room to see that the temperature is maintained between 80° and 85°F (26.6° to 29.4°C). Maintaining this environmental temperature reduces caloric losses through the skin and thus shivering and physiologic stress (Williams, Coffee, & Yurko, 2007).

13. Ms. Champlin has asked the nurses that no visitors be allowed in to see her. Briefly discuss Ms. Champlin's psychological reaction to her burn. How should the nurse respond? The client's psychological response to a burn injury may be significant. Clients are often in a state of shock or disbelief and may express anger over what has happened. The client with a burn injury, especially of the face, will experience a body image disturbance. This negative image of one's self may motivate a refusal to interact with others. The client may become withdrawn and easily irritated. The client's psychological state prior to the burn injury can have a significant effect on their emotional response to their condition. Ms. Champlin has a history of depression. She should be monitored carefully, particularly during the acute phase, for suicidal ideation. The nurse should recognize the client's request as an anticipated response to her injury, and that Ms. Champlin's efforts to protect herself and preserve her dignity may last for a week or more. Nursing interventions include respecting and supporting Ms. Champlin and her decision to limit visitors at this time. The nurse should acknowledge the client's loss of sense of self and difficulty coping at this time, and help the client to identify effective coping mechanisms she employed during other times in her life when faced with a significant challenge. A therapeutic and supportive nurse-client relationship will help to create a sense of comfort and understanding that will encourage Ms. Champlin to share her concerns and fears with the nurse (Green, 2007).

14. Ms. Champlin is being discharged. She will wear a custom molded hand and arm splint at home. Briefly describe the teaching points the nurse should address regarding limb assessment and proper use of the splint. Splints are custom-made devices molded directly to the client's limb to help prevent contracture and immobilize a joint in the anatomically correct position after grafting. Clients are instructed to wear the splint according to an established schedule and are given instructions

to do range of motion exercises to help maintain and enhance the function of the limb. The client should be provided with discharge teaching
that addresses how to assess for adequate circulation (capillary refill and
pulses), skin color and temperature, sensation, and movement. The client must be able to demonstrate how to apply and remove the splint and
convey an understanding of proper care and cleaning of the device. The
client should report impaired circulation, pain, signs of wound infection,
or areas of increased pressure from an improperly fitting splint. It is likely
that Ms. Champlin will experience itching as the skin heals. The itching
can be uncomfortable and anxiety provoking. Skin care creams can help
to minimize the discomfort (Abbott, 2004; Green, 2007).

**15. Ms. Champlin asks the nurse, "I have heard there is a cream you can
apply to decrease scarring." What types of cream might Ms. Champlin be
referencing?** Ms. Champlin might be referring to any number of creams
currently available in the consumer market that claim to decrease scar formation. She is most likely referring to Aloe Vera, Eucerin, vitamin E cream
and/or cocoa butter. Aloe Vera has been shown to hasten the healing process by stimulating the growth of new cells. Aloe Vera is most effective when
applied to minor (first-degree) burns. Aloe Vera gel is expressed from the
leaves of an aloe plant. The gel is applied to the skin three to four times
daily and left to heal in open air (Green, 2007). Eucerin cream is a mois-
turizer that contains urea as the active ingredient. Found naturally in the
skin, urea attracts water. By increasing the ability of the skin to absorb and
retain water, Eucerin rehydrates, softens, and soothes the skin and reduces
itching. Vitamin E cream has also been touted as useful in reducing the
risk of scar formation. Creams containing vitamin E are believed by some
to have anti-inflammatory effects and to moisturize the skin, speeding the
healing process and minimizing the appearance of scars following recovery. Cocoa butter cream also is suggested to help heal scars. Several products, such as Bioskincare cream and Mederma, can be found in stores and
on the Internet that assert they improve skin strength and elasticity, have
anti-inflammatory and antioxidant properties, and help regulate blood
vessel formation and oxygenation. Clients should be advised that the effect
of such skin care therapy is unproven, and results, if any, will vary for each
individual. Clients should be cautioned against spending a lot of money to
purchase products that claim to prevent scarring. The principal benefit of
any skin care cream is to moisten the skin and increase circulation to the
area by massaging the cream onto the site. Therefore, many clients can
achieve maximum benefit from relatively inexpensive store-brand products. Clients should be instructed not to apply creams to open wounds and
to follow the manufacturer's suggestions for safe use. The client should
discontinue using the cream if they develop contact dermatitis.

References

Abbott, P. (2004). Applying a splint. In G. B. Altman (Ed.), *Delmar's fundamental & advanced nursing skills* (pp. 1347–1353). Clifton Park, NY: Thomson Delmar Learning.

Ackley, B., & Ladwig, G. (2006). *Nursing diagnosis handbook: A guide to planning care.* St. Louis, MO: Mosby.

Centers for Disease Control (CDC). (2006). Tetanus. In *Pink Book* (pp. 69–78). Retrieved January 14, 2007, from www.cdc.gov.

Ehrlich, A., & Schroeder, C. L. (2005). Skin: The integumentary system. In *Medical terminology for health professions* (pp. 351–352). Clifton Park, NY: Thomson Delmar Learning.

Green, C. J. (2007). Burns. In *Phipps' medical-surgical nursing: Health and illness perspectives* (pp. 1910–1944). St. Louis, MO: Mosby Elsevier.

National Library for Health. (2006). *Clinical knowledge summaries: Burns and scalds.* Retrieved January 15, 2007, from www.prodigy.nhs.uk.

Rizzo, D. C. (2006). The integumentary system. In *Health assessment & physical examination* (p. 126). Clifton Park, NY: Thomson Delmar Learning.

Williams, T. D., Coffee, T., & Yurko, L. (2007). Burns: Nursing management. In R. Daniels, L. J. Nosek, & L. H. Nicoll (Eds.). *Contemporary medical-surgical nursing* (p. 1541). Clifton Park, NY: Thomson Delmar Learning.

Zator Estes, M. E. (2006). Skin, hair, and nails. In *Health assessment & physical examination* (p. 302). Clifton Park, NY: Thomson Delmar Learning.

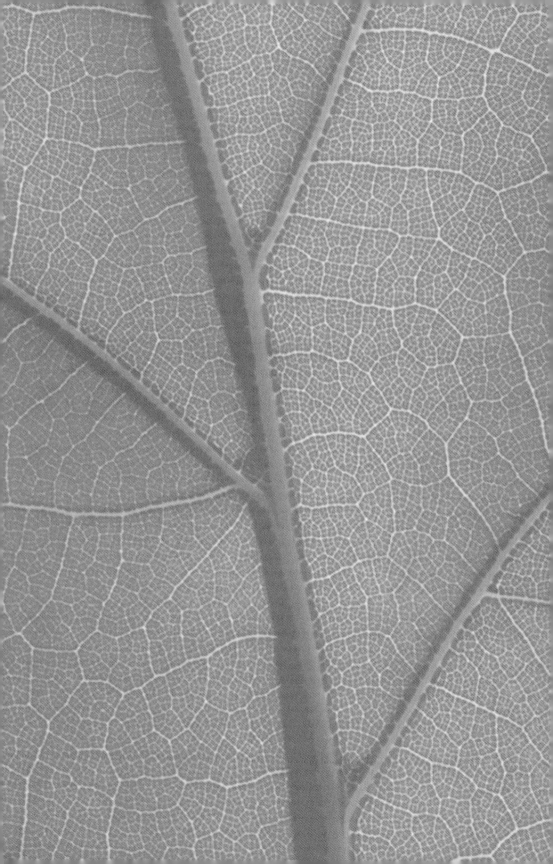

PART SEVEN

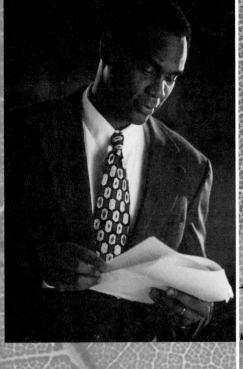

The Nervous/ Neurological System

CASE STUDY 1

Derek

GENDER

Male

AGE

21

SETTING

■ Hospital

ETHNICITY

■ White American

CULTURAL CONSIDERATIONS

PREEXISTING CONDITION

COEXISTING CONDITION

COMMUNICATION

■ Possible hearing loss

DISABILITY

■ Potential for permanent neurologic impairment and hearing loss

SOCIOECONOMIC

■ College student
■ Resides in a fraternity house on campus

SPIRITUAL/RELIGIOUS

PHARMACOLOGIC

■ Ceftriaxone sodium (Rocephin); dexamethasone sodium phosphate (Decadron Phosphate); acetaminophen (Tylenol); morphine sulfate (MS contin); meningococcal polysaccharide vaccine (MPSV4 or Menomune); meningococcal conjugate vaccine (MCV4 or MenactraT)

LEGAL

■ Local health department notification

ETHICAL

ALTERNATIVE THERAPY

■ Nonpharmacologic interventions to promote comfort

PRIORITIZATION

■ Respiratory isolation and seizure precautions

DELEGATION

■ Collaboration with university health services

THE NERVOUS/NEUROLOGICAL SYSTEM

Level of Difficulty: Easy

Overview: In this case, the nurse must recognize the clinical manifestations of meningitis and discuss further assessment and diagnostic testing to confirm the diagnosis. Precautions are implemented to maintain the client's safety as well as decrease the risk of transmitting the infection to others. Appropriate treatment for the client with bacterial meningitis is reviewed and nonpharmacologic nursing interventions to promote client comfort identified. The nurse generates priority nursing diagnoses to help develop a plan of care.

Client Profile

Derek is a 22-year-old male found by his roommate to be conscious but very lethargic and not responding to questions. Derek was transported to the emergency department (ED) by emergency medical personnel who began administering oxygen via a non-rebreather mask in route to the hospital. Upon arrival in the ED, Derek is conscious but unresponsive. Derek's roommate accompanied him to the ED. The roommate states, "I went into the TV room in the frat house this afternoon and Derek was lying on the sofa. I started talking to him. He just looked at me with a blank stare, and would not answer me. He was just lying there almost stiff looking. What in the world is wrong with him?"

Case Study

Derek's vital signs are blood pressure 132/56, heart rate 130, respiratory rate 20, and rectal temperature of 104.1°F (40°C). His oxygen saturation is 97% on oxygen. A 12-lead electrocardiogram (ECG, EKG) shows sinus tachycardia. Physical assessment findings include severe neck and joint stiffness and a petechial rash on his chest. Diagnostic tests prescribed include a computed tomography (CT) scan of Derek's head and then a lumbar puncture (LP). A complete blood count (CBC), urinalysis (U/A), urine culture and sensitivity (U/A C&S), basic metabolic panel (BMP), blood cultures × 2 sites (BC × 2), and a serum drug screen have been prescribed. Suspecting that Derek may have meningitis, the health care provider (HCP) prescribes ceftriaxone sodium 2 grams intravenous (IV) every twelve hours, with the first dose to be given after obtaining the blood cultures and doing the LP. Derek is admitted and assigned to a respiratory isolation room. IV fluids of normal saline are prescribed. Derek's white blood cells (WBC) are 15,300 cells/mm^3. The CT scan was negative for a cranial mass or bleeding. The cerebral spinal fluid (CSF) obtained during the LP appears cloudy. CSF analysis findings reveal a decreased glucose level, elevated protein level, and an elevated WBC count. The urinalysis, urine culture, blood cultures, and BMP are within normal limits. Derek's drug screen is negative.

Questions

1. Discuss the causes of meningitis and describe the pathophysiologic changes in the brain that result from this infection.

2. Describe the clinical manifestations of bacterial and viral meningitis.

3. The nurse assesses Derek for the *Kernig's sign* and *Brudzinski's sign*. Describe how each sign is assessed and what a positive result indicates.

Questions (continued)

4. Briefly discuss the incidence of bacterial meningitis. Which individuals are more often affected in terms of age and gender, and is there an increase in cases depending on the time of the year?

5. Derek is admitted to a respiratory isolation room. When can he be transferred to a regular hospital room?

6. The nurse applies pads to the bedside rails and makes sure that there is suction equipment, an airway, oxygen, and a padded tongue blade by Derek's bedside. Explain why the nurse has taken these precautions and any concerns you have about the precautions the nurse has implemented.

7. Explain why the HCP has prescribed a head CT scan and why the CT scan should be done prior to the lumbar puncture.

8. Briefly discuss why the HCP has requested that Derek have a lumbar puncture. What are the nurse's responsibilities in assisting the HCP during the lumbar puncture procedure?

9. What is the rationale for doing a serum drug screen as part of Derek's diagnostic workup?

10. Derek's roommate explained that Derek "just looked at me with a blank stare and would not answer me." Offer a brief explanation for why Derek did not answer his roommate.

11. A gram stain of the CSF reveals *Neisseria meningitidis*. Derek has bacterial meningitis (meningococcal meningitis). The HCP has already prescribed ceftriaxone sodium following the blood cultures and lumbar puncture. Additional medications prescribed are dexamethasone, acetaminophen, and morphine sulfate. Briefly discuss the rationale for each of these prescribed medications.

12. Identify at least three nonpharmacologic nursing interventions that the nurse can implement to promote comfort for the client with meningitis.

13. Identify three priority nursing diagnoses appropriate for inclusion in Derek's plan of care.

14. Considering Derek's living situation, discuss the precautions that should be taken.

Questions and Suggested Answers

1. Discuss the causes of meningitis and describe the pathophysiologic changes in the brain that result from this infection. A bacteria, virus, or fungi may cause meningitis. The causative organism of bacterial meningitis is often identified in the person's oropharynx. Viral meningitis, also called aseptic meningitis, is the most common form of meningitis and is often caused by enteroviruses (common viruses that enter the body) and mumps organisms. Viruses and bacteria can enter the central nervous system by a variety of routes and cause infections and inflammation. The infection targets the arachnoid and pia mater layers of the meninges (membranes that cover the brain and spinal cord) and the CSF. For example, in an individual with an upper respiratory tract infection, the bacteria in the nasopharynx can enter the bloodstream. The bloodstream carries the bacteria to the brain where the subarachnoid spaces, pia mater and arachnoid membranes, and CSF become infected. The infection can spread rapidly through the meninges and invade the ventricles of the brain. Purulent exudate is produced that clings to the meningeal layers and clogs the CSF, causing vascular congestion and obstruction. As the exudate coats the nerve sheath, there is cranial nerve dysfunction. Eventually, there is hyperemia (excess blood) of the meningeal blood vessels, edema of the brain tissue, increased intracranial pressure (ICP), and exudation of WBCs into the subarachnoid spaces as a result of the generalized inflammatory reaction (Forsyth & Garnett, 2007; NINDS, 2006).

2. Describe the clinical manifestations of bacterial and viral meningitis. Clinical manifestations of bacterial and viral meningitis include a severe headache, neck pain and stiffness (nuchal rigidity), restricted neck flexion, drowsiness, malaise, fever, nausea, and vomiting. Assessment of the client with meningitis often reveals an erythematous throat, heme-positive stools, photophobia (intolerance to light), cervical lymphadenopathy, hearing loss, an unsteady gait, and back pain upon lifting their legs (Kernig's sign). Clients with bacterial meningitis may have a petechial or hemorrhagic rash on the chest, arms, abdomen, and back. A headache occurs because of the stretching of meningeal membranes due to inflammation of the subarachnoid space. Meningitis headaches are generalized and severe and may radiate down the neck. Complications of meningitis include septic shock, vasomotor collapse, seizures, and cerebral edema. Cerebral edema can cause increased ICP, resulting in the symptoms of nausea and vomiting. An elevated ICP can also cause the client to be delirious or completely disoriented. The client's level of consciousness can decline rapidly from drowsiness to a coma. The elevated ICP can cause changes in cardiopulmonary function and lead to brainstem herniation, coma, and death. The onset of bacterial meningitis is often acute and can cause serious morbidity and mortality (15% of cases). Bacterial meningitis is a medical emergency because without treatment it can be fatal within hours to days. Many who survive bacterial meningitis have severe neurologic deficits such as ocular and facial palsies and deafness. Viral meningitis, also called aseptic meningitis, is a more benign and self-limiting illness than bacterial meningitis (CDC, 2005; Forsyth & Garnett, 2007; NMAUS, 2006).

3. The nurse assesses Derek for the *Kernig's sign* and *Brudzinski's sign*. Describe how each sign is assessed and what a positive result indicates. Positive Kernig's and Brudzinski's signs indicate irritation of the motor nerve roots passing through inflamed meninges. To assess Derek for the *Kernig's sign*, the nurse flexes Derek's leg at the hip holding the leg in a

90-degree angle. The nurse then attempts to extend the leg out straight. The nurse is concerned if Derek is unable to extend his leg at the knee while his thigh is flexed or if he exhibits pain or spasm in his hamstrings during extension of his leg. To check for the *Brudzinski's sign,* while Derek is lying in a supine position, the nurse passively flexes his head and neck looking to see if, in response, he flexes his hips and knees. This flexion is of concern (Forsyth & Garnett, 2007; Huffstutler, 2007).

4. Briefly discuss the incidence of bacterial meningitis. Which individuals are more often affected in terms of age and gender, and is there an increase in cases depending on the time of the year? In the United States over 17,000 cases of bacterial meningitis occur each year. Meningitis is most common in the very young and the very old and occurs more often in males than in females. Most cases of meningitis occur during the late winter into early spring and there is a decline during the summer months. Up to 20% of survivors have long-term disabilities, including brain damage, hearing loss, and limb amputations (Forsyth & Garnett, 2007; NMAUS, 2006; Wener, 2005).

5. Derek is admitted to a respiratory isolation room. When can he be transferred to a regular hospital room? Respiratory isolation is required for clients with meningococcal infections until a culture of the nasopharynx is negative for the causative pathogen. A negative culture is usually obtained 24 hours after antibiotic therapy has been initiated (Forsyth & Garnett, 2007).

6. The nurse applies pads to the bedside rails and makes sure that there is suction equipment, an airway, oxygen, and a padded tongue blade by Derek's bedside. Explain why the nurse has taken these precautions and any concerns you have about the precautions the nurse has implemented. In the client with meningitis, the inflammatory response to the infection produces purulent exudates that clings to the meningeal layers and clogs the CSF causing vascular congestion and obstruction. If this exudate blocks the small passages between the ventricles of the brain, acute hydrocephalus may result, and the client may experience a seizure (CDC, 2005; Forsyth & Garnett, 2007). Seizure precautions are taken to prevent the client from being injured during a seizure. Seizure precautions vary depending on agency policy. Recommendations include oxygen and suction equipment with an airway available at the client's bedside. Although side rails are rarely the source of significant injury during a seizure, most agency policies instruct that side rails should be in the up position. There exists debate regarding whether the use of padded side rails helps maintain safety, but padding is usually in place along the bedside rails. The nurse should also assess Derek's neurologic status at least every two hours to identify changes in his level of consciousness.

Of concern is that the nurse placed a padded tongue blade by Derek's bedside. Padded tongue blades are no longer used to prevent a client from biting their tongue, and should not be inserted in a client's mouth during a seizure. A client's jaw often clenches down during a seizure and forcing the tongue blade into the client's mouth may chip teeth and increase the risk of aspiration of tooth fragments that could obstruct the airway (Hausman, 2006).

7. Explain why the HCP has prescribed a head CT scan and why the CT scan should be done prior to the lumbar puncture. A head CT scan can identify cerebral edema, hydrocephalus, abscesses, and infection. A CT scan of the head is also used to rule out the possibility that Derek has an intracranial mass, cerebral hemorrhage, herniated disk, or other pathologic condition that is causing his symptoms. The CT scan is assessed prior to a lumbar puncture to help determine if there is increased ICP. Increased ICP is of concern because there is a risk of brain shift or herniation from a sudden change or decrease in ICP that occurs during the lumbar puncture procedure (NINDS, 2006).

8. Briefly discuss why the HCP has requested that Derek have a lumbar puncture. What are the nurse's responsibilities in assisting the HCP during the lumbar puncture procedure? A lumbar puncture helps to facilitate a definitive diagnosis of bacterial meningitis. A lumbar puncture procedure (also called a spinal tap) measures the opening pressure of the subarachnoid space and is used to obtain a sample of CSF to be cultured to identify the causative organism in the client with meningitis. The first CSF pressure measured with a manometer is called the opening pressure. A normal opening pressure is 6 to 13 mm Hg. Pressures that exceed 15 mm Hg are abnormal. The HCP will also assess for fluctuations in the manometer pressure readings. Normally CSF pressure fluctuates with coughing, straining, and changes in respiration. If there is a blockage in the spinal canal, the CSF pressure may not fluctuate. The CSF, which is clear in a healthy individual, is also tested to detect the presence of blood, elevated WBC count (a sign of infection), and to measure glucose levels, which will be below normal limits in the individual with bacterial or fungal meningitis. In the client with meningitis, the CSF is often cloudy (or turbid) because of the presence of a pyogenic (pus producing) organism, and an increased protein level in the CSF is noted (Forsyth & Garnett, 2007; NINDS, 2006; Petit, 2005).

The nurse's responsibilities in assisting the HCP during the LP procedure include:

- Obtain an LP tray.
- Assess the client's ability to understand and follow instructions necessary to assume and maintain the proper fetal position to avoid trauma of the spinal canal by the spinal needle.

- Provide the HCP performing the LP with assessment and CT scan documentation regarding increased intracranial pressure.
- Assess the client for allergies to antiseptic solution (povidone-iodine) and local anesthetic agent (1% to 2 % lidocaine).
- Check to see that the client has given informed consent for the LP.
- Assess the client's understanding of the procedure and provide additional education as needed.
- Assess baseline vital signs and neurologic status prior to the LP.
- Have the client void before the procedure to prevent interruption of the procedure.
- Prepare labels and test requisitions for the CSF specimen(s) collected during the procedure.
- Assist the client into the fetal position with his back facing you/the HCP and place a pillow between his knees to prevent the upper leg from rolling forward.
- Expose the client's back.
- While the qualified HCP performs the LP, provide assistance with maintaining position, provide verbal support, and observe him for neurologic changes, changes in respiratory status, and complaints of tingling, numbness, or pain in his legs or lower back.
- Don gloves and assist with the application of direct pressure and application of antibiotic ointment and a dressing to the puncture site.
- Complete documentation on the specimen labels and requisitions noting the name, date, time and order in which specimens were obtained (i.e., 1, 2, 3).
- Following the LP procedure, instruct the client to lie flat for the next 12 to 24 hours to help prevent a headache, which is the most common adverse reaction following a LP (10% to 25% of clients), and to decrease the risk of leakage from the puncture site, and to call for assistance the first time he ambulates after the procedure.
- Unless contraindicated, encourage fluid intake to replace fluid loss and manage pain as needed.
- Complete documentation of a nursing note in the client's record noting client education prior to the LP, vital signs pre- and post-procedure, date and time of LP, HCP, how client tolerated procedure, opening and/or closing CSF pressure(s), appearance of CSF, specimen(s) sent, condition of puncture site, any complaints by the client of headache, pain, tingling, or numbness.
- According to agency policy (e.g., every 15 minutes × 4, every 30 minutes × 4, and hourly × 4), assess the client for neurologic changes; changes in vital signs; complaints of tingling, numbness, or pain in his legs or lower back; ability to move lower extremities; and ability to void.

- Assess the puncture site every four hours for redness, swelling, drainage, and pain. Notify the HCP if there is leakage.

(Altman, 2004; Chernecky & Berger, 2004)

9. What is the rationale for doing a serum drug screen as part of Derek's diagnostic workup? A serum drug (toxicology) screen is prescribed by the HCP to rule out the possibility of substance abuse, which could have been the cause of Derek's clinical manifestations or may have been contributing to the clinical manifestations observed. Some of the common drugs included in this test are acetaminophen, alcohol, amphetamines, barbiturates, benzodiazepines, cannabinoids, cocaine, hypnotics, methadone, narcotics, and opiates (Chernecky & Berger, 2004).

10. Derek's roommate explained that Derek "just looked at me with a blank stare, and would not answer me." Offer a brief explanation for why Derek did not answer his roommate. Hearing loss is a classic indicator of meningeal irritation and cranial nerve dysfunction. Derek may not have responded to his roommate because of damage to his hearing (Forsyth & Garnett, 2007).

11. A gram stain of the CSF reveals *N. meningitidis.* **Derek has bacterial meningitis (meningococcal meningitis). The HCP has already prescribed ceftriaxone sodium following the blood cultures and lumbar puncture. Additional medications prescribed are dexamethasone, acetaminophen, and morphine sulfate. Briefly discuss the rationale for each of these prescribed medications.** Because acute bacterial meningitis is a life-threatening infection that can progress quickly, it is considered a medical emergency. The most important intervention for the client with bacterial meningitis is the administration of antibiotic therapy specific to the causative organism. Antibiotic therapy is usually prescribed for 10 to 14 days. *Ceftriaxone sodium* is a third-generation cephalosporin. This anti-infective is a broad spectrum antibiotic that is an effective empiric antibiotic therapy that can be initiated immediately based on clinical manifestations until the causative organism identified through a blood or CSF culture are known. The blood cultures and lumbar puncture to obtain a CSF sample should be done prior to initiation of the antibiotic to prevent masking the identification of the causative organism. Ceftriaxone sodium is an appropriate choice for adults who are suspected of having meningitis caused by *Streptococcus pneumoniae* or *N. meningitidis.*

Dexamethasone is a long-acting corticosteroid that is administered to control cerebral edema. Including dexamethasone in the treatment plan for the client with meningitis has been shown to decrease mortality.

Acetaminophen is a mild analgesic antipyretic medication prescribed to help decrease the client's fever and provide some relief of the client's headache.

Morphine sulfate is a narcotic analgesic prescribed to help provide relief of the moderate to, often, severe headache pain.

(CDC, 2005; Spratto & Woods, 2006)

12. Identify at least three nonpharmacologic nursing interventions that the nurse can implement to promote comfort for the client with meningitis. Nonpharmacologic nursing interventions to promote comfort for the client with meningitis include:

- Ice packs applied to the forehead to reduce headache pain
- Heat applied to decrease muscle aches
- Avoiding unnecessary touch and stimulation of the client
- Tepid baths to reduce fever
- A darkened room to decrease photophobia
- Minimizing light and noise

(Forsyth & Garnett, 2007).

13. Identify five priority nursing diagnoses appropriate for inclusion in Derek's plan of care. Priority nursing diagnoses appropriate for Derek's plan of care include:

- Acute pain related to (r/t) nuchal rigidity, inflammation of meninges, headache
- Disturbed sensory perception: hearing r/t central nervous system infection
- Disturbed thought processes r/t inflammation of brain, fever
- Excess fluid volume r/t increased ICP
- Ineffective tissue perfusion: cerebral r/t inflamed cerebral tissues and meninges, increased ICP
- Impaired comfort r/t central nervous stimulation
- Impaired mobility r/t neuromuscular/central nervous system insult
- Risk for infection r/t invasive procedure (LP)
- Risk for aspiration r/t seizure activity
- Risk for injury r/t seizure activity

(Ackley & Ladwig, 2006)

14. Considering Derek's living situation, discuss the precautions that should be taken. Two-thirds of bacterial meningitis cases are community acquired. *N. meningitidis* (meningococcal meningitis) is highly contagious and can be transmitted to others through close contact with contaminated secretions (or airborne droplets) such as with kissing, coughing, or sharing a cup or cigarette. Students living in dormitories are up to six times more likely to have meningitis than other people. Crowded living situations, such as a college fraternity house, pose the risk of an outbreak. Because of the severity of meningitis symptoms and potential for serious morbidity and mortality, federal and state regulations require that all cases of bacterial meningitis be reported to the local health department. Health services at the university that Derek attends should be made aware in order to facilitate cooperation in identifying students at risk of exposure, encourage antibiotic therapy for Derek's close contacts, and educate the university community about symptoms to report and ways to prevent transmission. The students who live in the fraternity house and Derek's other close contacts (such as a girlfriend or male partner) should be assessed for symptoms of meningitis. If not previously vaccinated, the students can be offered the meningococcal vaccine. The two vaccines available in the United States are the meningococcal polysaccharide vaccine (MPSV4 or Menomune) and the meningococcal conjugate vaccine (MCV4 or MenactraT). The meningococcal conjugate vaccine is the preferred vaccine for those 11 to 55 years of age and provides protection for up to 10 years. The limitation of this vaccine is that while the vaccine helps prevent most meningococcal meningitis infections, it does not prevent the B subtype. There are several strains of the meningococcal bacteria, and the B subtype accounts for two-thirds of all cases of meningococcal meningitis (CDC, 2005; Lazoff, 2005; NMAUS, 2006).

References

Ackley, B., & Ladwig, G. (2006). *Nursing diagnosis handbook: A guide to planning care*. St. Louis, MO: Mosby.

Altman, G. (2004). *Delmar's fundamental & advanced nursing skills* (pp. 1491–1496). Clifton Park, NY: Thomson Learning.

Centers for Disease Control and Prevention (CDC), Division of Bacterial and Mycotic Diseases. (2005). *Meningococcal disease*. Retrieved August 22, 2006 from www.cdc.gov.

Chernecky, C. C., & Berger, B. J. (2004). *Laboratory tests and diagnostic procedures*. Philadelphia, PA: Elsevier.

Forsyth, L. W., & Garnett, J. C. (2007). Traumatic and neoplastic problems of the brain. In F. Monahan, J. Sands, M. Neighbors, J. Marek, & C. Green (Eds.), *Phipps' Medical surgical nursing: Health and illness perspectives* (pp. 1394, 1416–1417). St. Louis, MO: Mosby Elsevier.

Hausman, K. A. (2006). Interventions for clients with problems of the central nervous system. In D. Ignatavicius & L. Workman (Eds.), *Medical-surgical nursing: Critical thinking for collaborative care* (p. 953). St. Louis, MO: Elsevier.

Huffstutler, S. Y. (2007). Assessment of the nervous system. In F. Monahan, J. Sands, M. Neighbors, J. Marek, & C. Green (Eds.), *Phipps' Medical-surgical nursing: Health and illness perspectives* (p. 1374). St. Louis, MO: Mosby Elsevier.

Lazoff, M. (2005). *Meningitis*. Retrieved August 22, 2006 from www.emedicine.com.

National Institute of Neurological Disorders and Stroke (NINDS). (2006). *Meningitis and encephalitis fact sheet*. Retrieved August 22, 2006 from www.ninds.nih.gov.

National Meningitis Association (NMAUS). (2006). *Meningococcal meningitis: Possible to prevent, dangerous to ignore*. Retrieved August 22, 2006 from www.nmaus.org,

Petit, J. (2005). Assessment of the neurologic system. In J. Black & J. Hawks (Eds.), *Medical-surgical nursing: Clinical management for positive outcomes* (pp. 2042–2044). St. Louis, MO: Elsevier.

Spratto, G. R., & Woods, A. L. (2006). *PDR nurse's drug handbook*. Clifton Park, NY: Thomson Delmar Learning.

Wener, K. (2005). *Meningitis*. Retrieved September 26, 2006 from www.nlm.nih.gov.

CASE STUDY 2

Mrs. Kahn

GENDER

Female

AGE

88

SETTING

- Hospital

ETHNICITY

- Arab American

CULTURAL CONSIDERATIONS

- Health care provider (HCP) gender preference.

PREEXISTING CONDITIONS

- Dementia, glaucoma, hypertension (HTN)

COEXISTING CONDITIONS

- Confusion, hemiplegia, nutrition via tube feeding

COMMUNICATION

- Primary language is Arabic, understands some English.

DISABILITY

SOCIOECONOMIC

- Widow for 10 years. Mother of two daughters (65 and 63 years old). Began having symptoms of dementia seven years ago and since then has lived with her younger daughter's family. Prior to admission, she needed assistance with bathing and dressing but was independent with feeding and toileting.

SPIRITUAL/RELIGIOUS

- Muslim

PHARMACOLOGIC

- Alteplase (tissue plasminogen activator; tPA); heparin sodium (heparin); enoxaparin (Lovenox)

LEGAL

- Advance directive

ETHICAL

ALTERNATIVE THERAPY

PRIORITIZATION

DELEGATION

- Collaboration with physical therapist (PT) and occupational therapist (OT)

MODERATE

THE NERVOUS/NEUROLOGICAL SYSTEM

Level of Difficulty: Moderate

Overview: This case requires that the nurse recognize the clinical manifestations of a stroke and convey an understanding of the pathophysiology of a stroke. Criteria for the use of tPA are reviewed. The case addresses the impact of a stroke on the client and family. Cognitive and physical disabilities resulting from the stroke have significantly decreased the client's quality of life. Her daughters disagree about what is best for their mother regarding continued care and code status. The benefits of an advance directive are considered. Priority nursing diagnoses are identified. Interventions appropriate for the client receiving tube feeding are reviewed.

Client Profile

Mrs. Kahn is an 88-year-old woman who lives with her daughter Rose's family. Two weeks ago, Rose went out to complete a few errands while her 12-year-old daughter stayed with Mrs. Kahn. Rose returned home at 1:00 P.M. to find Mrs. Kahn with slurred speech and facial drooping on her right side. When asked, the granddaughter states, "I noticed she was talking a little funny about two hours ago but I thought she was just more confused today. She did not say she felt sick. She just sat in her chair and seemed to want to watch television. Is she okay?" Rose called 9-1-1. Concerned that Mrs. Kahn was having a stroke, emergency personnel transported Mrs. Kahn to the emergency department (ED).

Case Study

In the ED, at 1:40 P.M., Mrs. Kahn is alert but confused. She is able to state her name but does not know where she is, the date, or the time of day. Her speech is slurred, and the right side of her face and right arm are flaccid. Her vital signs are blood pressure 190/114, heart rate 100, respiratory rate 32, and temperature 99.2°F (37.3°C). She is on 2 liters of oxygen with an oxygen saturation of 95%. The health care team initiates a stroke protocol. A computerized tomography (CT) scan shows a large ischemic infarction. Mrs. Kahn is not a candidate for tPA therapy. She is treated with intravenous (IV) heparin. A carotid venous study is negative for carotid stenosis.

It has been three weeks since her admission to the hospital. Mrs. Kahn continues to have right-sided hemiplegia. She has expressive aphasia and diminished proprioception. She is unable to communicate through writing. Her swallowing is impaired. She is being fed through a percutaneous endoscopic gastrostomy (PEG) tube, receiving Jevity at 50 mL per hour. She is incontinent, dependent for all of her activities of daily living, and requires two assists to be turned and repositioned. Mrs. Kahn's two daughters have been very attentive and visit daily, staying hours at a time. Mrs. Kahn is currently a "full code" status. She does not have an advance directive. The health care team's recommendation is that Mrs. Kahn be placed in a long-term nursing care facility. Her oldest daughter understands that this is best for her mother, but Rose believes that given a few more weeks in the hospital, Mrs. Kahn will start to speak again and be able to eat. "Our grandmother had a stroke and died in a nursing home. I do not want the same thing to happen to my mother. Once she is back to her old self, I can take her back home to live with me."

Questions

1. Briefly describe the pathophysiology by which a stroke occurs. Define the term "infarction." Explain the difference between the two types of stroke, an ischemic infarction and a hemorrhagic infarction. Which type of stroke is more common?

2. Upon arrival in the ED, Mrs. Kahn was confused, but she was alert and able to state her name. Now, Mrs. Kahn has expressive aphasia and is unable to communicate verbally or in writing. Explain the progressive nature of the severity of her communication deficits.

3. Briefly discuss four risk factors that contributed to Mrs. Kahn having a stroke. Which of these factors could have been modified?

4. Discuss six clinical manifestations that can indicate a person is having a stroke. Why is early recognition of the signs of a stroke important?

5. Following a stroke, a client may exhibit deficits in motor, elimination, communication, sensory-perceptual, and cognitive (or emotional) function. Identify the deficits that Mrs. Kahn is experiencing because of her stroke.

6. Describe the nursing considerations for positioning the client with hemiplegia and helping to increase mobility. Identify other members of the health care team with whom the nurse can collaborate to develop the client's plan of care.

7. What is the function of Broca's area and Wernicke's area, and how are these areas affected when a client has a stroke?

8. Based on Mrs. Kahn's deficits, which hemisphere has been affected by her stroke?

9. Mrs. Kahn's medical record notes that she is a "full code." What does this mean?

10. While speaking with the nurse about feeling pressured by the health care provider (HCP) and her sister to move Mrs. Kahn to a long-term care facility, Rose states, "It is the hospital's fault the stroke did so much damage to her. They should have given her that tPA medication I heard about that stops a stroke. They were negligent. If she had gotten that medicine, she would not just be lying there like she is." Explain the role tPA plays in the treatment of a client who is having a stroke and why tPA was not an appropriate treatment option for Mrs. Kahn.

11. Mrs. Kahn's daughters have differing opinions about what is best for their mother. The health care team has explained that Mrs. Kahn will not regain her independence and former quality of life. Mrs. Kahn's HCP has discussed changing Mrs. Kahn's code status to "do not resuscitate" (DNR). Rose is not willing to do this. Rose and her sister are overheard having an argument about changing Mrs. Kahn's code status. Discuss how this situation would likely be different if Mrs. Kahn had an advance directive.

12. In order of priority, identify five nursing diagnoses that are appropriate for Mrs. Kahn.

13. Briefly explain the appropriate nursing actions to help minimize the risk of aspiration for a client receiving tube feeding. What should the nurse do prior to changing Mrs. Kahn's bed linens?

14. Enoxaparin is prescribed for Mrs. Kahn. Discuss the indication for this medication and its potential adverse effects. What should the nurse monitor while Mrs. Kahn is receiving enoxaparin?

15. Discuss how Mrs. Kahn's culture and religion may play a role in her health care while in the hospital.

Questions and Suggested Answers

1. **Briefly describe the pathophysiology by which a stroke occurs. Define the term "infarction." Explain the difference between the two types of stroke, an ischemic infarction and a hemorrhagic infarction. Which type of stroke is more common?** A stroke, also called a "cerebrovascular accident" (CVA) or "brain attack," is the most common neurologic disorder in adults. It is estimated that in the United States an individual has a stroke every 45 seconds. It is the third leading cause of death, after heart disease and cancer (ASA, 2006). A stroke is "a group of sudden focal neurologic deficits resulting from interruption of cerebral blood flow. It is called a syndrome rather than a disease because it has more than one cause" (Flannery & Bulecza, 2007, p. 1422). Because the brain is unable to store oxygen or glucose, it relies on a constant supply of oxygen and nutrients from the blood. Two major pairs of arteries supply blood to the brain. The internal carotids supply blood to the anterior portions of the brain and the vertebrals supply the posterior portions. An *infarction* is a zone of tissue that is deprived of its blood supply (Smeltzer & Bare, 2004). The two major types of cerebrovascular infarction are ischemic and hemorrhagic. Both types of stroke reflect impaired oxygenation to a specific area of the brain and can result in temporary or permanent neurologic deficits.

An ischemic infarction is the more common type of stroke (85% of cases). An ischemic infarction involves a lack of blood supply to an area of the brain caused by the obstruction of a blood vessel by thrombi. Many ischemic infarcts (approximately 60%) occur during sleep. An ischemic infarction may be classified according to four developmental processes. The first, a transient ischemic attack (TIA), is a brief episode of neurological deficit that resolves within 24 hours (and often within minutes) without any residual deficits. A reversible ischemic neurologic deficit (RIND) is a condition that usually resolves within 48 hours, but may last up to three weeks. The third process is called a stroke in evolution. Deficits caused by this progressive stroke occur in a stepwise pattern. Finally, in a completed stroke symptoms develop abruptly or progress over a period of hours, depending on the amount of blood that is able to pass through an obstructed vessel. The cellular damage caused by a completed stroke is irreversible and results in a stable syndrome of deficits.

A hemorrhagic infarction is less common, but has a higher mortality rate than an ischemic stroke. This type of stroke most often results from a ruptured blood vessel caused by hypertension and typically occurs in the waking hours. A hemorrhagic stroke is classified by the location of the bleed. A person with a subarachnoid hemorrhagic stroke has bleeding in the subarachnoid space. This occurs in approximately 7% of all strokes. A person with an intracerebral hemorrhagic stroke has bleeding in the tissue of the brain itself (about 10% of all strokes). The degree of injury ranges from a small hemorrhage of 1 to 2 mL that is usually isolated in a cystlike formation called a lacuna, to an extensive hemorrhage (≤50 mL) that forms a hematoma and disrupts the blood-brain barrier causing increased intracranial pressure. A massive hemorrhage such as this is often fatal.

(Flannery & Bulecza, 2007; Smeltzer & Bare, 2004)

2. Upon arrival in the ED, Mrs. Kahn was confused, but she was alert and able to state her name. Now, Mrs. Kahn has expressive aphasia and is unable to communicate verbally or in writing. Explain the progressive nature of the severity of her communication deficits. Most strokes produce a stable syndrome of neurologic deficits within an hour, but the full extent of some clients' disability may take more than 72 hours to be realized. Secondary injury or cerebral edema resulting from ischemia further impedes the blood supply. The overall effect of cerebral edema may take 72 hours after the initial infarction to peak (Flannery & Bulecza, 2007).

3. Briefly discuss four risk factors that contributed to Mrs. Kahn having a stroke. Which of these factors could have been modified? The four factors that presented an increased risk of a stroke for Mrs. Kahn include her advanced age, heredity, hypertension, and to some degree, her gender. Approximately 88% of stroke deaths occur in adults over the age of 65 years. A person's risk doubles for each decade after the age of 55. There is a positive family history of Mrs. Kahn's mother having a stroke. HTN is a major risk factor for a stroke. Although the incidence of stroke in men is twice that of women, more deaths from a stroke occur in women. HTN is the only risk factor that is modifiable in Mrs. Kahn's case. Effective management of HTN significantly reduces a person's risk of a stroke. Those with a blood pressure below 120/80 mmHg reduce their lifetime risk of a stroke by half (Flannery & Bulecza, 2007; Smeltzer & Bare, 2004).

4. Discuss six clinical manifestations that can indicate a person is having a stroke. Why is early recognition of the signs of a stroke important? The progressive cellular changes that occur during a stroke present HCPs with a small window of opportunity to preserve neurologic function. Knowing the warning signs of a stroke facilitates early recognition and intervention. Clinical manifestations of a stroke include:

- Confusion or change in mental status
- Difficulty walking, dizziness, or a loss of balance or coordination
- Numbness or weakness of the face, arm, or leg, especially on one side of the body
- Sudden severe headache

- Trouble speaking or understanding speech
- Visual disturbances (decreased acuity, diplopia [double vision]), homonymous hemianopia (defective vision or blindness in half of the visual field)

(AHA, 2006; Smeltzer & Bare, 2004)

5. Following a stroke, a client may exhibit deficits in motor, elimination, communication, sensory-perceptual, and cognitive (or emotional) function. Identify the deficits that Mrs. Kahn is experiencing because of her stroke.

Mrs. Kahn is experiencing the following deficits:

Motor

- Dysphagia (difficulty swallowing)
- Hemiplegia (paralysis of one side of the body)

Elimination

- Incontinence

Communication

- Agraphia (inability to express self in writing)
- Alexia (inability to understand the written word)
- Expressive aphasia (also called nonfluent or motor aphasia) (difficulty or inability to express oneself verbally)

Sensory-Perceptual

- Diminished proprioception (knowledge of position of body parts)
- Constructional apraxia (inability to sequence a planned act necessary for activities of daily living)

Cognitive (Emotional)

- Loss of reasoning, judgment, and abstract thinking ability

(Flannery & Bulecza, 2007).

6. Describe the nursing considerations for positioning the client with hemiplegia and helping to increase mobility. Identify other members of the health care team with whom the nurse can collaborate to develop the client's plan of care. While providing nursing care for the client with paralysis of the face, arm, and leg, the nurse should place objects (such as the nursing call bell) within the client's reach on the nonaffected side. If the client is able to understand instruction, the nurse can provide teaching regarding range-of-motion exercises that will increase the strength

of the client's unaffected side of the body. The client's position should be changed every two hours. The amount of time the client lies on the affected side should be limited since there is impaired sensation. The affected side of the client's body should be aligned in a functional position. When voluntary control of the muscles is lost, the adductor muscles tend to be stronger than the abductors. This causes the affected arm to rotate internally, and the elbow and wrist tend to flex. The affected leg often rotates externally at the hip and flexes at the knee. Plantar flexion of the ankle leads to foot drop. To prevent adduction of the affected arm, a pillow is placed under the arm with the arm in a slightly flexed (neutral) position, with the elbow positioned higher than the shoulder and the wrist higher than the elbow. This position also helps to decrease edema. Fingers of the affected hand should be barely flexed and with palms facing upward. Splints or hand rolls are used to support positioning. Hand rolls should not be used however if the muscles of the upper limb are spastic, since a hand roll can stimulate the grasp reflex. When positioning the client, the nurse should assess for possible signs of pressure over bony prominences and use pillows or soft protectors to minimize the risk of pressure ulcer development. Footboards can help minimize foot drop. Passive range-of-motion exercises of the affected side help to decrease atrophy and contractures. Nursing interventions are enhanced through collaboration with a PT and OT who can also work with the client to increase the client's strength and function and foster increased independence with activities of daily living (Smeltzer & Bare, 2004).

7. What is the function of Broca's area and Wernicke's area, and how are these areas affected when a client has a stroke? The cerebral cortex is composed of two frontal lobes, two parietal lobes, two temporal lobes, and two occipital lobes. Each lobe, named for its overlying bone, carries out one or more functions. The cerebral cortex is divided into the right and the left hemisphere. A person's speech is a function of their brain's dominant hemisphere. For all right-handed and most of left-handed individuals, the dominant hemisphere is the left side. The brain has two speech centers, Broca's area and Wernicke's area. Broca's area is located in the lateral inferior portion of the frontal lobe. Broca's area is critical for the motor control of speech and controls a person's verbal, expressive speech. Wernicke's area is located in the posterior part of the superior temporal lobe and extends to adjacent portions of the parietal lobe. Wernicke's area controls one's auditory association facilitating the reception and understanding of language. When the dominant hemisphere is affected by a stroke, aphasia can result. Aphasia is a language disorder of which there are several forms. Expressive (or motor) aphasia is a motor disorder involving Broca's area that leaves a client with difficulty expressing thoughts. The client is able to understand the spoken words of others but may have difficulty finding a desired word or have oral responses restricted to the use of a single word. Receptive aphasia is a sensory disorder that results when Wernicke's area is affected. Clients with this form of aphasia can speak fluently but their language often has many errors. When the Broca's or Wernicke's area is affected, the client also may have difficulty expressing ideas in writing or have difficulty understanding the written word (Flannery & Bulecza, 2007; Huffstutler, 2007).

Other areas of the brain that control a person's ability to communicate include an area in the frontal lobe that controls the ability to write and an area in the occipital lobe that functions to interpret and understand written material. As with verbal communication ability after a stroke, a stroke that affects these areas of the brain will likely affect a person's ability to communicate through writing (Huffstutler, 2007).

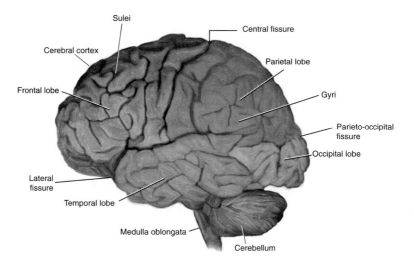

The lobes of the cerebral cortex

8. Based on Mrs. Kahn's deficits, which hemisphere has been affected by her stroke? Mrs. Kahn's left hemisphere has been affected by her stroke. Based on her deficits, the left hemisphere was her dominant hemisphere.

9. Mrs. Kahn's medical record notes that she is a "full code." What does this mean? The term "full code" indicates that if this client should have a respiratory or cardiac arrest, resuscitation efforts will be administered in an attempt to restore respiratory and cardiovascular function. HCPs will

perform rescue breathing, deliver chest compressions, perform defibrilla-
tion, administer medications, and place the client on a mechanical ventila-
tor to provide respiratory support.

**10. While speaking with the nurse about feeling pressured by the HCP and
her sister to move Mrs. Kahn to a long-term care facility, Rose states, "It
is the hospital's fault the stroke did so much damage to her. They should
have given her that tPA medication I heard about that stops a stroke. They
were negligent. If she had gotten that medicine, she would not just be
lying there like she is." Explain the role tPA plays in the treatment of a client who is having a stroke and why tPA was not an appropriate treatment
option for Mrs. Kahn.** Similar to the ischemia that occurs in a myocardial
infarction (MI), a stroke occurs when a lack of oxygen causes cerebral cells
to die, creating a core of necrotic tissue. In addition, as with an MI, the
lack of blood supply to a zone of the brain also results in a second area of
tissue damage that renders cells temporarily unable to function, but still
viable. This secondary area of infarction is called the "penumbra." The
function of the penumbra cells can be restored with timely intervention.
If reperfusion is restored within three hours, blood flow and metabolism
in the ischemic cells may be returned to normal. tPA is a thrombolytic
agent that converts plasminogen to plasmin that digests the fibrin threads
and fibrinogen in blood clots. Alteplase lyses the clot(s) causing an acute
ischemic stroke. This therapeutic effect removes the obstruction, restores
blood flow to the affected area, and decreases neurological sequelae resulting from a stroke. Approved in 1996 to reverse the effects of an ischemic
stroke, alteplase must be administered within a three-hour treatment window from the onset of the first clinical manifestation of a stroke. Rapid
diagnosis of a stroke and initiation of thrombolytic therapy decreases the
size of the stroke and improves the overall functional outcome after three
months. Timing is critical since revascularization of necrotic tissue begins
to develop after three hours and increases the risk of cerebral edema and
hemorrhage. Although there is always the risk of cerebral hemorrhage, the
risk is lowest when alteplase is administered within the three-hour window
and preferably within 60 minutes of the client presenting to the ED. The
client must meet strict eligibility criteria. An individual is excluded as a
candidate for thrombolytic therapy with tPA if they have contraindications
to the administration of this medication. The clinical indications and contraindications for tPA include:

Mrs. Kahn was excluded as a candidate for treatment with tPA based on
her blood pressure of 190/114 and the time lapse of greater than three
hours since the onset of her symptoms (Deglin & Vallerand, 2007; Flannery
& Bulecza, 2007; Hickey & McCoy, 2007; Smeltzer & Bare, 2004).

Clinical Indications and Contraindications for tPA in Stroke Clients

Indications	Acute onset of neurological symptoms
	Onset less than three hours
	18 years or older
	No evidence of cerebral hemorrhage, sulcal edema, or swelling on CT scan
Clinical contraindications	Onset of stroke greater than three hours
	Rapid improvement of symptoms
	Mild stroke symptoms
	Obtunded or comatose state (involving middle cerebral artery stroke)
	Seizure activity at stroke onset or within three hour window prior to tPA
	Symptoms suggesting subarachnoid hemorrhage
	Uncontrolled hypertension (systolic blood pressure greater than 185 mm Hg or diastolic blood pressure greater than 110 mm Hg)
	Less than 18 years old
History contraindications	Minor ischemic stroke within 30 days
	Major ischemic stroke or head trauma within last three months
	History of intracerebral bleed
	Untreated cerebral aneurysm, arteriovenous malformation (AVM), or brain tumor
	GI or GU hemorrhage within last three weeks
	Lumbar puncture within last 3 days or arterial puncture (at noncompressible site) within last 7 days
	Patients with international normalized ratio (INR) greater than 1.7 and taking oral anticoagulants
	Patients receiving heparin within last 48 hours and with elevated activated partial thromboplastin time (aPTT)
	Patients receiving low molecular weight heparin within last 24 hours

(Continues)

Clinical Indications and Contraindications for tPA in Stroke Clients (*continued*)

	Pregnant or anticipated pregnant female
	Known coagulation disorder
	Received tPA within last 7 days
Laboratory contraindications	Glucose less than 50 or greater than 400 mg/dL
	Platelet count less than 100,000 mm^3
	Prothrombin time greater than 15 or INR greater than 1.7
	Elevated APT
	Positive pregnancy test
Radiological contraindications	Intracranial hemorrhage
	Findings suggesting a new or evolving stroke
	Intracranial tumor, aneurysm, or AVM

Adapted from Institute for Clinical Systems Improvement. (2003). *Diagnosis and initial treatment of ischemic stroke.* Retrieved June 13, 2006, from www.guideline.gov.

11. Mrs. Kahn's daughters have differing opinions about what is best for their mother. The health care team has explained that Mrs. Kahn will not regain her independence and former quality of life. Mrs. Kahn's HCP has discussed changing Mrs. Kahn's code status to DNR. Rose is not willing to do this. Rose and her sister are overheard having an argument about changing Mrs. Kahn's code status. Discuss how this situation would likely be different if Mrs. Kahn had an advance directive. An advanced directive is a document that defines the care that an individual deems acceptable should they become incapacitated and unable to express their wishes. A living will provides written direction about the medical care that a person desires in order to guide care in the event that the individual becomes unable to express these decisions personally. A living will outlines the individual's wishes regarding medical care, artificial nourishment, resuscitation measures, and life support. A health care proxy or durable power of attorney (POA) is authorization that a competent individual gives to another person so that the designated person may exercise decision-making authority on the individual's behalf. An individual completes an advance care medical directive in consultation with an HCP, relative, or personal advisor. This document provides instruction for the type of care the individual wants and/or does not want in different scenarios. If Mrs. Kahn had completed an advance directive prior to having her stroke, her wishes regarding end of life care, code status, and desire to have a feeding tube may have been known. Mrs. Kahn also could have appointed a health care proxy or durable POA. Discussing her wishes with her health care proxy would allow this appointed person to speak on her behalf when she became unable. An advance directive must be completed while the individual is still competent. Therefore, Mrs. Kahn would have had to make these decisions prior to her dementia (Kozier, et al., 2004; Marek & Boehnlein, 2007).

12. In order of priority, identify five nursing diagnoses that are appropriate for Mrs. Kahn. Appropriate nursing diagnoses to consider for Mrs. Kahn in order of priority include:

- Ineffective tissue perfusion (cerebral) related to (r/t) interruption of blood flow
- Risk for aspiration r/t impaired swallowing secondary to neuromuscular dysfunction
- Incontinence (reflex) r/t loss of feeling to void, confusion, and difficulty communicating
- Risk for impaired skin integrity r/t hemiplegia, immobility, and incontinence
- Impaired verbal communication r/t pressure damage and decreased circulation to brain in speech center informational sources
- Impaired physical mobility r/t hemiplegia, loss of balance and coordination, and brain injury
- Self-care deficit (feeding, bathing/hygiene, toileting) r/t decreased strength and endurance, and hemiplegia
- Interrupted family processes r/t catastrophic illness and caregiver burdens
- Risk for disuse syndrome r/t hemiplegia
- Impaired social interaction r/t limited physical mobility and limited ability to communicate

(Ackley & Ladwig, 2006; Flannery & Bulecza, 2007; Smeltzer & Bare, 2004)

13. Briefly explain the appropriate nursing actions to help minimize the risk of aspiration for a client receiving tube feeding. What should the nurse do prior to changing Mrs. Kahn's bed linens? To help minimize the risk of aspiration, the nurse monitors for correct placement of the percutaneous endoscopic gastrostomy (PEG) feeding tube, gastric residual, decreased gastric motility, and maintenance of the client in high Fowler's position. Placement of the PEG tube is assessed before administering any liquids through the tube. Mrs. Kahn is receiving continuous gastric feeding, and therefore placement is assessed every four hours. Gastric contents are aspirated to assess for gastric residual. Aspirated gastric contents should be returned to the stomach to prevent fluid and electrolyte imbalance. Auscultation for bowel sounds helps to determine gastric motility. If proper placement cannot be confirmed, the residual amount is greater than 100 mL, or if bowel sounds are hypoactive or absent, the nurse should be concerned about decreased absorption. The tube feeding should be stopped, and the HCP notified. The head of the client receiving a tube feeding should always be in the high Fowler's position and never lower than 30 degrees. Prior to lowering the head of Mrs. Kahn's bed to change the bed linens, the tube feeding pump should be stopped so that the Jevity is not being administered while the head of the bed is lower than thirty degrees (Altman, 2004). Since Mrs. Kahn will be in a high Fowler's position, the nurse should assess the client for pressure sores in her coccyx area.

14. Enoxaparin is prescribed for Mrs. Kahn. Discuss the indication for this medication and its potential adverse effects. What should the nurse monitor while Mrs. Kahn is receiving enoxaparin? Enoxaparin is a low molecular weight heparin administered through a subcutaneous injection. This anticoagulant prevents the conversion of fibrinogen to fibrin and prothrombin to thrombin. It is prescribed as prophylaxis of a deep vein thrombosis (DVT). A client with severely restricted mobility, such as Mrs. Kahn, is at risk for developing a DVT, which can lead to pulmonary embolism. Potential adverse effects include thrombocytopenia, hypochromic anemia, hemorrhage, confusion, fever, nausea, and edema. At the site of the injection, mild local irritation, pain, hematoma, or erythema may be noted. The nurse should monitor for signs of bleeding by monitoring the client's complete blood count, coagulation studies, and occult blood in the stool. The client should be assessed for bleeding gums, petechiae, ecchymosis, hematuria, and epitaxis. Vital signs are monitored for increased body temperature and decreased blood pressure. Any indication of bleeding in the client should be reported to the HCP immediately (Skidmore-Roth, 2005; Spratto & Woods, 2006).

15. Discuss how Mrs. Kahn's culture and religion may play a role in her health care while in the hospital. It is important to recognize that not everyone of a particular ethnic background or religion will conform to a set of expected behaviors. However, a client's cultural and religious beliefs are an important consideration in providing holistic nursing care. The nurses may be perceived by Mrs. Kahn and her family as helpers, but not health care professionals. If this is the case, the nurse's suggestions may not be respected. The HCP may need to explain the nurse's role to the client and family. Individuals of Arab heritage value nonverbal expressions as an important part of communication. Titles are valued, and the nurse should ask how the client or family members prefer to be addressed. Shaking hands is an acceptable form of introduction, but a male should not initiate a handshake with a female. The right hand only is used for shaking hands because the left hand is the hand used for toileting and is therefore considered dirty. Same gender HCPs are strongly preferred. The client may be reluctant to share sensitive information with a person of the opposite gender. Arabs are not accustomed to the professional role of a social worker. Arab individuals rely on their families, other relatives, and friends for help and support. This may result in difficulty arranging discharge placement for Mrs. Kahn if the family does not understand the role of the social worker in offering suggestions for long-term care.

The Muslim religion prohibits alcohol. Medications prescribed for the client should not contain alcohol. The nurse should be aware that many Muslims observe prayer five times a day. Mrs. Kahn's daughters may bring an amulet for her to wear, to be pinned to her hospital gown or placed by her bed. Ramadan is a holy month that begins with the sighting of the new moon, which begins September 13 and ends October 13 in 2007. During Ramadan, fasting is required from sunup until sundown. Mrs. Kahn's daughters may request that medications, IV therapy, and the tube feeding be held during this observance. However, fasting is not required for Muslims during illness. It may be helpful for HCP to explain the rationale and therapeutic effect of medications, IV therapy, and the tube feeding if the daughters are struggling between the devout Muslim beliefs and Mrs. Kahn's treatment plan. The month of Ramadan is a time for spiritual reflection and prayer. Nursing staff should accommodate the family's requests regarding time to visit with family and pray together. Throughout Mrs. Kahn's hospital stay, she will likely have many visitors since it is considered a social obligation for friends and family to visit and bring gifts.

Should Mrs. Kahn's condition worsen and death is imminent, her bed should be positioned to face Mecca, which is located northeast from the United States. Organ donation is an acceptable option. Some Muslims prefer to bury the person's body on the day death occurs (Ahmad, 2004; Fernandez & Fernandez, 2005).

The nurse should avoid making assumptions, but being aware of common beliefs shared by members of a culture or religion can help the nurse care for the client as an individual and serve as a client advocate. The nurse should clarify Mrs. Kahn's personal beliefs, practices, and preferences with her daughters. For example, the nurse might assess this by asking, "It is my understanding that individuals who are of Arab heritage prefer same gender health care providers. Do you think that Mrs. Kahn would prefer that only female staff provide her care?" The nurse might also ask, "Is there something that I have not asked you or that you request that will make a difference in how I plan your mother's care?"

References

Ackley, B., & Ladwig, G. (2006). *Nursing diagnosis handbook: A guide to planning care*. St. Louis, MO: Mosby.

Ahmad, N. M. (2004). *Arab-American culture and health care*. Retrieved September 18, 2006, from www.case.edu.

Altman, G. (2004). *Delmar's fundamental & advanced nursing skills* (pp. 742–743). Clifton Park, NY: Thomson Learning.

American Heart Association (AHA). (2006). *Heart attack, stroke and cardiac arrest warning signs*. Retrieved September 16, 2006, from www.americanheart.org.

American Heart Association (ASA). (2006). *Learn about stroke*. Retrieved September 16, 2006, from www.strokeassociation.org.

Deglin, J. H., & Vallerand, A. H. (2007). *Davis's drug guide for nurses*. Philadelphia, PA: F. A. Davis.

Fernandez, V. M., & Fernandez, K. M. (2005). *Transcultural nursing: Basic concepts and casestudies*. Retrieved September 18, 2006, from www.culturaldiversity.org.

Flannery, J., & Bulecza, S. (2007). Vascular and degenerative problems of the brain. In F. Monahan, J. Sands, M. Neighbors, J. Marek, & C. Green (Eds.), *Phipps' Medical-surgical nursing: Health and illness perspectives* (pp. 1421–1439). St. Louis, MO: Mosby Elsevier.

Hickey, B., & McCoy, C. A. (2007). Dysfunction of the brain: Nursing management. In R. Daniels, L. J. Nosek, & L. H. Nicoll (Eds.), *Contemporary medical-surgical nursing* (pp. 1171–1182). Clifton Park, NY: Thomson Delmar Learning.

Huffstutler, S. Y. (2007). Assessment of the nervous system. In F. Monahan, J. Sands, M. Neighbors, J. Marek, & C. Green (Eds.), *Phipps' Medical-surgical nursing: Health and illness perspectives* (pp. 1355–1356). St. Louis, MO: Mosby Elsevier.

Kozier, B., Erb, G., Berman, A., & Snyder, S. J. (2004). Loss, grieving, and death. In *Fundamentals of nursing: Concepts, process, and practice.* (pp. 1043–1044). Upper Saddle River, NJ: Pearson Education.

Marek, J., & Boehnlein, M. (2007). Preoperative nursing. In F. Monahan, J. Sands, M. Neighbors, J. Marek, & C. Green (Eds.), *Phipps' Medical-surgical nursing: Health and illness perspectives* (p. 241). St. Louis, MO: Mosby Elsevier.

Skidmore-Roth, L. (Ed.) (2005). *Mosby's drug guide for nurses* (pp. 309–310). St. Louis, MO: Mosby.

Smeltzer, S., & Bare, B. (2004). Management of patients with cerebrovascular disorders. In L. Brunner & D. Suddarth (Eds.), *Textbook of medical-surgical nursing* (pp. 1887–1909). Philadelphia, PA: Lippincott Williams & Wilkins.

Spratto, G. R., & Woods, A. L. (2006). *PDR nurse's drug handbook* (pp. 476–478). Clifton Park, NY: Thomson Delmar Learning.

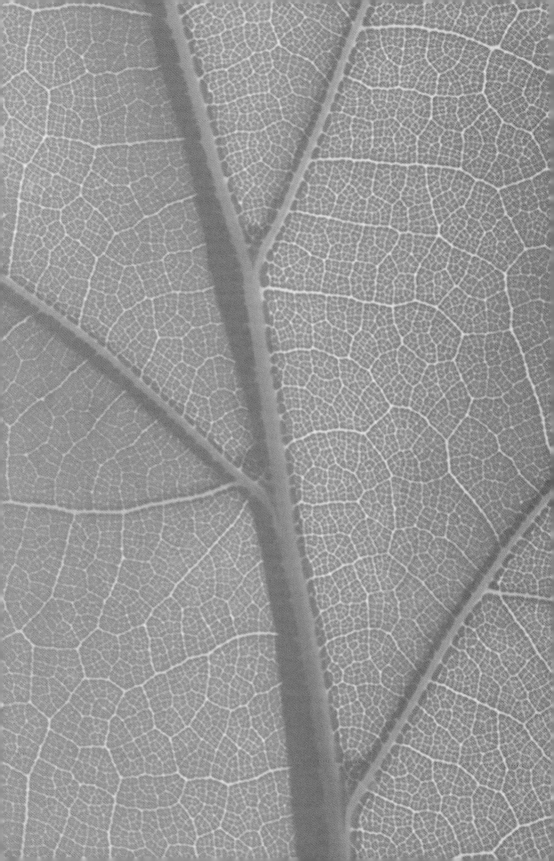

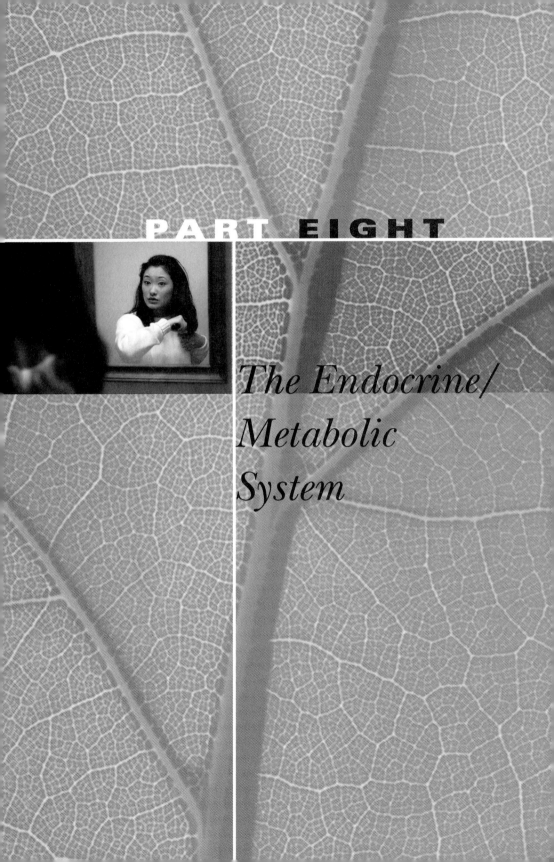

PART EIGHT

The Endocrine/ Metabolic System

CASE STUDY 1

Mrs. Duarte

EASY

GENDER

Female

AGE

40

SETTING

■ Primary Care

ETHNICITY

■ White American

CULTURAL CONSIDERATIONS

PREEXISTING CONDITION

COEXISTING CONDITIONS

■ Goiter
■ Exophthalmos

COMMUNICATION

DISABILITY

SOCIOECONOMIC

■ Married
■ Preschool teacher

SPIRITUAL/RELIGIOUS

PHARMACOLOGIC

■ Levothyroxine sodium (Levothroid, Synthroid)

LEGAL

ETHICAL

ALTERNATIVE THERAPY

PRIORITIZATION

DELEGATION

THE ENDOCRINE/METABOLIC SYSTEM

Level of Difficulty: Easy

Overview: This client in this case presents to her primary health care provider (HCP) with concern about a lump that she has noticed on the left side of her neck. The client's fear that the lump is indicative of cancer proves unwarranted. However, her HCP is concerned that she has thyroid disease. Diagnostic testing prescribed to confirm the diagnosis is reviewed. Client education regarding radioiodine iodine therapy and a newly prescribed medication is provided. Nursing diagnoses appropriate for this client are identified, and a plan of care is created for the priority nursing diagnosis.

197

Client Profile

Mrs. Duarte is a 40-year-old woman who has scheduled an appointment with her primary HCP to assess a lump that has developed on the left side of her neck.

Case Study

Mrs. Duarte explains to her HCP that she has noticed a swollen area on the left side of her neck that has been increasing in size. She states, "I am really afraid I have cancer. I eat plenty but seem to be losing weight. I have lost 10 pounds in less than 2 months. I have been very agitated and irritable. Perhaps I am nervous about the possibility that this lump is cancer." Her vital signs are blood pressure 142/64, pulse 128, respiratory rate 24, and temperature 98.8°F (37°C). The HCP notes that Mrs. Duarte's hands have a fine tremor, and she has mild periorbital edema indicative of exophthalmos. On physical assessment, the HCP palpates a smooth, soft, enlarged left lobe of the thyroid gland. The HCP places the bell of the stethoscope over the swollen area and auscultates a bruit. Further discussion reveals that Mrs. Duarte has been having difficulty sleeping, thinning hair, and loose bowel movements. Concerned that Mrs. Duarte has a thyroid disorder, the HCP prescribes serum laboratory testing to assess the client's levels of thyroid stimulating hormone (TSH) and free tetraiodothyronine (thyroxine or T_4), and schedules the client for a radioactive iodine uptake test.

Questions

1. Describe the anatomy of the thyroid gland, its hormone production, and briefly discuss its function.

2. Does the HCP suspect that Mrs. Duarte has hypothyroidism or hyperthyroidism? Identify the clinical manifestations that support your answer.

3. Identify three nursing diagnoses appropriate for Mrs. Duarte.

4. Referring to the diagnoses identified in question #3, what is the priority nursing diagnosis for Mrs. Duarte? Write two outcome goals for the client related to this diagnosis, and generate at least three nursing interventions to include in her plan of care.

5. The HCP heard a bruit over Mrs. Duarte's thyroid gland. Is this a normal or abnormal finding? Explain what a bruit is and what it indicates.

6. Mrs. Duarte is noted to have mild periorbital edema. What causes this edema? What are the potential complications that can arise? What suggestions can the nurse offer for minimizing the potential complications and discomfort if the edema worsens?

7. Briefly explain what the TSH and free T_4 tests measure and provide the normal range for each. What TSH and free T_4 test results will confirm the suspected thyroid disease identified in question # 2?

Questions (continued)

8. Identify the chief component in the synthesis of T$_3$ and T$_4$, and discuss how most individuals obtain adequate amounts of this component to support the body's normal thyroid function.

9. Explain to Mrs. Duarte how the radioactive iodine uptake test is conducted and how the results will help the HCP confirm Mrs. Duarte's diagnosis.

10. Mrs. Duarte does not have cancer. Explain what is causing the "lump" in Mrs. Duarte's neck.

11. The HCP suggests that Mrs. Duarte have radioactive iodine (RAI) therapy. Briefly explain this therapy to Mrs. Duarte and the precautions she should take regarding contact with others in the days following RAI therapy.

12. What potential adverse effect of the initial dose of RAI therapy is considered a medical emergency? Briefly discuss the clinical manifestations that should be monitored to detect this adverse effect.

13. To insure that Mrs. Duarte is an appropriate candidate for RAI therapy, explain which laboratory test will be performed prior to beginning treatment.

14. Mrs. Duarte develops hypothyroidism following her RAI therapy. Her HCP prescribes levothyroxine sodium. She asks the nurse, "What is this medication for, and how long will I need to take it?" Provide the client with teaching regarding the rationale for the prescribed levothyroxine sodium and respond to Mrs. Duarte's question regarding the length of treatment.

Questions and Suggested Answers

1. Describe the anatomy of the thyroid gland, its hormone production, and briefly discuss its function. The term *thyroid* comes from the Greek word for "shield." The thyroid gland is a butterfly-shaped gland located in the front of the neck just below the thyroid cartilage of the larynx (voice box). The gland is approximately 5 cm long and 3 cm wide and consists of two lobes connected by a band of tissue called the isthmus. One lobe is situated on the right side and one on the left side of the trachea. The thyroid tissue is composed of follicular and parafollicular cells. The majority of the gland is composed of follicular cells, which secrete iodine-containing hormones called triiodothyronine (T$_3$) and thyroxine (T$_4$). T$_3$ and T$_4$ are referred to collectively as thyroid hormone (TH). The parafollicular cells secrete the hormone calcitonin. Homeostasis of the level of thyroid hormone (TH) in the body is maintained by a negative feedback mechanism regulated by the hypothalamus and pituitary glands. When low levels of TH are detected, the hypothalamus, a small part of the brain located above the pituitary gland, produces thyrotropin releasing hormone (TRH). The TRH stimulates the pituitary, a gland located at the base of the brain, to release TSH. An increased level of TSH in turn stimulates the thyroid gland to increase its uptake of iodine and produce more TH, thus restoring the level of TH in the body to homeostasis (Carroll, 2005; Rizzo, 2006).

The T_3 and T_4 hormones of the thyroid gland function to regulate the metabolism of carbohydrates, fats, and proteins. Thyroid hormones are required for normal growth and development in children and for maturation of the nervous system. Thyroid hormones cause an increase in the rate of carbohydrate and lipid breakdown, which generates energy molecules and increases the rate of protein synthesis. This increased metabolic rate helps the body acclimate to environmental changes in temperature. Calcitonin works with the parathyroid hormones to regulate serum and tissue calcium levels by moving calcium into storage in the bones and teeth (Carroll, 2005; Rizzo, 2006).

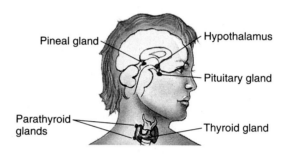

Structures of the endocrine system

2.   Does the HCP suspect that Mrs. Duarte has hypothyroidism or hyperthyroidism? Identify the clinical manifestations that support your answer. The HCP suspects that Mrs. Duarte has hyperthyroidism. Hyperthyroidism is the second most prevalent endocrine disorder after diabetes mellitus. The most common type of hyperthyroidism is Graves' disease. This disease is eight times more common in women than in men, and the onset is usually in the second and fourth decades of life. Graves' disease is caused by abnormal stimulation of the thyroid gland by circulating immunoglobulins, which results in hypersecretion of thyroid hormone. Graves' disease is believed to be an autoimmune disorder, characterized by a variable degree of opthalmopathy (eye disease), goiter (enlarged thyroid gland), and sometimes an infiltrative dermopathy (skin disease). Mrs. Duarte has presented with mild exophthalmos (abnormal protrusion of the eyes) and goiter, which are two of the characteristic signs of Graves' disease. In a client with hyperthyroidism, elevated levels of circulating TH cause the body processes to "speed up." Consistent with this response to increased TH, Mrs. Duarte has tachycardia, and an elevated systolic blood pressure, and is complaining of progressive weight loss, agitation, and irritability; difficulty sleeping; and loose bowel movements. She is also noted to have thinning hair and a fine hand tremor. These are all clinical manifestations of hyperthyroidism (Larson, 2005; Smeltzer & Bare, 2004; Ulchaker, 2007).

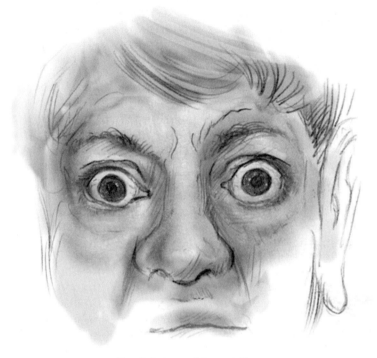

Exophthalmos of Graves' disease

3. Identify three nursing diagnoses appropriate for Mrs. Duarte. Possible nursing diagnoses for this client (in alphabetical order) include:

- Anxiety related to (r/t) increased stimulation and loss of control
- Diarrhea r/t increased gastric motility
- Disturbed sleep pattern r/t anxiety and excessive sympathetic discharge
- Imbalanced nutrition: Less than body requirements r/t increased metabolic rate and increased gastrointestinal (GI) activity
- Risk for altered body temperature (hyperthermia) r/t accelerated metabolic rate
- Risk for disturbed sensory perception (visual) r/t exophthalmos
- Risk for ineffective coping r/t irritability and emotional instability
- Risk for injury: Eye damage r/t exophthalmos

(Ackley & Ladwig, 2006; Larson, 2005; Smeltzer & Bare, 2004; Ulchaker, 2007).

4. Referring to the diagnoses identified in question #3, what is the priority nursing diagnosis for Mrs. Duarte? Write two outcome goals for the client related to this diagnosis, and generate at least three nursing interventions to include in her plan of care. The priority nursing diagnosis for Mrs. Duarte is *Imbalanced nutrition: Less than body requirements r/t increased metabolic rate, increased gastrointestinal activity.*

Expected client outcomes include:

- Mrs. Duarte will gain weight to within five pounds of her ideal body weight for height within a month.
- Mrs. Duarte will be free of signs of malnutrition (brittle hair that is easily plucked, dry skin, pale skin and conjunctiva, smooth red tongue, bruises, and muscle wasting).
- Mrs. Duarte will identify high-calorie, high-protein foods and foods to avoid following client education.
- Mrs. Duarte will avoid GI stimulants following client education.
- Mrs. Duarte will report decreased episodes of diarrhea.

Nursing interventions include:

- Encourage increased nutrient intake with a high-calorie, high-protein, and high-carbohydrate diet with foods selected from all the food groups.
- Encourage the client to consume six small meals a day to provide a consistent intake of nutrients throughout the day to meet metabolic demands.
- Avoid foods that irritate the GI tract and increase the incidence of diarrhea, such as highly seasoned foods as well as GI stimulants such as tea, coffee, colas, and alcohol.
- Monitor and document food intake, recording the percentage of each meal that the client eats. Consult with a dietician to determine actual calorie count as needed.
- Monitor the client's weight at least weekly. This helps to determine if nutritional needs are being met and if further intervention is needed.
- Monitor laboratory values for serum albumin, total protein, hemoglobin, electrolytes, and lymphocyte levels to determine if nutrition is adequate to meet the client's metabolic needs.
- Monitor for signs of malnutrition including brittle hair, dry skin, bruises, pale skin and conjunctiva, muscle wasting, and smooth red tongue.

(Ackley & Ladwig, 2006; Smeltzer & Bare, 2004; Ulchaker, 2007)

5. The HCP heard a bruit over Mrs. Duarte's thyroid gland. Is this a normal or abnormal finding? Explain what a bruit is and what it indicates. A bruit is an intermittent swooshing or musical sound heard during auscultation with the bell of the stethoscope. When heard over the thyroid gland, a bruit is an abnormal assessment finding. It indicates increased turbulence in a vessel and results from increased blood flow through the thyroid gland that has become enlarged due to diffuse toxic goiter (Smeltzer & Bare, 2004).

6. Mrs. Duarte is noted to have mild periorbital edema. What causes this edema? What are the potential complications that can arise? What suggestions can the nurse offer for minimizing the potential complications and discomfort if the edema worsens? In the client with periorbital edema, the connective tissue and extraocular muscle volume expand because of fluid retention. The accumulation of fluid in the fat pads and muscles behind the eyes forces the eyeballs forward. Periorbital and eyelid edema put pressure on the optic nerve, and the enlarged and stretched extraocular muscles do not function at their optimal level, often resulting in diplopia (blurred vision). Clients may complain of photophobia (intolerance to light). The client with exophthalmos may experience irritation and excessive tearing and a feeling of pressure behind the eyes. Some clients are unable to close their eyelids. Exposure and excess drying can lead to a corneal ulceration and infection. If the optic nerve is involved, the client may develop optic neuropathy, which causes a loss of vision (Larson, 2005; Ulchaker, 2007).

The nurse can suggest that Mrs. Duarte use moisturizing eye drops to decrease the dryness and irritation. Blinking will also help lubricate the eye and minimize debris that can cause corneal irritation. Dark sunglasses reduce eye discomfort and photophobia and provide protection against dust and dirt. Taping the eyes closed or a sleeping mask worn at night can offer protection as long as the client does not notice that the mask shifts during the night, increasing the chance of scratching the eye. Elevating the head of the bed at night also helps to decrease the discomfort of the edema. The HCP may prescribe prednisone to reduce inflammation of the periorbital tissues or a diuretic to decrease the periorbital edema. In addition, the nurse should suggest that the client follow a low sodium diet. The client should be informed that the exophthalmos may or may not resolve with treatment of the client's hyperthyroidism (Larson, 2005).

7. Briefly explain what the TSH and free T_4 tests measure and provide the normal range for each. What TSH and free T4 test results will confirm the suspected thyroid disease identified in question #2? *TSH* is a diagnostic test used to measure the levels of circulating thyroid-stimulating hormone and detect abnormal thyroid activity resulting from excessive pituitary stimulation. The high sensitivity of this test (greater than 95%) makes it an excellent screening tool for thyroid function (Larson, Anderson, & Koslawy, 2000). Its primary function is to differentiate thyroid versus pituitary involvement. The normal range of TSH is 0.4 to 4.2 µU/mL. A client with hyperthyroidism will have a TSH level that is below normal limits (Chernecky & Berger, 2004).

Free tetraiodothyronine (thyroxine or T_4) is abbreviated as such because his hormone contains four iodine atoms. This test is prescribed to confirm an abnormal TSH. It measures the amount of unbound thyroxine. The normal range of free T_4 is 0.58 to 1.64 ng/dL. A client with hyperthyroidism will have an elevated T_4 level (Chernecky & Berger, 2004).

8. Identify the chief component in the synthesis of T_3 and T_4, and discuss how most individuals obtain adequate amounts of this component to support the body's normal thyroid function. The chief component in the synthesis of T_3 and T_4 is iodine. Most individuals obtain adequate amounts of iodine through the intake of water, food, and iodized table salt in their diet. Iodide ingested in the diet is absorbed into the blood in the GI tract. The thyroid gland takes the iodide from the blood and converts it to iodine molecules that react with an amino acid to produce thyroid hormones (Smeltzer & Bare, 2004).

9. Explain to Mrs. Duarte how the RAI uptake test is conducted and how the results will help the HCP confirm Mrs. Duarte's diagnosis. An RAI reuptake test measures the rate of iodine uptake by the thyroid gland. This test measures the amount of radioactivity in the thyroid after the client receives a relatively small dose of RAI in either intravenous or pill form. The thyroid gland absorbs iodine and uses it to make hormones. Therefore, the amount of RAI detected in the thyroid gland corresponds with the amount of thyroid hormone the client's thyroid is producing.

Mrs. Duarte will be given a tracer dose of a radionuclide such as iodine-123 (^{123}I). Using an instrument called a scintillation counter, the HCP administering the test will scan over her thyroid gland to detect the amount of radioactive iodine still present in the thyroid gland at various time intervals following the administered dose. Since the amount of radioactive iodine detected corresponds to the amount of thyroid hormone the thyroid is producing, a client with hyperthyroidism will exhibit a high uptake of the iodine-123 (as high as 90%) (Chernecky & Berger, 2004; Smeltzer & Bare, 2004).

10. Mrs. Duarte does not have cancer. Explain what is causing the "lump" in Mrs. Duarte's neck. Hyperthyroidism results from an immunoglobulin that stimulates the TSH receptor on the thyroid gland. This causes hypertrophy of the thyroid gland and overproduction of TH. The lump that Mrs. Duarte presents with is the physical enlargement of the left lobe of the thyroid gland, often called a goiter. The gland can grow to three or four times its normal size (Larson, 2005).

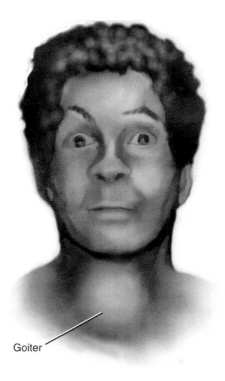

Goiter

Goiter of Graves' disease

11. The HCP suggests that Mrs. Duarte have RAI therapy. Briefly explain this therapy to Mrs. Duarte and the precautions she should take regarding contact with others in the days following RAI therapy. RAI therapy is a long-term treatment option for adult clients with hyperthyroidism resulting from Graves' disease. RAI therapy is also referred to as a chemical thyroidectomy. This therapy involves the oral administration of radioactive iodine, such as ^{123}I or ^{131}I, used to destroy thyroid cells, and consequently a portion of the thyroid gland, thus diminishing thyroid hormone secretion. The radioiodine is colorless and tasteless. The dose of iodine administered is prescribed based on the size of the client's thyroid and results of the 24-hour iodine uptake test. It will take several weeks for the radioactive iodine to destroy the exposed thyroid cells and approximately six weeks to six months for the client to achieve a normal thyroid hormone level (euthyroid state). Seventy to 85% of clients are cured with one dose of RAI.

Others require a repeat dose of RAI therapy to achieve a euthyroid state (Larson, 2005; Smeltzer & Bare, 2004; Ulchaker, 2007).

Almost all of the RAI that enters the body becomes concentrated in the thyroid gland. The RAI is eliminated from the body over the course of a few days, primarily through the urine. Small amounts of the RAI will also appear in saliva. For several days following therapy, Mrs. Duarte should avoid sharing food, beverages, and eating utensils with others. She should also refrain from kissing and minimize close contact with children. Mrs. Duarte is a preschool teacher. As a precaution, she should request an absence from her place of employment for a week following her RAI therapy.

12. What potential adverse effect of the initial dose of RAI therapy is considered a medical emergency? Briefly discuss the clinical manifestations that should be monitored to detect this adverse effect. Although rare, the initial dose of RAI may cause an acute release of TH that can cause clinical manifestations referred to as a thyroid storm (thyroid crisis or thyrotoxicosis). A client experiencing this life-threatening condition will exhibit an increased severity of the clinical manifestations of hyperthyroidism. A high fever and diaphoresis are often the earliest manifestations of a thyroid crisis. The client should be monitored for a change in vital signs from their baseline. Increased tachycardia, palpitations, a cardiac dysrhythmia, increased blood pressure, and/or increased respiratory rate are signs of a thyroid storm. The client should be assessed for weight loss, worsening diarrhea, tremors, and/or restlessness. As well, the client is monitored for a change in mental state, such as somnolence, delirium, paranoia, and possibly coma. Clients with thyroid storm require intensive care, including respiratory support, fever reduction, and interventions to address hemodynamic instability (Campbell, 2007; Smeltzer & Bare, 2004; Ulchaker, 2007).

13. To ensure that Mrs. Duarte is an appropriate candidate for RAI therapy, explain which laboratory test will be performed prior to beginning treatment. RAI therapy is contraindicated in pregnancy and nursing mothers because the radioiodine crosses the placenta and is secreted in breast milk. Mrs. Duarte is not breastfeeding. The HCP should not rely on the client's report of her last menstrual period as an indication of pregnancy since hyperthyroidism can cause a change in menses. A serum pregnancy test will need to be conducted to confirm that she is not pregnant before initiating the therapy (Smeltzer & Bare, 2004).

14. Mrs. Duarte develops hypothyroidism following her RAI therapy. Her HCP prescribes levothyroxine sodium. She asks the nurse, "What is this medication for, and how long will I need to take it?" Provide the client with teaching regarding the rationale for the prescribed levothyroxine sodium, and respond to Mrs. Duarte's question regarding the length of treatment. Because the RAI destroys thyroid cells, more than 80% of clients in the first year and over 90% of clients within five years of RAI therapy, will develop hypothyroidism. TH replacement is necessary to treat this condition. Levothyroxine is a synthetic thyroid hormone prescribed to compensate for lost thyroid function. Mrs. Duarte's hormone supplementation with levothyroxine sodium will be lifelong (Deglin & Vallerand, 2007; Smeltzer & Bare, 2004).

References

Ackley, B., & Ladwig, G. (2006). *Nursing diagnosis handbook: A guide to planning care.* St. Louis, MO: Mosby.

Campbell, J. (2007). Endocrine dysfunction: Nursing management. In R. Daniels, L. J. Nosek, & L. H. Nicoll (Eds.), *Contemporary medical-surgical nursing* (pp. 1887–1888). Clifton Park, NY: Thomson Delmar Learning.

Carroll, R. G. (2005). The metabolic systems. In J. M. Black & J. H. Hawks (Eds.), *Medical-surgical nursing: Clinical management for positive outcomes* (pp. 1146, 1150). St. Louis, MO: Elsevier.

Chernecky, C. C., & Berger, B. J. (2004). *Laboratory tests & diagnostic procedures.* Philadelphia, PA: Elsevier.

Deglin, J. H., & Vallerand, A. H. (2007). *Davis's drug guide for nurses.* Philadelphia, PA: F. A. Davis.

Larson, A. M. (2005). Management of clients with thyroid and parathyroid disorders. In J. M. Black & J. H. Hawks (Eds.), *Medical-surgical nursing: Clinical management for positive outcomes* (pp. 1191–1193, 1198–1206). St. Louis, MO: Elsevier.

Larson, J., Anderson, E. H., & Koslawy, M. (2000). Thyroid disease: A review for primary care. *Journal of the American Academy of Nurse Practitioners, 12* (6), 226–232.

Rizzo, D. C. (2006). *Fundamentals of anatomy & physiology.* Clifton Park, NY: Thomson Delmar Learning.

Smeltzer, S., & Bare, B. (2004). Assessment and management of patients with endocrine disorders. In L. Brunner & D. Suddarth (Eds.), *Textbook of medical-surgical nursing* (pp. 1212–1227). Philadelphia, PA: Lippincott Williams & Wilkins.

Ulchaker, M. M. (2007). Pituitary, thyroid, parathyroid, and adrenal gland problems. In F. Monahan, J. Sands, M. Neighbors, J. Marek, & C. Green (Eds.), *Phipps' medical-surgical nursing: Health and illness perspectives* (pp. 1073–1080). St. Louis, MO: Mosby Elsevier.

CASE STUDY 2

Mr. Kiley

GENDER

Male

AGE

33

SETTING

- Hospital

ETHNICITY

- Black American

CULTURAL CONSIDERATIONS

PREEXISTING CONDITIONS

- Type 1 diabetes mellitus
- Bipolar II disorder

COEXISTING CONDITION

- Hypothermia

COMMUNICATION

DISABILITY

SOCIOECONOMIC

- Lives with sister
- Employed as an auto mechanic

SPIRITUAL/RELIGIOUS

PHARMACOLOGIC

- Regular insulin (Humulin R, Novolin R); lithium; 50% dextrose (D50); glucagon (GlucaGen)

LEGAL

ETHICAL

ALTERNATIVE THERAPY

PRIORITIZATION

- Medical stabilization

DELEGATION

- Collaboration between client's admitting health care provider (HCP) and treating psychiatrist

MODERATE

THE ENDOCRINE/METABOLIC SYSTEM

Level of Difficulty: Moderate

Overview: The client in this case has been noncompliant with his lithium. His altered mental status has affected his ability to manage his diabetes and maintain control of his blood glucose. The nurse must recognize the clinical manifestations of hypoglycemia and appropriate emergency interventions. The client's coexisting psychiatric disorder is reviewed. The nurse generates appropriate nursing diagnoses for the client's plan of care. Lastly, the impact of the client's illness on his family member is acknowledged.

Client Profile

Mr. Kiley is a 33-year-old male who presents to the emergency department after losing consciousness at work. The emergency medical technicians (EMTs) report that Mr. Kiley was unconscious when they arrived at the auto shop, and a finger stick blood glucose could not be measured on the glucometer (Accucheck) because it was so low. A fellow employee recounted the event for the EMTs stating, "He was fine all day. In fact, he was in a great mood, talking nonstop and telling me how he stayed up all night surfing the Internet and buying hundreds of dollars of Elvis memorabilia for his collection. Then for a time he was quiet. He was working under the car. When I asked him a question and he didn't answer, I pulled him out from under the car and he was sweating buckets. He wouldn't talk to me. We know he is diabetic, so we tried to give him juice. But he wouldn't swallow." The client's vital signs when the EMTs arrived were blood pressure 140/70, pulse 122, respiratory rate of 38, and temperature of 89°F (31.7°C). En route to the hospital, the client was covered with blankets, an intravenous (IV) access was established, and the client was given an ampule of 50% dextrose (D50) by IV bolus.

Case Study

Upon arrival in the emergency department, the client's skin is cold, and he is diaphoretic. He is having seizure activity. The client's vital signs are blood pressure 146/74, pulse 118, respiratory rate 34, and temperature 90°F (32.2°C). His blood glucose is 24 mg/dL. A second IV access is established to allow for the simultaneous administration of medication and 5% dextrose in water (D5W) as prescribed by the HCP. Warm blankets and warming lights are used to help raise the client's body temperature. The client is given a second ampule of D50. Oxygen is administered via nasal cannula, and the client is monitored for potential cardiac dysrhythmias. The client begins to regain consciousness. His seizure activity has subsided. His serum glucose is 84 mg/dL, and his temperature has risen to 93°F (33.9°C).

Mr. Kiley's sister has arrived in the emergency department. She tells the nurse that her brother is bipolar. She states, "He is usually very good about taking his medication and keeps his sugars in good control. This happened to him once before. He stopped taking his lithium and lost track of when he had taken his insulin. Last time this happened, he took way too much insulin and I found him unconscious in our apartment. I was away on a business trip this past week. It is my fault. If I had called more often while I was away and checked on him I could have noticed in his voice that he was off his med." When asked, Mr. Kiley reveals that he has not been taking his lithium and did not eat today. When asked, the client denies ingesting alcohol, engaging in vigorous exercise, smoking marijuana, or taking other recreational drugs or prescription medications. Mr. Kiley is admitted to the intensive care unit (ICU), and his treating psychiatrist is notified of the admission so that the admitting HCP can collaborate with the psychiatrist to plan the client's medical care.

Questions

1. Define hypoglycemia. What are hypoglycemic blood glucose values in an adult?

2. Describe the clinical manifestations of hypoglycemia. How low does a client's blood glucose need to fall before the client exhibits clinical manifestations?

3. Provide a rationale for why the HCP asked the client about alcohol intake, vigorous exercise, marijuana, the use of recreational drugs, and prescription medications.

4. Briefly define hypothermia, and explain why the client with hypoglycemia is often hypothermic.

5. If an IV access site could not be established, could the 50% dextrose (D50) be administered intramuscularly? What is another medication that the HCP might prescribe to treat the client's hypoglycemia, and what is that medication's most common adverse effect?

6. Briefly discuss bipolar disorder and the distinguishing feature of bipolar II disorder. What are the characteristic manifestations of the manic and depressive episodes experienced by a client with bipolar disorder? Briefly discuss the clinical manifestations of bipolar disorder that the client exhibited in the past 24 hours.

7. Discuss how Mr. Kiley's bipolar disorder contributed to his hypoglycemia.

8. Mr. Kiley's sister told the nurse that the client usually maintains good control of his blood glucose. The client's hemoglobin A1C (HbA_{1C}) is 5%. What does an HbA_{1C} value represent, and does the client's value indicate good control?

9. Help the nurse identify three priority nursing diagnoses to include in Mr. Kiley's plan of care.

10. The ICU nurse notices that the skin around the IV access site on Mr. Kiley's left hand is inflamed and warm. What is the most appropriate nursing intervention?

11. Although his fellow employees were trying to help Mr. Kiley, why was their attempt to give him juice an inappropriate intervention?

12. Briefly discuss how Mr. Kiley's bipolar disorder has had an impact on his sister's life, and identify a nursing diagnosis that acknowledges the challenges of her role as a caregiver.

Questions and Suggested Answers

1. Define hypoglycemia. What are hypoglycemic blood glucose values in an adult? Hypoglycemia (also called an insulin reaction in a known diabetic) is an abnormally low glucose level. In a healthy adult under 60 years of age, the normal range of blood glucose is between 70 and 105 mg/dL. In an older adult (over 60 years old), the normal range of blood glucose is between 80 and 115 mg/dL. Hypoglycemia is defined as a blood glucose level below 50 mg/dL in adult men and below 45 mg/dL in adult women (Chernecky & Berger, 2004; McLeod, 2006).

2. Describe the clinical manifestations of hypoglycemia. How low does a client's blood glucose need to fall before the client exhibits clinical manifestations? The clinical manifestations of hypoglycemia can be divided into two sets of symptoms. The initial adrenergic symptoms occur when the sympathetic nervous system is activated and epinephrine increases in response to a drop in blood glucose. More severe reactions manifest as a neuroglycopenic response in which there is a decreased supply of glucose to the brain and depression of the central nervous system (CNS). Adrenergic manifestations represent a mild reaction and often include hunger, tremors, shaking, irritability, palpitations, tachycardia, pallor, and diaphoresis. Clients with low blood glucose levels are often nervous or anxious, but are capable of recognizing the signs and symptoms and treating themselves to restore their blood glucose to within a normal range. If the client does not or cannot respond to the adrenergic symptoms to raise their glucose level, the client experiences neuroglycopenic manifestations. The body's neuroglycopenic response manifests as a decrease in cognitive function as exhibited by a headache, dizziness, lethargy, inability to concentrate, slurred speech, paresthesias, and blurry vision. This more severe hypoglycemic reaction can advance to confusion, convulsions, seizure, loss of consciousness, and possibly coma. Clients with severe hypoglycemic reactions often require emergency treatment initiated by another person. Prolonged or untreated hypoglycemia may result in impaired learning ability, memory loss, permanent brain damage, paralysis, and death (Fain, 2005; Ulchaker, 2007).

The onset of a client's clinical manifestations is rapid (minutes to hours). A client will usually exhibit clinical manifestations of hypoglycemia when the blood glucose level is less than 60 mg/dL. If the level continues to drop below 45 mg/dL, the symptoms progress to neuroglycopenic manifestations. However, the exact blood glucose level at which a client will have clinical manifestations is highly variable (Fain, 2005; Ulchaker, 2007). In addition, some clients with long-standing type 1 diabetes mellitus develop hypoglycemic unawareness in which they no longer experience the warning symptoms of an impending hypoglycemic reaction. "Hypoglycemic unawareness occurs in about 25% of diabetic clients and about 50% of all clients who have had type 1 diabetes for 30 years or longer" (McLeod, 2006, p. 1539).

3. Provide a rationale for why the HCP asked the client about alcohol intake, vigorous exercise, marijuana, the use of recreational drugs, and prescription medications. Alcohol intake and vigorous exercise without additional carbohydrate compensation can cause a hypoglycemic reaction.

Hypoglycemia is an adverse effect of some prescription medications, such as sulfonamides, salicylates, and monoamine oxidase (MAO) inhibitors. The client is assessed for marijuana and recreational drug use since, as with alcohol, these substances can impair a client's recognition of the early clinical manifestations of hypoglycemia. The HCP asks about alcohol, recreational drugs, and prescription medications because clients with bipolar disorder often abuse these substances as a coping strategy during manic or depressive episodes. Excessive exercise lowers the level of sodium in the client's body, which can cause lithium to build up and lead to toxicity. Clinical manifestations of lithium toxicity include drowsiness, mental dullness, slurred speech, confusion, and muscle twitching. Since these manifestations and those exhibited by the client are similar, ruling out the possibility of lithium toxicity is important to help determine an accurate diagnosis and plan appropriate medical treatment (Deglin & Vallerand, 2007; Spearing, 2007; Ulchaker, 2007).

4. Briefly define hypothermia, and explain why the client with hypoglycemia is often hypothermic. A decrease in a person's body temperature to below 95°F (35°C) is considered hypothermic. Primary hypothermia occurs because of exposure to cold. Secondary hypothermia occurs in the client with a disease state that causes an inability of the body to maintain thermoregulation. Human beings maintain a uniform body temperature through the internal generation of heat. A stable body temperature is achieved through a balance between internal heat production and the loss of body heat into the environment. The CNS processes input from central and peripheral thermal sensors to regulate body temperature. CNS function depends on a continuous supply of glucose in the blood. Clients with diabetes mellitus are at greater risk of secondary hypothermia. The client with hypoglycemia does not have an adequate supply of glucose to support CNS function, and inadequate thermoregulation results in a decrease in body temperature. Hypoglycemia produces hypothermia by inhibiting the shivering response, which occurs when a client's blood glucose falls below 45 mg/dL, and increasing the loss of heat through involuntary diaphoresis. When the client's body temperature falls below 95°F (35°C), the body becomes less capable of generating heat. Without intervention, the individual's body temperature will continue to drop. Clients with a body temperature below 89.6°F (32°C) are at an increased risk of developing ventricular dysrhythmias and should be carefully monitored (CDC, 2006).

5. If an IV access site could not be established, could the 50% dextrose (D50) be administered intramuscularly? What is another medication that the HCP might prescribe to treat the client's hypoglycemia and what is that medication's most common adverse effect? No. If an IV access could not be established, the ampule of D50 should not be given intramuscularly

(IM) nor subcutaneously (SC). If an IV access cannot be established, the HCP could prescribe 1 mg of glucagon to be administered IM or SC. The nurse should be aware that vomiting is a common adverse effect of glucagon. To prevent aspiration, especially in the client with a decreased level of consciousness, the nurse should position the client on their side following the administration of glucagon and have suction equipment available (Deglin & Vallerand, 2007; McLeod, 2006).

6. **Briefly discuss bipolar disorder and the distinguishing feature of bipolar II disorder. What are the characteristic manifestations of the manic and depressive episodes experienced by a client with bipolar disorder? Briefly discuss the clinical manifestations of bipolar disorder that the client exhibited in the past 24 hours.** Bipolar disorder is a mood disorder formerly called manic-depressive disorder or manic-depressive illness. Bipolar disorder is characterized by cycling mood changes that cause shifts in an individual's energy levels and ability to function. Clients with bipolar disorder fluctuate between severe highs (mania) and severe lows (depression). Cycles often are predominantly manic or depressive with periods of normal mood and behavior between cycles. These cycles of mood changes may occur within hours or days of one another, or the cycles can be separated by months or years. A client with bipolar II disorder never develops severe mania, but instead experiences milder episodes called hypomania. These episodes of hypomania usually alternate with episodes of depression. The severity of the mood changes and behaviors will vary. During episodes of depression, the client exhibits sadness, persistent negative thinking (pessimism), guilt, hopelessness, crying, and decreased socialization, energy, and motivation. The client often experiences changes in sleep pattern, appetite (increased or decreased), and sexual interest. The depressed client may experience suicidal ideations. When the client is experiencing a manic episode, they often exhibit excessive cheerfulness, an unrealistic, optimistic attitude toward their accomplishments, and an overabundance of energy. The manic client is often very talkative. Their speech pattern is rapid and excessive and they are easily distracted. Manic clients may engage in impulsive acts that are dangerous or socially inappropriate, such as driving erratically or engaging in spending sprees or promiscuous behavior. Some clients are irritable, restless, and experience decreased sleep and a change in appetite (Shoemaker, 2005; Spearing, 2007).

In the past 24 hours, Mr. Kiley appears to have been exhibiting manifestations of a manic episode. A mild to moderate level of mania (hypomania) may be associated with the ability to continue to function and be productive. Mr. Kiley appears to have been able to continue to function in his role as an auto mechanic. A fellow employee recounts, however, that Mr. Kiley exhibited an overabundance of energy today and was very talkative. Mr. Kiley experienced decreased sleep, and spent large sums of money on collectibles. The client also reports a change in his appetite. It is likely that this manic episode began days ago. Without proper treatment, hypomania can progress to severe mania or could switch to a state of depression (Spearing, 2007).

7. Discuss how Mr. Kiley's bipolar disorder contributed to his hypoglycemia. Mr. Kiley's bipolar disorder has complicated the self-management of his diabetes mellitus. The client's psychiatric illness was exacerbated when he discontinued his lithium. As a result, Mr. Kiley experienced a hypomanic episode. During this phase, it appears that he may have increased the frequency of his insulin administration and/or made an error in the insulin dosage. It is likely that he did not monitor his blood glucose levels on a regular schedule during his manic episode. In addition, the client has had a change in appetite and reports having skipped meals today. These are all common causes of hypoglycemia.

8. Mr. Kiley's sister told the nurse that the client usually maintains good control of his blood glucose. The client's hemoglobin A1C (HbA$_{1C}$) is 5%. What does an HbA$_{1C}$ value represent, and does the client's value indicate good control? The HbA$_{1C}$ laboratory test helps to determine the degree of long-term glucose control in a diabetic. The majority (97% to 98%) of a healthy adult's hemoglobin is hemoglobin A (HbA). About 4% to 6% of HbA consists of hemoglobin molecules that have been somewhat modified by the attachment of glucose onto the beta chain. This modified hemoglobin is called glycosylated hemoglobin. Higher blood glucose levels result in high levels of this glycosylated hemoglobin, also called hemoglobin A1C or HbA$_{1C}$. The HbA$_{1C}$ represents, in a percentage, the client's average blood glucose during the previous three months. High levels indicate inadequate diabetic control. The normal range in a nondiabetic is 3.5% to 6%. In the diabetic client, the goal is to maintain optimal long-term glucose control as expressed by an HbA$_{1C}$ below 7%. Mr. Kiley's HbA$_{1C}$ of 5% indicates good control of his blood glucose levels during the past three months (Chernecky & Berger, 2004; Daniels, 2002; Fain, 2005).

9. Help the nurse identify three priority nursing diagnoses to include in Mr. Kiley's plan of care. Priority nursing diagnoses for Mr. Kiley's plan of care include:

- Disturbed thought processes related to (r/t) insufficient blood glucose to the brain and inaccurate interpretations of environment (mania)
- Hypothermia r/t hypoglycemia
- Imbalanced nutrition: Less than body requirements r/t imbalance of glucose and insulin level

- Disturbed sleep pattern r/t mania and hyperagitated state
- Self-care deficit (feeding) r/t cognitive impairment (mania) and impaired perception
- Ineffective health maintenance r/t deficient knowledge regarding disease process and self-care
- Noncompliance r/t complexity of therapeutic regimen and denial of illness
- Ineffective coping r/t situational crisis

(Ackley & Ladwig, 2006).

10. The ICU nurse notices that the skin around the IV access site on Mr. Kiley's left hand is inflamed and warm. What is the most appropriate nursing intervention? The client has phlebitis at the site of the D50 administration. The IV cannula should be removed, and a warm compress applied to help decrease the swelling. Early recognition of phlebitis, no longer administering medications through the IV access, and removing the access from the client's hand is essential to help prevent further damage to the site and possible extravasation. Extravasation occurs when a medication escapes into the subcutaneous tissue and causes tissue damage (McLeod, 2006).

11. Although his fellow employees were trying to help Mr. Kiley, why was their attempt to give him juice an inappropriate intervention? Mr. Kiley had a decreased level of consciousness and was unable to swallow the juice. In a client that is in a stupor, unable to swallow, or unconscious, liquids should not be given because of the risk of aspiration (inhalation of fluids into the respiratory tract).

12. Briefly discuss how Mr. Kiley's bipolar disorder has had an impact on his sister's life and identify a nursing diagnosis that acknowledges the challenges of her role as a caregiver. Like many serious and chronic illnesses, having a family member with bipolar disorder is difficult for spouses, children, and siblings. Mr. Kiley's sister has taken on the role of caregiver. Mr. Kiley lives with his sister, and she has accepted responsibility for monitoring the client and assessing for changes in behavior that could indicate a need for intervention. Family members of a client with bipolar disorder must cope with unpredictable changes in the client's behavior and potentially dangerous situations that can be life threatening for the client (or others). The client's family may often feel responsible for resolving the consequences of the client's behavior (e.g., financial). A nursing diagnosis that acknowledges the challenges inherent in the role of caregiver is risk for caregiver role strain related to unpredictability of condition and mood swings (Ackley & Ladwig, 2006).

References

Ackley, B., & Ladwig, G. (2006). *Nursing diagnosis handbook: A guide to planning care*. St. Louis, MO: Mosby.

Centers for Disease Control and Prevention (CDC). (2006). Hypothermia-related deaths: United States, 1999–2002 and 2005. *Morbidity and Mortality Weekly Report, 55* (10), 282–284. Retrieved January 27, 2007, from www.cdc.gov.

Chernecky, C., & Berger, B. (2004). *Laboratory tests and diagnostic procedures*. Philadelphia, PA: Elsevier.

Daniels, R. (2002). *Delmar's guide to laboratory tests and diagnostic tests*. Albany, NY: Delmar.

Deglin, J. H., & Vallerand, A. H. (2007). *Davis's drug guide for nurses*. Philadelphia, PA: F. A. Davis.

Fain, J. A. (2005). Management of clients with diabetes mellitus. In J. Black & J. Hawks (Eds.), *Medical-surgical nursing: Clinical management for positive outcomes* (pp. 1243–1288). St. Louis, MO: Elsevier.

McLeod, M. E. (2006). Interventions for clients with diabetes mellitus. In D. Ignatavicius & L. Workman (Eds.), *Medical-surgical nursing: Critical thinking for collaborative care* (pp. 1539–1542). St. Louis, MO: Elsevier Saunders.

Shoemaker, N. (2005). Clients with psychosocial and mental health concerns. In J. Black & J. Hawks (Eds.), *Medical-surgical nursing: Clinical management for positive outcomes* (pp. 530–535). St. Louis, MO: Elsevier.

Spearing, M. (2007). *Bipolar disorder*. Retrieved January 27, 2007, from www.nimh. nih.gov.

Ulchaker, M. M. (2007). Diabetes mellitus and hypoglycemia. In F. Monahan, J. Sands, M. Neighbors, J. Marek, & C. Green (Eds.), *Phipps' Medical-surgical nursing: Health and illness perspectives* (pp. 1135–1136). St. Louis, MO: Mosby Elsevier.

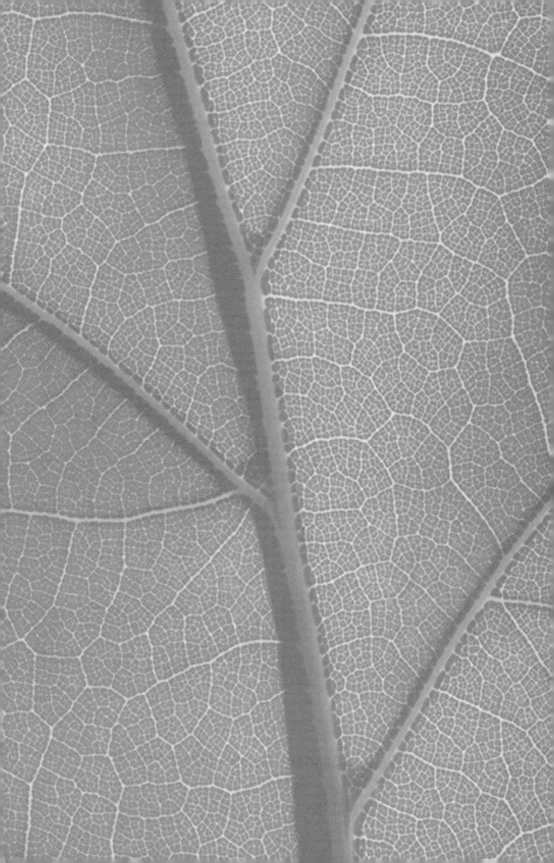

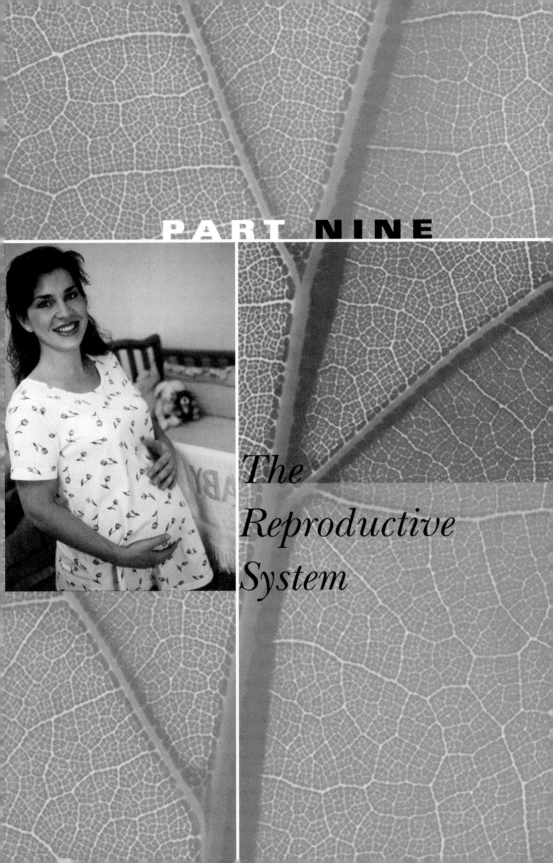

PART NINE

The Reproductive System

CASE STUDY 1

Ms. Swan

GENDER

Female

AGE

19

SETTING

- Walk-in Health Care Center

ETHNICITY

- Black American

CULTURAL CONSIDERATIONS

PREEXISTING CONDITIONS

- Sexually active since age 15
- Seven male sex partners in lifetime

COEXISTING CONDITION

COMMUNICATION

DISABILITY

SOCIOECONOMIC

- Student
- Covered under mother's health insurance

SPIRITUAL/RELIGIOUS

PHARMACOLOGIC

- Valacyclovir hydrochloride (Valtrex)

LEGAL

- Sexually transmitted disease (STD) reporting to the national Centers for Disease Control and Prevention (CDC)

ETHICAL

- Partner notification

ALTERNATIVE THERAPY

- Herpevac Trail for Women

PRIORITIZATION

- Client education regarding spread of sexually transmitted diseases

DELEGATION

- Urine testing by trained ancillary personnel

THE REPRODUCTIVE SYSTEM

Level of Difficulty: Easy

Overview: The client has contracted an STD. The nurse assists the health care provider (HCP) to determine the client's diagnosis and rule out other coexisting conditions. The client's risk factors for contracting an STD and lifestyle considerations to help prevent the spread of an STD are reviewed. The psychological impact of being diagnosed with an STD is acknowledged. The nurse provides the client with teaching regarding a newly prescribed medication and the need for additional pharmacologic treatment in the future. Nursing diagnoses appropriate for this client are prioritized. Finally, the HCP's responsibility for reporting the client's case to the health department for national CDC reporting is discussed.

Client Profile

Ms. Swan is a 19-year-old female who presents to the community walk-in health care center. She explains to the nurse, "I think I have a very bad urine infection. It burns really, really, bad when I go to the bathroom. I haven't looked down there, but it must be very raw because it hurts when I wipe and it is very itchy. The burning and itching have been bothering me for about a week now. On a couple of nights, I was burning up with a fever. I had chills and my whole body ached. I just feel awful. My mom's doctor is closed today so I came here. My friend said she had a urine infection once and that you could give me antibiotics or something to get rid of it." The client's vital signs are blood pressure 116/54, pulse 76, respiratory rate 18, and temperature 99.4°F (37.4°C). Ms. Swan states that the first day of her last menstrual period was "about a month ago. I can't remember the exact date, but I am due to get it any day now." She denies a sore throat, abdominal pain, and has not noticed any abnormal vaginal discharge.

Case Study

Further nursing assessment reveals that Ms. Swan has been sexually active since the age of 15 years and has had seven male partners. She recently ended a relationship. Her last sexual intercourse was three weeks ago. When the nurse asks if Ms. Swan uses condoms, she replies, "Sure. Most of the time." She denies having had an STD in the past and does not take an oral contraceptive or use another form of birth control. The nurse learns that this will be Ms. Swan's first gynecologic examination. Ms. Swan explains, "My mother brought me to her doctor once before but I was too nervous and scared to have the exam. I cried so much, that the doctor couldn't do it. I never went back." The nurse explains that the HCP's examination will likely involve the use of a speculum and reassures the client that she will be in the room to hold her hand and provide support throughout the examination. The nurse asks the client to provide a urine sample prior to undressing. The nurse provides the client with a sterile urine container labeled with the client's name and explains how to collect a clean-catch specimen. The client states an understanding of the instructions and an ability to control her stream of urine to collect a midstream specimen. The nurse escorts the client to the bathroom, shows Ms. Swan where to leave the urine specimen when she has finished, and provides her with privacy.

Questions

1. The nurse has instructed Ms. Swan to collect a clean-catch urine specimen. Help Ms. Swan recall the steps in the proper order.

— Wash hands.

— Wash hands.

— Use the thumb and forefinger to separate the labia.

— Wipe with toilet paper.

— Sit with legs separated on the toilet.

— Place the sterile lid onto the container and close tightly. Clean and dry the outside of the container with a towelette.

— With the labia separated, use a downward stroke (from the top of the labia toward the rectal area), and cleanse one side of the labia with a towelette. Discard the towelette and repeat the procedure on the other side of the labia with another towelette, keeping the labia separated at all times. With the third towelette, use a downward stroke from the top of the urethral opening to the bottom and discard.

— Open the specimen collection kit and/or three antiseptic towelettes and place on a firm surface.

— Begin to urinate in the toilet. After the stream starts with a good flow, place the collection cup under the stream of urine. Avoid touching the skin with the container. Fill the container half to three-quarters full with urine (30 to 60 cc) and remove the container before urination ends.

— Leave the specimen for the nurse as instructed.

— Open the sterile container, placing the lid with the sterile side up on a firm surface.

2. Why has the nurse requested that Ms. Swan collect a clean-catch urine specimen prior to being seen by the HCP? Briefly explain which urine tests the nurse anticipates the HCP will request. Which of these tests can be processed by the nurse (or trained ancillary personnel, such as a certified nursing assistant) for immediate results? Which tests must be sent to a laboratory for processing? Can all of the tests be processed directly from the clean-catch specimen in the sterile container?

3. Upon visual examination of Ms. Swan's genital area, the HCP diagnoses Ms. Swan with genital herpes. Describe what the HCP observed during the examination. What test can be performed to confirm the diagnosis?

4. Provide an explanation for the clinical manifestations that Ms. Swan assumed were indicative of a urinary tract infection.

5. Ms. Swan comments, "I can't believe my last boyfriend had this and didn't tell me. How could he have sex with me knowing I would catch it too?" Did the client contract the herpes virus in her most recent sexual relationship? Discuss your answer.

6. During the gynecologic examination, the HCP collects a vaginal and endocervical swab culture to test for gonorrhea and Chlamydia. Briefly describe what bacteria cause these two diseases and the clinical manifestations of each in women.

7. The HCP prescribes 1 g of valacyclovir hydrochloride (Valtrex) by mouth twice a day for seven days. Provide the client with teaching regarding the medication's mechanism of action, how long to take the medication, and the common adverse effects she may experience.

Questions (continued)

8. What should the nurse tell Ms. Swan regarding sexual activity, hygiene, and the use of feminine hygiene products while she is being treated for genital herpes?

9. Ms. Swan comments, "I am so ashamed. Is this something that a future boyfriend could catch?" How should the nurse respond?

10. Discuss why Ms. Swan should be offered testing for the human immuno-deficiency virus (HIV) while she is at the health center.

11. Identify the factors and lifestyle choices that have placed Ms. Swan at increased risk for contracting herpes simplex virus (HSV).

Ms. Swan's urine dipstick and pregnancy test are negative. The nurse provides Ms. Swan with literature about STDs and methods of birth control. A follow-up appointment is scheduled for one week to see how Ms. Swan is feeling and to discuss the results of her HIV test. The gonorrhea and Chlamydia cultures will be back within 48 to 72 hours, and the nurse will call Ms. Swan if the results are positive so that she can be seen earlier for treatment. The nurse suggests that Ms. Swan read the educational materials prior to her next visit and write down any questions she has, to be answered at the next appointment. The nurse also provides Ms. Swan with a list of HCPs in the area. The nurse reassures Ms. Swan that she can always seek care in the community walk-in center. However, the nurse encourages her to speak with her mother and make an appointment with one of the HCPs on the list, or perhaps return to her mother's HCP if she feels comfortable, in order to establish a relationship with a primary HCP.

12. Prioritize five nursing diagnoses for Ms. Swan.

Ms. Swan returns to the community health center the following week. The results of her HIV test and gonorrhea and Chlamydia cultures are negative. The client's herpes blisters are healing, and she has been taking her medication as prescribed with no adverse effects. Ms. Swan states she feels much better and is relieved her other tests are negative. "It has been a hard week worrying that I could be HIV positive. I guess I have been pretty stupid. You never think something like this will happen to you." Ms. Swan has reviewed the educational materials the nurse gave her and informs the nurse that she has scheduled an appointment with a new HCP to discuss starting on a birth control pill.

13. Ms. Swan asks "How long before I am cured?" What should the nurse tell her?

14. The HCP gives Ms. Swan a prescription for valacyclovir hydrochloride to fill the next time she has an outbreak. How often should Ms. Swan anticipate having outbreaks? What information should the nurse provide regarding the clinical manifestations Ms. Swan should monitor to detect an outbreak, possible triggers, and when to start taking her valacyclovir hydrochloride.

15. Ms. Swan comments to the nurse, "I was reading online that herpes is very common, especially in people my age. It's too bad there isn't a shot we could all get to prevent spreading it." What news can the nurse share about current research regarding a herpes vaccine?

16. Does the HCP need to report Ms. Swan's genital herpes diagnosis to the national CDC? If the client's HIV, gonorrhea, or Chlamydia results had been positive, would those need to be reported?

Questions and Suggested Answers

1. The nurse has instructed Ms. Swan to collect a clean-catch urine specimen. Help Ms. Swan recall the steps in the proper order.

<u>1</u> Wash hands.

<u>10</u> Wash hands.

<u>5</u> Use the thumb and forefinger to separate the labia.

<u>8</u> Wipe with toilet paper.

<u>4</u> Sit with legs separated on the toilet.

<u>9</u> Place the sterile lid onto the container and close tightly. Clean and dry the outside of the container with a towelette.

<u>6</u> With the labia separated, use a downward stroke (from the top of the labia toward the rectal area), and cleanse one side of the labia with a towelette. Discard the towelette and repeat the procedure on the other side of the labia with another towelette, keeping the labia separated at all times. With the third towelette, use a downward stroke from the top of the urethral opening to the bottom and discard.

<u>2</u> Open the specimen collection kit and/or three antiseptic towelettes and place on a firm surface.

<u>7</u> Begin to urinate in the toilet. After the stream starts with a good flow, place the collection cup under the stream of urine. Avoid touching the skin with the container. Fill the container half to three quarters full with urine (30 to 60 cc) and remove the container before urination ends.

<u>11</u> Leave the specimen for the nurse as instructed.

<u>3</u> Open the sterile container, placing the lid with the sterile side up on a firm surface.

(Bouska Lee & Altman, 2004)

2. Why has the nurse requested that Ms. Swan collect a clean-catch urine specimen prior to being seen by the HCP? Briefly explain which urine tests the nurse anticipates the HCP will request. Which of these tests can be processed by the nurse (or trained ancillary personnel, such as a certified nursing assistant) for immediate results? Which tests must be sent to a laboratory for processing? Can all of the tests be processed directly from the clean-catch specimen in the sterile container? Based on the client's presenting clinical manifestations, the nurse anticipates that the HCP will request a urine dipstick and possibly a urinalysis (UA) with culture and sensitivity (C&S) to rule out a urinary tract infection, and a urine pregnancy test. To minimize discomfort during the physical examination, the nurse suggests that Ms. Swan empty her bladder. In anticipation of the HCP requesting urine tests, the nurse asks Ms. Swan to collect a midstream clean-catch specimen when she uses the bathroom prior to being seen by

the HCP, since waiting until after her visit may result in the client being unable to provide a urine sample.

The nurse (or trained ancillary personnel, such as a certified nursing assistant) can perform the urine dipstick and urine pregnancy test in the health care center for immediate results. The manufacturer's instructions will indicate what the nurse (or ancillary personnel) is to observe to determine a positive or negative pregnancy test. The urine dipstick is a preliminary screening test that uses a reagent strip impregnated with chemicals that react with substances in the urine and change color when abnormalities are present. The nurse (or ancillary personnel) will pay particular attention to the pH of the urine. A pH value above 7 indicates alkaline urine and possible urinary tract infection. Positive leukocyte esterase, nitrites, and blood should be noted, since these results are also indicative of a urinary tract infection. The nurse should assess the urine for an abnormal color, cloudy appearance, and/or foul odor, which suggest an infection. Results of the urine dipstick are reported to the HCP before the client is seen to provide data to help make an accurate diagnosis. If the dipstick is positive for an infection, the UA and C&S are sent to a laboratory for more thorough microscopic processing. A urine culture and sensitivity identifies the bacterium that has caused the infection and helps determine to which antibiotic the bacterium is most sensitive. If the urine specimen will not arrive in the laboratory within 30 minutes, it can be refrigerated for up to four hours (Anunciado, 2004; Daniels, 2002).

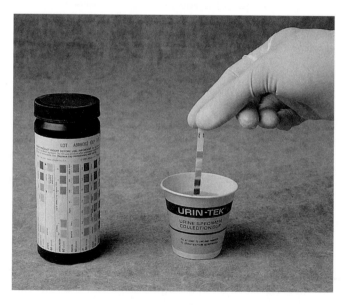

Urine dipstick

The nurse should pour a small sample of the urine collected in the sterile specimen container into a clean container (or second sterile container) to be used to conduct the dipstick and pregnancy test. Separating the sample maintains the integrity of the clean-catch specimen for processing the urinalysis and culture and sensitivity, by preventing contamination of the sample with microorganisms from the dipstick reagent strip and/or pipette collection device used to obtain a sample for the pregnancy test.

3. Upon visual examination of Ms. Swan's genital area, the HCP diagnoses Ms. Swan with genital herpes. Describe what the HCP observed during the examination. What test can be performed to confirm the diagnosis? Women with genital herpes present with one or more lesions on or around the genital area, thighs, buttocks, and/or rectum that appear as vesicles (or blisters). Lesions also may be visualized on the cervix. The lesions begin as small red raised sores that develop into blisters. When the blisters break, painful open ulcers remain. The sores develop a crust and then heal without leaving a scar. The HCP also may have observed that the skin of the perineal area is reddened and irritated. During a primary infection (the first outbreak of herpes simplex virus), the lesions will become worse in the first 10 to 15 days and then crust over and heal (Warshaw, 2007).

Genital herpes is an STD caused by either HSV type 1 (HSV-1) or type 2 (HSV-2). Most cases of genital herpes are caused by HSV-2, whereas HSV-1 usually causes cold sores, which some call "fever blisters." However, since oral-genital transmission is possible, HSV-1 may affect the genital area, and HSV-2 may produce a sore in the area of the mouth. A culture confirms the viral infection. The herpes lesion(s) is/are swabbed and processed in a laboratory to confirm growth of the HSV. A blood test cannot show if a client is having an outbreak, but can reveal if the client is infected with HSV. Type-specific blood tests are also available to identify if the client has HSV-1 or HSV-2. In Ms. Swan's case, the HCP will likely swab the affected area to obtain a culture sample to confirm HSV infection (Centers for Disease Control and Prevention, 2004; National Institutes of Health, 2005).

4. Provide an explanation for the clinical manifestations that Ms. Swan assumed were indicative of a urinary tract infection. The primary infection (or initial outbreak) of genital herpes is the first infection a client experiences, and often is the most severe. While some individuals are asymptomatic during their primary infection, many experience significant disease characterized by several days of feeling ill, during or after which they have itching, burning, dysuria, and/or nonspecific vaginal or urethral discomfort soon followed by the appearance of genital lesions (blisters or sores). There is dull perineal pain, and the perineal tissue feels irritated or raw. Many women complain of "yeast infection" symptoms. Other clinical manifestations include local inflammation, swollen glands, back pain, a stiff neck, generalized signs of infection such as photophobia, headache, and flulike symptoms of chills, fever, muscle aches, and malaise. Some women have a vaginal discharge and may complain of a feeling of pressure in their lower abdomen. Women tend to have more severe clinical manifestations with the primary infection than do men (Division of STD Prevention, CDC, 2005; Massachusetts Department of Public Health, 2007; Warshaw, 2007).

5. Ms. Swan comments, "I can't believe my last boyfriend had this and didn't tell me. How could he have sex with me knowing I would catch it too?" Did the client contract the herpes virus in her most recent sexual relationship? Discuss your answer. It is not possible to determine with certainty if Ms. Swan contracted the herpes virus during her most recent sexual relationship. The symptoms of a primary infection (initial outbreak) usually occur within two weeks of sexual contact with an infected person. However, it is possible for a person to carry the virus without knowing they have it. Since up to 80% of individuals infected with HSV-2 are not aware they have it, it is possible that Ms. Swan unknowingly transmitted the infection to her partner. The client may have contracted the virus from any of her previous sexual partners, perhaps even several years ago. HSV can remain inactive for long periods before it causes symptoms (Division of STD Prevention, CDC, 2005; Warshaw, 2007).

6. During the gynecologic examination, the HCP collects a vaginal and endocervical swab culture to test for gonorrhea and Chlamydia. Briefly describe what bacteria cause these two diseases and the clinical manifestations of each in women. Gonorrhea and Chlamydia are highly contagious STDs. *Gonorrhea* is caused by the bacterium *Neisseria gonorrhoeae*. The infection can be present without noticeable signs. The clinical manifestation of gonorrhea in women often begins as an asymptomatic inflammation of the cervix (cervicitis). Some women are diagnosed when they seek treatment for painful urination, frequency, vaginal bleeding with intercourse, an abnormal (bloody or yellow) vaginal discharge, and/or vague complaint of pelvic or abdominal discomfort. However, many women are not treated until the gonorrhea is diagnosed through screening or after a partner has symptoms and is diagnosed. *Chlamydia* is a disease caused by the *Chlamydia trachomatis* bacterium. It is the most frequently reported bacterial STD in the United States (CDC, 2004). The majority of women (75%) are asymptomatic. Women who are symptomatic have cervicitis, pelvic inflammatory disease (PID), and report increased vaginal discharge or bleeding, burning during urination, irritation of the area around the vagina, vaginal bleeding with intercourse, and lower abdominal pain. Early treatment with antibiotics is essential since untreated STDs can result in devastating complications for women, including PID, infertility, sterility, increased susceptibility to other diseases, and fetal deformities and complications during pregnancy (Ehrlich & Schroeder, 2005; Warshaw, 2007).

7. **The HCP prescribes 1 g of valacyclovir hydrochloride (Valtrex) by mouth twice a day for seven days. Provide the client with teaching regarding the medication's mechanism of action, how long to take the medication, and the common adverse effects she may experience.** Valacyclovir hydrochloride is an antiviral medication that is converted to acyclovir. Acyclovir acts by inhibiting the replication of viral DNA. By inhibiting viral replication, antiviral medication eases the symptoms of HSV, decreases viral shedding, reduces the time it takes for the lesions to heal, and helps to suppress future outbreaks. Ms. Swan should fill the prescription that day and begin taking the medication as soon as possible. She should finish all of the medication prescribed even if she begins to feel better or notices that the lesions are healing. Common adverse effects include headache, nausea, dizziness, constipation, and diarrhea (Deglin & Vallerand, 2007; NIH, 2005; Spratto & Woods, 2006).

In the future, Ms. Swan may be prescribed daily valacyclovir hydrochloride if she has frequent (more than six) outbreaks per year. Daily suppressive therapy with valacyclovir hydrochloride has been shown to reduce the risk of transmission of genital herpes. Antiviral medication, especially when combined with the use of condoms, can decrease the risk of passing herpes to uninfected sexual partners (NIH, 2005; Spratto & Woods, 2006).

8. **What should the nurse tell Ms. Swan regarding sexual activity, hygiene, and the use of feminine hygiene products while she is being treated for genital herpes?** Ms. Swan should abstain from sexual activity until the lesions are completely healed. Her risk of transmitting HSV to a partner is greatest during an outbreak, and sexual activity prolongs the time it takes the lesions to heal. She should wipe from front to back and wash her hands well after voiding, touching the affected area, and handling feminine napkins or tampons. She should try not to touch the lesions and keep the affected area clean and dry. Although HSV is not likely to be transmitted to others from a bath towel, the client should use her own bath towel as a precaution, and prevent spreading the active disease to other parts of her body by drying her genital area last. Her laundry does not need to be done separately from the rest of the family's. Douching at any time is not advised since this disturbs the natural vaginal and cervical environments and can predispose women to infection. Ms. Swan should be instructed to wear cotton underwear (instead of nylon or silk), and avoid wearing pantyhose because these garments trap moisture and prevent circulation of air to the genitalia. Unless a topical ointment or cream has been prescribed as treatment, lotions and creams should not be applied to the affected area (Warshaw, 2007).

9.   Ms. Swan comments, "I am so ashamed. Is this something that a future boyfriend could catch?" How should the nurse respond? Ms. Swan's expression of shame and grief upon learning that she has contracted an STD is understandable. As with other STDs, there is a negative stigma attached to genital herpes. The physical consequences of the HSV infection are often far outweighed by the emotional consequences the diagnosis evokes. Many who are infected with an STD, especially a lifelong disease such as herpes, experience psychological distress. Clients often feel betrayal, anger, guilt, and fear of rejection. The nurse should provide support and reassurance that genital herpes is a common virus with outbreaks that are treatable. Millions of Americans (more than 45 million), age 12 and older have genital herpes, with approximately a million new cases diagnosed each year. Genital herpes is more common than diseases such as diabetes and asthma. The virus, particularly HSV-2, is more common in women (one out of four) than men (one out of five). Anyone who is sexually active, even with just one person and only one time can get genital herpes. HSV is spread through close skin-to-skin contact and through the many forms of sexual contact. HSV is more easily transmitted from men to women. The virus can be transmitted through vaginal or anal intercourse, oral-genital or oral-anal contact, kissing, and when using sexual toys. Herpes is most contagious when a person has open sores, but the disease is often transmitted in the absence of recognizable symptoms. HSV is rarely spread by contact with objects such as a toilet seat or in a hot tub. In the future, before a relationship becomes sexual, the client should speak honestly with her partner about the virus since it can be transmitted through sexual contact, and it is both partners' responsibility to use safe sexual practices every time they engage in sexual contact. When Ms. Swan experiences an outbreak, she should refrain from sexual activity of any kind to decrease the risk of transmitting the herpes virus to her partner. The nurse should reinforce that while condoms are the recommended method of protection secondary to abstinence, condoms offer no guarantee against passing on or acquiring any STD since a condom cannot cover all infected areas (CDC, 2004; Division of STD Prevention, CDC, 2005; NIH, 2005; Warshaw, 2007).

10. Discuss why Ms. Swan should be offered testing for the HIV while she is at the health center. A client diagnosed with a primary infection of herpes should be screened for other STDs and for HIV. Clients infected with the HSV-2 are at increased risk of HIV since genital herpes causes open sores through which the HIV may pass. Ms. Swan has had multiple sex partners and inconsistent use of condoms. Her risk factors are significant, and an HIV test is recommended (Massachusetts Department of Public Health, 2007).

11. Identify the factors and lifestyle choices that have placed Ms. Swan at increased risk for contracting HSV. It is estimated that approximately 19 million new cases of an STD occur in the United States each year. Almost half of these cases are among individuals between the ages of 15 and 24 years (CDC, 2004). In Ms. Swan's case, the following factors and lifestyle choices have increased her risk of contracting HSV:

- The client is female. Herpes is more common in women (infecting approximately one of four) than in men (one of five).
- She is a black American. Black Americans are more likely to test positive for HSV-2. Caucasians, however, have a higher incidence of experiencing active genital symptoms. Over the past few years, the greatest increase in HSV-2 has been noted in Caucasian adolescents.
- She is 19 years old. Since the late 1970s, the number of people with genital herpes has increased 30% nationwide. The largest increase has been among teens and young adults.
- She engaged in early sexual activity. Anyone who is sexually active is at risk for HSV infection. In one study, nearly 22% of Americans over the age of 12 years were infected with HSV-2.
- She has had multiple sex partners. The risk of HSV infection increases with the number of sexual partners.
- There is a normal developmental tendency for risk-taking behaviors among 15 to 24-year-olds.
- She reports inconsistent use of barrier contraceptive methods that offer some protection against STDs. Women have an 80% to 90% chance of contracting HSV-2 after unprotected sexual activity with an infected partner.
- She has deficient knowledge regarding the transmission of STDs.
- She has deficient knowledge regarding the symptoms of an STD.
- She does not have a primary HCP, routine gynecologic care, or have routine screening for STDs.

(CDC, 2004; NIH, 2005; Warshaw, 2007).

12. Prioritize five nursing diagnoses for Ms. Swan. Priority nursing diagnoses for Ms. Swan include:

1. Acute pain related to (r/t) active herpes lesions
2. Risk for infection r/t transmission of STD to partners
3. Impaired tissue integrity r/t active herpes lesions
4. Impaired urinary elimination r/t pain with urination
5. Ineffective health maintenance r/t deficient knowledge regarding diagnosis, treatment, and preventing the spread of disease
6. Situational low self-esteem r/t expressions of shame or guilt

(Ackley & Ladwig, 2006).

13. Ms. Swan asks "How long before I am cured?" What should the nurse tell her? There is no cure for HSV. She will have the disease in her body for the rest of her life. With regard to her current outbreak, the lesions should heal in about three to four weeks. This outbreak has run its course when all of the lesions are completely healed, there are no scabs present, and new skin has formed where the lesions were located (Division of STD Prevention, CDC, 2005; Warshaw, 2007).

14. The HCP gives Ms. Swan a prescription for valacyclovir hydrochloride to fill the next time she has an outbreak. How often should Ms. Swan anticipate having outbreaks? What information should the nurse provide regarding the clinical manifestations Ms. Swan should monitor to detect an outbreak, possible triggers, and when to start taking her valacyclovir hydrochloride? Symptoms of herpes are called "outbreaks." Herpes is a lifelong disease marked by unpredictable recurrent outbreaks. When the virus is no longer active, it remains in an inactive state within the nerves of the spinal column. Many clients experience a recurrence of symptoms in the weeks or months following their initial outbreak. This second outbreak is often less severe and shorter than the initial outbreak. HSV-2 genital infections are more likely to result in recurrences than HSV-1 genital infections. Some individuals experience monthly outbreaks, others have several outbreaks a year and still others have only one or two outbreaks in a lifetime. The severity of the outbreaks and number of outbreaks tend to decrease over a period of years. Individuals with weakened immune systems can experience frequent outbreaks that are severe and longer lasting. Ms. Swan should inspect her skin, genital area, and mouth for lesions and monitor for any vaginal discharge. Self-examination will help the client to recognize the signs and symptoms of a herpes outbreak and indications of other STDs. Outbreaks may be triggered by illness, stress, anxiety, depression, exposure to sunlight or cold temperatures (more so with HSV-1), poor nutrition, being overtired or fatigued, consumption of acidic foods, during menstruation, or by trauma to the area affected by lesions. Some outbreaks are signaled by a prodromal phase characterized by tingling and itching, vaginal discharge, and a burning feeling or pain in the genital or anal area. These symptoms may or may not be followed by a breakout of skin lesions, or the lesions may be small and easily overlooked. Ms. Swan should fill her prescription and begin taking the valacyclovir hydrochloride within a day of noting the reappearance of symptoms. The medication is most effective when started within 48 hours after the onset of symptoms. Individuals who experience six or more outbreaks per year are often prescribed daily suppressive medication. Sometimes the virus becomes active, but the client is asymptomatic. When this occurs, small amounts of the virus may be shed at or near the area of the primary outbreak. Clients are often

unaware of this asymptomatic shedding, but can still infect sexual partners during this time. The likelihood of recurrent episodes of asymptomatic shedding emphasizes the importance of consistent safe sex practices to prevent unknowingly transmitting the disease to another person. Ms. Swan should also inspect any sexual partner for signs of an STD before engaging in sexual intercourse (CDC, 2004; Division of STD Prevention, CDC, 2005; NIH, 2005; Spratto & Woods, 2007; Warshaw, 2006).

15. Ms. Swan comments to the nurse, "I was reading online that herpes is very common, especially in people my age. It's too bad there isn't a shot we could all get to prevent spreading it." What news can the nurse share about current research regarding a herpes vaccine? Several vaccines are currently in various stages of development and testing. The National Institute of Allergy and Infectious Diseases (NIAID) and GlaxoSmithKline are sponsoring a large clinical trial in women testing an experimental vaccine that may help prevent the transmission of genital herpes. The trial, called the "Herpevac Trail for Women," is being conducted in over 35 sites in the United States. The nurse can provide Ms. Swan with the Web site address where she can learn more (herpesvaccine.nih.gov) (NIH, 2005).

16. Does the HCP need to report Ms. Swan's genital herpes diagnosis to the national CDC? If the client's HIV, gonorrhea, or Chlamydia results had been positive, would those need to be reported? Cases of genital herpes are not reported nationally; whereas gonorrhea and Chlamydia are reportable STDs. Reporting the client's HIV status would depend upon the state.

In every state in the United States, syphilis, gonorrhea, Chlamydia, and acquired immunodeficiency syndrome (AIDS) are reportable to the CDC through local health department reporting methods. HIV infection and chancroid are reportable in many states. Genital herpes, trichomoniasis, and human papillomavirus (HPV) infection are not nationally reportable. It is important that nurses and HCPs are familiar with their local requirements for reporting STDs (Warshaw, 2007).

References

Ackley, B., & Ladwig, G. (2006). *Nursing diagnosis handbook: A guide to planning care.* St. Louis, MO: Mosby.

Anunciado, C. J. (2004). Diagnostic testing. In R. Daniels (Ed.), *Nursing fundamentals: Caring & clinical decision making* (p. 708). Clifton Park, NY: Delmar Learning.

Bouska Lee, C. A., & Altman, G. B. (2004). Collecting a clean-catch, midstream urine specimen. In G. B. Altman (Ed.), *Delmar's fundamental & advanced nursing skills* (pp. 99–105). Clifton Park, NY: Thomson Delmar Learning.

Centers for Disease Control and Prevention (CDC). (2004). *Genital herpes, CDC fact sheet.* Retrieved January 20, 2007 from www.cdc.gov.

Daniels, R. (2002). *Delmar's guide to laboratory and diagnostic tests*. Albany, NY: Delmar.

Deglin, J. H., & Vallerand, A.H. (2007). *Davis's drug guide for nurses* (pp. 1179–1180). Philadelphia, PA: F. A. Davis.

Division of STD Prevention, Centers for Disease Control and Prevention. (2005). *Genital herpes*. Retrieved January 20, 2007 from www.womanshealth.gov.

Ehrlich, A., & Schroeder, C. L. (2005). The reproductive systems. In *Medical terminology for health professions* (pp. 400–401). Clifton Park, NY: Thomson Delmar Learning.

Massachusetts Department of Public Health. (2007). *Public health fact sheet: Genital herpes (herpes simplex virus—HSV)*. Retrieved April 22, 2007 from www.mass.gov.

National Institutes of Health (NIH). (2005). *Genital herpes*. Retrieved January 20, 2007 from www.niaid.nih.gov.

Spratto, G. R., & Woods, A. L. (2006). *PDR nurse's drug handbook* (pp. 1446–1448). Clifton Park, NY: Thomson Delmar Learning.

Warshaw, M. K. (2007). Sexually transmitted diseases. In F. Monahan, J. Sands, M. Neighbors, J. Marek, & C. Green (Eds.), *Phipps' Medical-surgical nursing: Health and illness perspectives* (pp. 1780–1792). St. Louis, MO: Mosby Elsevier.

CASE STUDY 2

Mr. Benjamin

GENDER		**SOCIOECONOMIC**	
Male		**SPIRITUAL/RELIGIOUS**	
AGE			
70		**PHARMACOLOGIC**	
SETTING		■ Finasteride (Proscar)	
■ Primary Care		**LEGAL**	
ETHNICITY		■ Informed consent	
■ White American		**ETHICAL**	
CULTURAL CONSIDERATIONS			
		ALTERNATIVE THERAPY	
PREEXISTING CONDITION		■ Lycopene (Rhodopurpurin); serenoa repens (saw palmetto, dwarf palm)	
COEXISTING CONDITION		**PRIORITIZATION**	
		■ Monitoring for postoperative complications	
COMMUNICATION		**DELEGATION**	
DISABILITY			

THE REPRODUCTIVE SYSTEM

Level of Difficulty: Moderate

Overview: The client in this case presents to his primary health care provider (HCP) with vague complaints of a change in his urinary pattern. The nurse further evaluates the client's symptoms using a symptom questionnaire. Diagnostic tests useful in making a definitive diagnosis are reviewed. Pharmacologic treatment options and the nurse's responsibilities when surgical intervention is necessary are discussed. Priority nursing diagnoses for a postoperative transurethral resection of the prostate (TURP) client are identified. Alternative treatment options are considered.

Client Profile

Mr. Benjamin is a 70-year-old male who has scheduled an appointment with HCP. He explains to the nurse, "I came in because over the last few months I have noticed that every time I go to the bathroom I have to really strain to go. Even though I feel like my bladder is full, only a little comes out. The next thing I know I am back in the bathroom trying like heck to go again. It is like it's clogged up there or something." The nurse gives Mr. Benjamin a copy of The American Urological Association BPH Symptom Index Questionnaire to complete while he waits for the HCP to see him. The nurse explains that based on the problems that he has described, this questionnaire will provide the HCP with additional information to help determine what may be causing his symptoms.

Case Study

Mr. Benjamin's HCP reviews the completed BPH Symptom Index Questionnaire. Mr. Benjamin's score is 12 out of 35. Physical exam reveals that Mr. Benjamin has an enlarged prostate. The HCP would like him to have a few tests to help make a definitive diagnosis. The HCP prescribes a urinalysis and culture and sensitivity (U/A C&S), complete blood count (CBC), serum blood urea nitrogen (BUN) and creatinine (creat) levels, and a prostate-specific antigen (PSA). Mr. Benjamin is also scheduled to have a cystography and bladder ultrasound.

Questions

1. Briefly explain the function of the prostate.

2. Discuss benign prostatic hypertrophy (BPH). What anatomical changes in the prostate result in BPH, and what are the clinical manifestations that result from the pathophysiologic changes caused by BPH?

3. The following diagnostic tests were prescribed by Mr. Benjamin's HCP: (a) U/A C&S, (b) CBC, (c) BUN and creatinine, (d) PSA, (e) cystography, and (f) bladder ultrasound. Provide a brief rationale for each test.

4. Discuss three diagnostic tests not prescribed in this case that could also be used

to help rule out differential diagnoses and make a definitive diagnosis of BPH.

5. The nurse asked Mr. Benjamin to complete The American Urological Association BPH Symptom Index Questionnaire. What are the seven questions asked on this assessment tool and describe what the client's score indicates.

6. Mr. Benjamin's HCP tells Mr. Benjamin, "I am glad you came in to see me to evaluate your symptoms. BPH is a very common problem and treatment can help prevent complications." What are the potential complications of BPH?

7. Discuss finasteride as a preferred pharmacologic treatment option for the client

Questions (continued)

with BPH. How does this medication work, what are the limitations of its use, and what potential adverse effects should the client be educated about prior to initiating therapy? Can you identify two other medications that may be prescribed to treat BPH?

8. Mr. Benjamin asks his HCP, "Is there any herbal or natural remedies for this problem? I am not a fan of taking pills. For 70 years, I have managed to avoid having to take pills every day and don't like having to start now." What two alternative therapies might the HCP suggest?

9. Mr. Benjamin's symptoms continue despite treatment and he has had recurrent urinary tract infections. He is scheduled to have a TURP. What is accomplished by this procedure? Does this require the client's informed consent?

10. Following his TURP, Mr. Benjamin is admitted to a surgical nursing unit. He has a three-way urinary catheter inserted

for continuous bladder irrigation. What clinical manifestations should the nurse monitor that indicate postoperative complications?

11. Describe continuous bladder irrigation and its purpose. What will the nurse document to help the surgeon determine when this intervention can be discontinued?

12. Postoperatively, Mr. Benjamin has on sequential compression devices (SCDs). Provide the rationale for why SCDs have been prescribed.

13. Identify three priority nursing diagnoses that are appropriate to consider while caring for Mr. Benjamin following his TURP.

14. Mr. Benjamin expresses concern to his nurse stating, "I heard that after this procedure, sometimes things don't always work right down there." Provide Mr. Benjamin with an explanation of the potential erectile dysfunction he may experience.

Questions and Suggested Answers

1. **Briefly explain the function of the prostate.** The prostate is a walnut-sized gland that is located below the bladder and in front of the rectum, and surrounds the urethra. The urethra carries urine from the bladder to the penis. Reliant upon male hormone for growth and function, the gland produces ejaculatory fluid that supports the viability and motility of sperm and modifies the pH of the female vagina to help protect the sperm (American Urological Association, 2002; Warshaw, 2007).

2. **Discuss benign prostatic hypertrophy (BPH). What anatomical changes in the prostate result in BPH, and what are the clinical manifestations that result from the pathophysiologic changes caused by BPH?** Growth of the prostate is rapid during puberty and tapers around the age of 30. The prostate once again undergoes changes in size and firmness after age 50. It is during this later stage of growth that symptoms of BPH occur. Cell growth is stimulated by an increase in the hormones androgen and estrogen, and an

increase in the enzyme 5-alpha reductase, which further stimulates prostate growth. Benign prostatic hypertrophy (also called hyperplasia or BPH) is the benign enlargement of the prostate and a change in the consistency of the tissue within the prostate. Portions of the prostate may become large or nodular and other portions may atrophy. These changes most often affect the inner core (transitional zone) of the prostate, which surrounds the urethra. These changes can result in problems with urination and can compromise kidney function (Warshaw, 2007).

BPH, formerly known as prostatism, occurs in at least 50% of all men over the age of 60, in 75% of men over 70, and in 90% of men over 80 years of age. Men with a family history of BPH are at greater risk. Symptomatic BPH is most often experienced by men in their mid-60s and can occur in men as young as 30 years old, although not every man with an enlarged prostate will have symptoms. Enlargement of the prostate and changes in the consistency of the tissue within the transitional zone of the prostate impinge on the urethra and cause the urethra to elongate and compress. This results in an obstruction in the bladder outlet and impairs urinary flow. The flow of urine is weak, and the man must strain to empty his bladder. Over time, the bands of bladder muscles within the bladder wall hypertrophy (enlarge, thicken), and contouring of the bladder wall increases creating pockets for urinary retention. As the muscles thicken, the capacity of the bladder decreases, and the bladder is less compliant, resulting in a feeling of increased pressure as the bladder fills. A prolonged exposure to this increased pressure can lead to hydronephrosis and atrophy of the kidneys. As bladder muscle tone diminishes over time, the bladder is not able to empty completely with each void. This post void residual becomes alkaline and is an ideal medium for bacteria growth and infection. The urethral and bladder changes in a male with BPH, cause him to experience symptoms of obstruction and irritation. The client will often report a decrease in urinary stream with less force of the stream on urination and often dribbling at the end of voiding. He may also complain of hesitancy, a difficulty initiating a urine stream, and an intermittent flow or inability to maintain a constant urine stream. The client may express the feeling that he is not able to empty his bladder completely. Nocturia from incomplete emptying is a common symptom. Clients may express that their daily activities are compromised due to the need to be near a bathroom. Symptoms of a urinary tract infection (dysuria, urgency, and urge incontinence) are caused by a loss of muscle tone in the bladder, changes in the angle of the bladder neck, and incomplete bladder emptying, posing an increased risk of infection. Blood vessels enlarge as the prostate enlarges. When the client strains to urinate, these blood vessels can break and hematuria may be noted (AUA, 2002; Warshaw, 2007).

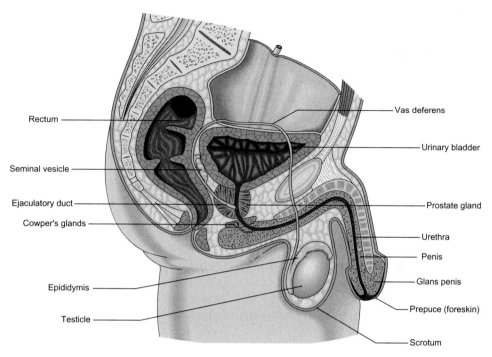

Rectum

Seminal vesicle

Ejaculatory duct

Cowper's glands

Epididymis

Testicle

Vas deferens

Urinary bladder

Prostate gland

Urethra

Penis

Glans penis

Prepuce (foreskin)

Scrotum

The male reproductive organs

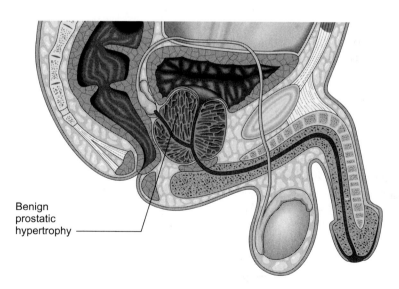

Benign
prostatic
hypertrophy

*Benign prostatic hypertrophy. The enlarged prostate presses against the bladder
and slows the flow of urine through the urethra*

3. The following diagnostic tests were prescribed by Mr. Benjamin's HCP: (a) U/A C&S, (b) CBC, (c) BUN and creatinine, (d) PSA, (e) cystography, and (f) bladder ultrasound. Provide a brief rationale for each test.

(a) A U/A C&S are used to screen for blood, detect the presence of proteinuria, and rule out a urinary tract infection (Daniels, 2002; Warshaw, 2007).

(b) A CBC is a blood test that consists of several tests that allow the HCP to evaluate different cellular components of the blood. The HCP will look to see if Mr. Benjamin's white blood cell (WBC) count is increased, which indicates infection. The HCP will also look for a decreased red blood cell (RBC) count, hemoglobin (Hgb), and hematocrit (Hct) to detect anemia (Daniels, 2002; Warshaw, 2007).

(c) Serum BUN and creatinine (creat) levels assess renal function. BUN and creatinine reflect the kidneys' ability to excrete the waste products of protein metabolism. Abnormal values indicate impaired kidney function (Daniels, 2002; Warshaw, 2007).

(d) A PSA test is a blood test to rule out prostate cancer. The PSA blood test is often evaluated annually in men 50 years and older, and may be used as an annual screening in men as young as 40 years old. It provides an estimate of the volume of the prostate gland. Two values are reported: the free PSA and the combined PSA, and then a total PSA score is obtained using these two values. The total PSA in a healthy male should be <1 ng/mL. An enlarged prostate will cause an elevated PSA. The percentage of free PSA helps to determine whether the elevated PSA is due to BPH or prostate cancer. A free PSA of 18% or greater is desirable since men with such values are more likely to have BPH than cancer (Charnow, 2006; Daniels, 2002; Warshaw, 2007).

(e) A cystography is an X-ray test of the lower urinary tract that instills contrast dye into the bladder via a catheter to assess the anatomy, integrity, and function of the bladder and urethra. This invasive procedure is used to assess for outflow obstruction, to measure the length of the urethra, and to visualize the extent of bladder involvement (Daniels, 2002; Warshaw, 2007).

(f) A bladder ultrasound is a noninvasive exam that uses ultrasound waves to examine the bladder's position, shape, and size. In the bladder of the client with BPH, contouring of the bladder wall (called trabeculation) leads to the development of pockets for urinary retention. This trabeculation and any post void residual can be visualized on an ultrasound (Daniels, 2002; Warshaw, 2007).

4. Discuss three diagnostic tests not prescribed in this case that could also be used to help rule out differential diagnoses and make

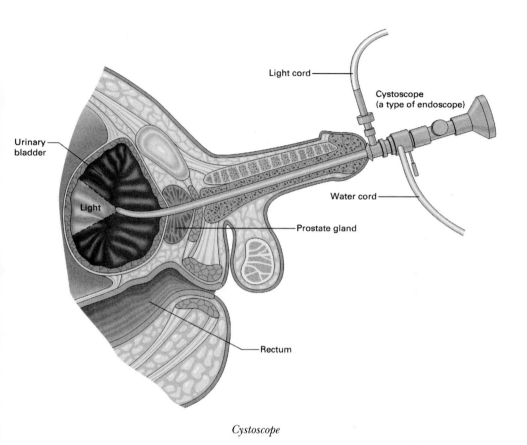

Cystoscope

a definitive diagnosis of BPH. A urinary catheter may be inserted to assess post void residual. This invasive assessment is less favorable than the noninvasive use of an uroflowmeter that evaluates bladder emptying, or a bladder ultrasound to estimate post void residuals. Urodynamics is a computerized test that measures bladder pressures and is helpful in diagnosing an obstruction and any bladder decompensation. Although not routinely prescribed for evaluating a suspected case of BPH, a male with complaints of hematuria usually will have an intravenous pyelogram (IVP) done. An IVP is performed to visualize the outline of the urinary tract and then assess the anatomy of the upper urinary tract by taking sequential X-rays. An IVP checks for calculi (stones) and evaluates the degree of bladder emptying (AUA, 2002; Daniels, 2002; Warshaw, 2007).

5. The nurse asked Mr. Benjamin to complete The American Urological Association BPH Symptom Index Questionnaire. What are the seven questions asked on this assessment tool and describe what the client's

score indicates. The American Urological Association BPH Symptom Index Questionnaire is used to determine the severity of a client's BPH. The seven questions follow.

Over the past month or so, how often have you:

1. had a sensation of not emptying your bladder completely after urinating?
2. had to urinate again less than two hours after you finished urinating?
3. stopped and started again several times when you urinate?
4. found it difficult to postpone urination?
5. had a weak urinary stream?
6. had to push or strain to begin urination?
7. over the last month, how many times did you usually get up to urinate from the time you went to bed at night until the time you got up in the morning?

For each of the seven symptom-related questions, the client's response is scored on a 5-point scale with 0 indicating a response of "never" to the question and 5 indicating the client "almost always" experiences the symptom. The sum of the seven scores results in a total score. A total symptom score of 0 to 7 indicates mild BPH. A score of 8 to 19 identifies the client with moderate BPH (as in Mr. Benjamin's case), and a score of 20 to 35 is found in clients with severe BPH (AUA, 2002; Warshaw, 2007).

6. Mr. Benjamin's HCP tells Mr. Benjamin, "I am glad you came in to see me to evaluate your symptoms. BPH is a very common problem and treatment can help prevent complications." What are the potential complications of BPH? Urinary retention can lead to recurrent urinary tract infections, pyelonephritis, and possibly sepsis. Complications of BPH also include kidney disorders caused by the pressure and backflow of urine. Men with severe blood loss or with renal insufficiency may become anemic (Warshaw, 2007).

7. Discuss finasteride as a preferred pharmacologic treatment option for the client with BPH. How does this medication work, what are the limitations of its use, and what potential adverse effects should the client be educated about prior to initiating therapy? Can you identify two other medications that may be prescribed to treat BPH? Medications can be prescribed to reduce the size of the prostate and/or relax the bladder neck and open the internal urethral sphincter to promote a more normal flow of urine. Finasteride inhibits the activity of 5-alpha-reductase so that this enzyme is unable to convert testosterone into dihydrotestosterone and subsequently begins to decrease the size of the prostate. The therapeutic effects of finasteride are most effective on very large prostates, but effects are often not seen for several months since it will take a considerable change in the size of the prostate to result in a noticeable decrease in the client's symptoms. In some clients, a decrease in symptoms is not achieved at all due to an inability of the finasteride to shrink the nodular growth in the transitional zone, which continues to compress the urethra and inhibit the flow of urine. Potential adverse effects of finasteride include a decreased libido, impotence, testicular pain, and ejaculation disorders. Finasteride can also interfere with an accurate evaluation of future PSA values while Mr. Benjamin is being treated for BPH since this medication lowers the PSA levels by 50% and can result in a false-negative PSA result, thus posing the risk of delayed recognition of prostate cancer (Spratto & Woods, 2006; Warshaw, 2006).

Other medications prescribed to decrease straining and relax bladder muscles include selective and nonselective alpha-blockers. These medications are effective because when alpha-receptors found in the bladder neck are stimulated, they help store urine. Therefore, by blocking these receptors, medications promote urination. Tamsulosin hydrochloride (Flomax) is particularly effective as a selective alpha-blocker for the bladder. This medication is a common choice of HCPs since it has fewer adverse effects than other alpha-blockers. Other medications that are somewhat less selective blockers, but may be prescribed include prazosin hydrochloride (Minipress), doxazosin mesylate (Cardura), and terazosin (Hytrin). The most common adverse effects of these medications are orthostatic (postural) hypotension and fatigue (Warshaw, 2007).

8. Mr. Benjamin asks his HCP, "Is there any herbal or natural remedies for this problem? I am not a fan of taking pills. For 70 years, I have managed to avoid having to take pills every day and don't like having to start now." What two alternative therapies might the HCP suggest? Some dietary supplements and herbs are reported to reduce the size of the prostate and provide relief of BPH symptoms. Two such alternative therapies are lycopene and saw palmetto. Naturally found in red tomatoes, watermelon, and pink grapefruit, giving these foods their color, lycopene is an antioxidant believed to help prevent or slow the growth rate of prostate, lung, and stomach cancer. The antioxidant effects of lycopene are thought to be at least twice as beneficial as beta-carotene, another carotenoid thought to be an effective cancer-preventing nutrient, because lycopene is not converted into vitamin A after eaten, which weakens the antioxidant properties. Lycopene is also available as a dietary supplement (American Cancer Society, 2005; Warshaw, 2007).

Saw palmetto is a low-growing palm tree found in the West Indies and in coastal regions of the southeastern United States. The berries of the tree are used in herbal remedies. There is evidence that saw palmetto relieves some of the symptoms of BPH, such as frequency, urgency, nocturia, and difficulty urinating. Its efficacy has been compared with that of finasteride but less effective that prazosin. Relief of symptoms appears to be provided by chemicals in the berries called sterols, which interfere with the ability of male hormones to promote prostate cell growth. Saw palmetto is not believed, however, to help prevent or treat prostate cancer. Saw palmetto is available as an herbal extract, tea, or in tablet/capsule form. If Mr. Benjamin chooses to take saw palmetto, his HCP should be aware since this herb can cause lower PSA values (ACS, 2005; Charnow, 2006; Deglin & Vallerand, 2007; Warshaw, 2007).

9. Mr. Benjamin's symptoms continue despite treatment, and he has had recurrent urinary tract infections. He is scheduled to have a TURP. What is accomplished by this procedure? Does this require the client's informed consent? Approximately 30% of men with symptomatic BPH will require surgical intervention. A TURP is a surgical procedure that removes the nodular gland tissue within the prostate but leaves the capsule of the prostate gland intact. Men who have a TURP are usually symptom free for at least eight years following surgery. Up to 15% of men will require retreatment for BPH in the future. Informed consent must be obtained from the client (Warshaw, 2007).

10. Following his TURP, Mr. Benjamin is admitted to a surgical nursing unit. He has a three-way urinary catheter inserted for continuous bladder irrigation. What clinical manifestations should the nurse monitor that indicate postoperative complications? Complications after a TURP include bleeding, infection, accidental displacement of the urinary catheter, stenosis of the urethra or bladder neck, and water intoxication and cerebral edema. Immediately following surgery, the nurse should monitor vital signs and urinary drainage closely. Frequent documentation of vital signs, urine output, urine color, and the presence of any blood clots in the urine is required. Persistent bladder discomfort, bladder spasms, failure of the catheter to drain properly, or bright red bleeding despite an increased rate of irrigation can be a sign of hemorrhage and clot retention within the bladder, displacement of the catheter, or that the bladder was perforated during surgery. These clinical manifestations warrant immediate medical attention and notification of the HCP. Another potential complication of the TURP procedure is water intoxication and cerebral edema. The bladder and urethra are continuously irrigated during a TURP. Because of this excessive irrigation being absorbed by the body, clients may develop water intoxication (also called transurethral resection syndrome or TUR syndrome). Cerebral edema can result, which is a medical emergency. The nurse should monitor Mr. Benjamin for signs of confusion and agitation, elevated blood pressure and respiratory rate, decreased pulse, and nausea and vomiting, which are signs of cerebral edema. Hyponatremia and other electrolyte imbalances may also be noted in the client with water intoxication. Any of these symptoms should be reported to the HCP immediately (Gray, 2005; Warshaw, 2007).

11. Describe continuous bladder irrigation and its purpose. What will the nurse document to help the surgeon determine when this intervention can be discontinued? After a TURP, if a significant amount of bleeding is anticipated, a large three-way catheter is inserted into the client's bladder. This large catheter helps to maintain urethral patency and allows clots to be removed from the bladder. Constant bladder irrigation prevents excessive clotting and the retention of blood clots in the bladder. An intravenous drip apparatus using an isotonic genitourinary irrigation solution attached to one of the three lumens of the catheter irrigates the bladder. The nurse should document the color of the urine that drains into the catheter collection bag as well as the clarity, and any debris noted. The color of the urine should change from bright red initially to pink and then to a normal amber (or straw) color. The nurse is responsible for regulating the flow rate of the irrigation solution. The surgeon may prescribe the rate of the irrigant or agency policy may dictate that the nurse regulate the flow based on the color and consistency of the urine output to maintain the urine light red to pink. If the urine is a dark red color, the flow of the irrigation solution should be increased. The nurse should not reduce the rate of irrigation without a prescription since premature reduction of the irrigation can predispose the client to the stasis of debris or blood, which can cause a blockage of the catheter. The client's intake and output is carefully documented. The catheter drainage bag should be emptied when it is three-quarters full to avoid interruption of urinary drainage. The volume of irrigation solution administered is subtracted from the amount of drainage output to

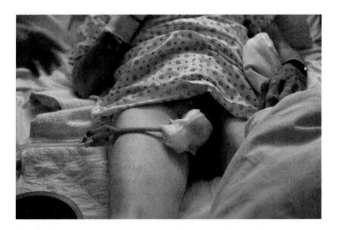

Three-way Foley catheter

determine the true urine output. The client's true urine output should be at least 50 mL per hour greater than the hourly flow of irrigation solution. A urinary output less than 50 mL/hour can indicate a possible obstruction. The surgeon will discontinue the bladder irrigation when there is progression of the urine color to within normal limits and when blood clots are no longer noted to be draining from the bladder. Discontinuing the irrigation is usually possible 24 to 48 hours after surgery (Altman, 2004; Gray, 2005; Warshaw, 2007).

12. Postoperatively, Mr. Benjamin has on SCDs. Provide the rationale for why SCDs have been prescribed. Venous thromboembolism (VTE) includes both thrombus and embolus complications. A thrombus (also called a thrombosis) is a blood clot that results from venous stasis, hypercoagulability, or endothelial injury. These three elements are referred to as Virchow's triad, and one or more element may cause a thrombosis. Surgery activates blood coagulation. Postoperative clients are at increased risk for a thrombus since they experience a change in their body's fibrinolytic activity, which varies with the extent of the surgery. Beginning 24 hours after surgery, a client's fibrinolytic activity decreases, and it is least active during the third postoperative day. The endothelial lining of a blood vessel is normally smooth. When there is injury to the endothelial lining, the lining becomes rough, causing platelet aggregation and adhesion as well as triggering clotting factors. Microtears in the lining of a blood vessel occur because of distension and venous stasis, as well as from direct trauma such as a surgical procedure. General anesthesia also contributes to the risk by decreasing vascular tone and disrupting the endothelial lining. This typically occurs when the patient is under general anesthesia for more than 30 minutes. During the TURP procedure, which may last over an hour, Mr. Benjamin was placed in the lithotomy position. This position places pressure on the popliteal space and blood vessels and presents the risk of thrombophlebitis and deep vein thrombosis (DVT). Intermittent pneumatic compression with SCDs, also called compression boots, apply intermittent external pressure to help prevent venous stasis, hypercoagulability, and endothelial injury (Blach & Ignatavicius, 2006; Maxwell-Thompson & Reid, 2007).

13. Identify three priority nursing diagnoses that are appropriate to consider while caring for Mr. Benjamin following his TURP. Priority nursing diagnoses that are appropriate for consideration in Mr. Benjamin's case include:

- Risk for injury related to (r/t) presence of urinary catheter, hematuria, and irrigation
- Acute pain r/t bladder spasms, incision, and irritation from catheter
- Risk for deficient fluid volume r/t fluid loss and possible bleeding
- Risk for excess fluid volume r/t surgical procedure (TUR syndrome)

- Risk for infection r/t invasive procedure (surgical removal of prostate gland) and route for bacteria entry (catheter)
- Risk for urinary retention r/t obstruction of urethra or catheter with blood clot

(Ackley & Ladwig, 2006; Gray, 2005; Warshaw, 2007)

14. Mr. Benjamin expresses concern to his nurse stating, "I heard that after this procedure, sometimes things don't always work right down there." Provide Mr. Benjamin with an explanation of the potential erectile dysfunction he may experience. If nerves are damaged during surgery, erectile dysfunction can result. This affects approximately 5% to 10% of men following a TURP. Clients experience retrograde (backward) ejaculation during which semen goes into the bladder when ejaculated and is then expelled with urination, causing cloudy urine. The client should be reassured that, while this will affect fertility potential, it is harmless and should not interfere with libido or erectile function (Gray, 2005).

References

Ackley, B., & Ladwig, G. (2006). *Nursing diagnosis handbook: A guide to planning care*. St. Louis, MO: Mosby.

Altman, G. (2004). *Delmar's fundamental & advanced nursing skills* (p. 804). Clifton Park, NY: Thomson Delmar Learning.

American Cancer Society (ACS). (2005). *Lycopene*. Retrieved August 22, 2006 from www.cancer.org.

American Urological Association (AUA). (2002). *Adult conditions: Prostate*. Retrieved August 22, 2006 from www.urologyhealth.org.

Blach, D. A., & Ignatavicius, D. D. (2006). Interventions for clients with vascular problems. In D. Ignatavicius & L. Workman (Eds.), *Medical-surgical nursing: Critical thinking for collaborative care* (pp. 812–816). St. Louis, MO: Elsevier.

Charnow, J. (2006). Understanding the facts about PSA testing. *Clinical Advisor*, 37–40.

Daniels, R. (2002). *Delmar's guide to laboratory and diagnostic tests*. Albany, NY: Delmar.

Deglin, J. H., & Vallerand, A. H. (2007). *Davis's drug guide for nurses*. Philadelphia, PA: F. A. Davis.

Gray, M. (2005). Management of men with reproductive disorders. In J. Black & J. Hawks (Eds.), *Medical-surgical nursing: Clinical management for positive outcomes* (pp. 1014–1027). St. Louis, MO: Elsevier.

Maxwell-Thompson, C. L., & Reid, K. B. (2007). Vascular problems. In F. Monahan, J. Sands, M. Neighbors, J. Marek, & C. Green (Eds.), *Phipps' Medical-surgical nursing: Health and illness perspectives* (pp. 885–892). St. Louis, MO: Mosby Elsevier.

Spratto, G. R., & Woods, A. L. (2006). *PDR nurse's drug handbook* (pp. 570–572). Clifton Park, NY: Thomson Delmar Learning.

Warshaw, M. K. (2007). Male reproductive problems. In F. Monahan, J. Sands, M. Neighbors, J. Marek, & C. Green (Eds.), *Phipps' Medical-surgical nursing: Health and illness perspectives* (pp. 1726–1734). St. Louis, MO: Mosby Elsevier.

CASE STUDY 3

Ms. Dalton

GENDER

Female

AGE

25

SETTING

- GYN primary care

ETHNICITY

- White American

CULTURAL CONSIDERATIONS

PREEXISTING CONDITION

- Gravida 0

COEXISTING CONDITION

COMMUNICATION

- Hard of hearing, reads lips

DISABILITY

SOCIOECONOMIC

- Employed as an accountant

SPIRITUAL/RELIGIOUS

PHARMACOLOGIC

- Current medications: Yasmin daily; multivitamin daily; acetaminophen as needed for headache
- Ethinyl estradiol 30 µg/drospirenone 3 mg (Yasmin 28-day); podofilox 0.5% (Condylox); imiquimod 5% (Aldara)

LEGAL

ETHICAL

ALTERNATIVE THERAPY

PRIORITIZATION

- Client education about transmission of sexually transmitted diseases (or illnesses) (also called STDs or STIs)

DELEGATION

THE REPRODUCTIVE SYSTEM

Level of Difficulty: Moderate

Overview: The client in this case has been diagnosed with cervical dysplasia and the human papillomavirus (HPV). Appropriate follow-up testing is reviewed. The potential health concerns for women and men with HPV are discussed. The role the new HPV vaccine will play in cancer prevention is acknowledged.

Client Profile

Ms. Dalton is a 25-year-old single female recently seen by her gynecologist for a routine annual exam. Her first sexual encounter was at age 14. She has had four lifetime partners. She is currently sexually active with one male partner and uses Yasmin as her form of contraception. She has taken oral contraceptives since she was 18 years old.

Case Study

Results of Ms. Dalton's annual Pap smear (Papanicolaou test) were abnormal, revealing that Ms. Dalton has cervical dysplasia. Her HPV testing was positive for the human papillomavirus-16 (HPV-16). She has returned to the gynecologist's office today for a colposcopy.

Questions

1. Discuss HPV. In your discussion, address how HPV is transmitted, clinical manifestations, the relationship between HPV and cancer, and what can be done to minimize a person's risk of HPV infection.

2. Identify at least five risk factors for cervical cancer. Indicate which factors have increased Ms. Dalton's risk.

3. Ms. Dalton is very anxious. She asks the nurse to explain what she is going to have done today. Describe a colposcopy to Ms. Dalton.

4. During the colposcopy procedure, the health care provider (HCP) asks the nurse to stand at the head of the examination table to assist during the procedure. What will be the nurse's primary responsibility during the procedure?

5. Provide Ms. Dalton with postprocedure instructions, prepare her for how she may feel in the 24 hours following the colposcopy, and educate her about the symptoms to report.

6. Before Ms. Dalton leaves the GYN office, she comments to the nurse, "Men have it so easy. They don't have to worry about things like HPV." How should the nurse reply?

7. Results of the colposcopy indicate that Ms. Dalton has CIN I. Her HCP schedules Ms. Dalton for a cone biopsy. Briefly explain what "CIN I" indicates and why the HCP is recommending a cone biopsy.

8. Ms. Dalton has a cone biopsy that successfully removes the cancerous region and its borders. How will her follow-up regarding routine Pap tests be different as compared with her prior diagnosis of cervical dysplasia and CIN I? What is a potential concern if she becomes pregnant in the future?

9. Ms. Dalton asks, "What should I tell my boyfriend? Should he be treated too?" How should the nurse respond?

10. Identify three priority nursing diagnoses appropriate for Ms. Dalton.

11. A few weeks after her cone biopsy, Ms. Dalton calls her HCP and asks, "I saw on television that there is a new vaccine for HPV. Can I schedule an appointment to come in and get the vaccine?" What information should the HCP share with Ms. Dalton regarding the benefits of the HPV vaccine, its administration, cost, potential adverse effects, and if she is a candidate for the vaccine?

Questions and Suggested Answers

1. **Discuss HPV. In your discussion, address how HPV is transmitted, clinical manifestations, the relationship between HPV and cancer, and what can be done to minimize a person's risk of HPV infection.** HPV is the most common STD (or STI) in the United States. It is estimated that 50% to 75% of sexually active men and women will acquire genital HPV infection at some point in their lifetime. The virus may manifest itself as genital warts, but the majority of individuals infected are asymptomatic. More than 100 different types of HPV have been identified, but most HPV infections in women present a low risk and resolve on their own. More than 30 HPV types are sexually transmitted and can infect the genital area of men and women. Almost all cases of cervical cancer are associated with the presence of one of 18 types of HPV. Testing with the HC2 high-risk HPV DNA test can identify 13 high-risk types of HPV associated with the development of cervical cancer. The HPV test is performed at the same time as the Pap test. The HPV-16 or HPV-18 type of the virus causes most cervical cancers. HPV causes cervical dysplasia (alteration in size, shape, and organization of cells), which can lead to invasive cervical cancer. Any individual who engages in sexual activity that involves genital contact with a person infected with HPV is at risk of becoming infected. Limiting the number of sexual partners, choosing a partner who has had no or few prior sex partners, remaining in a monogamous relationship with an uninfected partner, and using a condom all help to decrease a person's risk of HPV infection. Individuals should be aware that HPV infection could occur in both male and female genital areas that are not covered by a latex condom (Centers for Disease Control, 2004; Erikson & Field, 2007; Lowdermilk, 2006).

2. **Identify at least five risk factors for cervical cancer. Indicate which factors have increased Ms. Dalton's risk.** Risk factors for cervical cancer include:

- Age
  The average age of women newly diagnosed with cervical cancer is between 50 and 55 years old. Cervical cancer rarely occurs in girls younger than 15 and begins to appear in women in their 20s (American Cancer Society, 2006).
- Cigarette smoking
- Compromised immunity, such as human immunodeficiency virus (HIV)
- Deficiencies of vitamins A and C
- Diabetes
- Early age at first pregnancy
- Family history of cervical cancer

- First sexual intercourse (coitus) before age 16
- Folic acid metabolism disorder
- Frequent douching
- High-risk male partner
- History of an STD, such as Chlamydia
- HPV infection
- Intrauterine exposure to diethylstilbestrol (DES)

  DES is a synthetic form of estrogen that was prescribed for women from 1938 until 1971 to help prevent premature delivery or miscarriage in women who previously had such complications in pregnancy. In 1971, the U.S. Food and Drug Administration (FDA) advised that DES no longer be prescribed when studies revealed that DES could interfere with the reproductive system of a fetus (ACS, 2005).
- Low socioeconomic status (inadequate access to health care services)
- Multiparity (two or more pregnancies resulting in a live offspring), especially for African Americans, Hispanic Americans, and Native Americans
- Multiple sexual partners
- Nulliparity (no births)
- Prostitution
- Use of oral contraceptives (OC)

  No definitive evidence exists linking the use of OCs with cervical cancer. There is some statistical evidence that long-term use may slightly increase a woman's risk. Some research suggests an increased risk of more than 50% after five years of OC use (ACS, 2006; Smith, 2003 as cited in Linhart, 2007).

(ACS, 2006; Linhart, 2007).

The known risk factors in Ms. Dalton's case are:

- First sexual intercourse (coitus) before age 16 (Ms. Dalton's first sexual intercourse was at age 14.)
- HPV infection
- Multiple sexual partners (Ms. Dalton has had four lifetime partners.)
- Nulliparity (The term "gravida" means pregnancy. Gravida 0 indicates Ms. Dalton has never been pregnant.)
- Use of oral contraceptives (Ms. Dalton has been taking OCs for seven years.)

3. **Ms. Dalton is very anxious. She asks the nurse to explain what she is going to have done today. Describe a colposcopy to Ms. Dalton.** When the results of a Pap smear are abnormal, it indicates that there are changes in the cells of the cervix that could indicate a risk of cancer. The

recommended follow-up is a sterile procedure called a colposcopy to take a closer, three-dimensional magnified look at the changes in the cells of the cervix. The HCP performs the colposcopy by inserting a vaginal speculum as done during a Pap smear and viewing the vagina and cervix through a special lighted microscope (called a stereoscopic binocular microscope or colposcope). The HCP will often collect a Pap smear sample. Then a solution similar to vinegar (3% acetic acid) is applied to the cervix, which makes the areas of concern more visible by accentuating the difference between normal and abnormal cell patterns. A colposcopy is useful in identifying suspicious lesions, but a definitive diagnosis requires a biopsy. During the colposcopy, a biopsy will be taken of any area of the cervix (lesions) of concern to the HCP in order to obtain more detailed information about these abnormal cells. These tissue samples are sent to a pathology laboratory where a better determination can be made regarding the risk that the abnormal cells are an indication of a cancerous lesion on the cervix. The procedure lasts approximately 20 minutes, and there may be mild discomfort. Prior to the colposcopy, an analgesic can be prescribed to promote comfort and in some cases, a mild sedative is given (ACS, 2006; Chernecky & Berger, 2004; Daniels, 2002; Lowdermilk, 2006).

4. During the colposcopy procedure, the HCP asks the nurse to stand at the head of the examination table to assist during the procedure. What will be the nurse's primary responsibility during the procedure? Ms. Dalton is hard of hearing and uses lip-reading as a method of communication. She is able to read the speech of another person from the movement of their lips and mouth. This method (also called speech reading) includes the reading of facial expressions and body language. Ms. Dalton will be lying flat (in the lithotomy position) on the examination table and unable to see the HCP who will be at the foot of the table. The nurse should stand at the head of the examination table so that Ms. Dalton can see the nurse's face clearly. The nurse should repeat any instructions and information that the HCP offers during the procedure. The nurse should also provide verbal support and perhaps offer to hold Ms. Dalton's hand as a gesture of comfort while the colposcopy is performed.

5. Provide Ms. Dalton with postprocedure instructions, prepare her for how she may feel in the 24 hours following the colposcopy, and educate her about the symptoms to report. Following a colposcopy, the client may feel vaginal or abdominal discomfort that is similar to premenstrual cramping. Over-the-counter pain medication can be taken as needed. She should rest for 24 hours after the procedure. A bloody or brown, coffee ground-like vaginal discharge may be noted for up to a week. This discharge is to be expected. The coffee-ground drainage is from dried blood, staining by

Lugol's iodine solution that may have been applied to the cervix to help visualize any abnormality if the areas were not sufficiently revealed by the 3% acetic acid, and/or Monsel's solution that is applied to the cervix to stop any bleeding. She should change sanitary pads frequently. Ms. Dalton should notify her HCP if she has heavy bleeding (more than a normal menses) or signs of infection, such as fever, foul smelling or a yellow-colored vaginal discharge, or increased abdominal pain. She should avoid lifting anything heavy, abstain from intercourse, and not insert anything into her vagina (such as a tampon) until healing of the biopsy is confirmed at a follow-up postprocedure appointment (usually in two weeks) (Chernecky & Berger, 2004; Daniels, 2002; Lowdermilk, 2006).

6. Before Ms. Dalton leaves the GYN office, she comments to the nurse, "Men have it so easy. They don't have to worry about things like HPV." How should the nurse reply? HPV does affect men. HPV can be transmitted in sexually active heterosexual and homosexual men. HPV can cause precancerous dysplasia of the anal canal as well as condyloma (elevated wartlike lesions) in the genital area. HPV-16 and HPV-18 can cause anal and penile cancer in men. Screening is available for men with cytological screening using the anal Pap test. It is recommended that men have this screening test every two to three years (CDC, 2004; Linhart, 2007).

7. Results of the colposcopy indicate that Ms. Dalton has CIN I. Her HCP schedules Ms. Dalton for a cone biopsy. Briefly explain what "CIN I" indicates and why the HCP is recommending a cone biopsy. A precancerous noninvasive stage of cervical cancer, called cervical carcinoma in situ, is the most common form diagnosed. The incidence of carcinoma in situ peaks between the ages of 25 and 35 years of age. The majority of cervical cancers (95%) are squamous cell, arising from the epidermal layer of the cervix. Cell dysplasia indicates the presence of a precursor lesion. These lesions, called cervical intraepithelial neoplasia (CIN), are classified according to three stages: CIN I (mild to moderate dysplasia), CIN II (moderate to severe dysplasia), and CIN III (severe dysplasia to carcinoma in situ). The client will not have any symptoms because of dysplasia. It is diagnosed only through cytology (Pap test). CIN I indicates that Ms. Dalton has a form of cancer (carcinoma) that is strictly confined to the cervix. Cervical conization (cone biopsy) is used therapeutically to remove the entire cervical lesion of a microinvasive cervical cancer. In this procedure, a cone-shaped piece of tissue is removed from the cervix. The base of the cone is formed by the ectocervix (outer portion of the cervix), and the point of the cone is from the endocervical canal (inner portion of the cervix). This method captures the transformation zone within the cone, which is the area of the cervix where precancers and cancers are most likely to develop. This surgical procedure is valuable in preserving a woman's fertility (ACS, 2006; Linhart, 2007; Novak, 2006).

8. Ms. Dalton has a cone biopsy that successfully removes the cancerous region and its borders. How will her follow-up regarding routine Pap tests be different as compared with her prior diagnosis of cervical dysplasia and CIN I? What is a potential concern if she becomes pregnant in the future? In healthy women, an annual Pap smear is recommended for all sexually active women. Early detection of preinvasive lesions (precancers) improves the chances of successful treatment and prevents early cervical cell dysplasia from becoming cancerous. Between 60% and 80% of American women newly diagnosed with invasive cervical cancer have not had a Pap test in the past five years. Routine screening begins within three years of the onset of sexual activity or at age 21. Screening should be done every year with the conventional Pap test or every two years using the newer liquid-based Pap test. Some HCPs may recommend less frequent Pap smears (every two to three years) once a woman is 30 years old or is in a monogamous relationship and has three consecutive normal Pap test results. Less frequent screenings are felt to be appropriate since the likelihood of viral acquisition is greatly reduced in these individuals. Since Ms. Dalton has been infected with HPV and has been diagnosed with CIN, she will be monitored closely with regular Pap tests and a colposcopy as needed. She should return for follow-up Pap tests every four to six months as recommended by her HCP. Once several Pap tests are within normal limits, the HCP will recommend how often to schedule future Pap tests. Rare, but potential concerns following a cone biopsy that may pose risks if Ms. Dalton becomes pregnant include a narrowing of the cervix (cervical stenosis) and the inability of the cervix to remain closed during pregnancy (incompetent cervix). Cervical stenosis can cause infertility. An incompetent cervix can cause pregnancies to end in miscarriage or cause premature labor (ACS, 2006; Gupta, 2006; Linhart, 2007; Nissl, 2005).

9. Ms. Dalton asks, "What should I tell my boyfriend? Should he be treated too?" How should the nurse respond? Yes. Her boyfriend should be examined by his HCP and treated if necessary. HPV is an STD that is passed from one person to another through any sexual activity that involves genital contact with a person infected with HPV. It is possible to contract HPV without having sexual intercourse. Many contract HPV within the first two to three years of becoming sexually active and often do not know that they have the virus. Approximately 30 types of HPV affect the genital area, and 10 of these types can lead to the development of cervical cancer. The two types that pose the greatest risk of cervical cancer are HPV-16 and HPV-18. Very rarely HPV infection results in anal or genital cancers. Low-risk types (HPV-6 and -11) can cause genital warts (condylomata acuminate). Genital warts are not life threatening but can cause emotional discomfort. Genital warts are soft flesh-colored growths or bumps that can be raised or flat. They appear on the external genital area (on or around the penis) or near the anus. They may produce burning, itching, or pain. If Ms. Dalton's boyfriend has genital warts, treatment is available in the form of podofilox 0.5% (Condylox) or imiquimod 5% (Aldara) which are both topical medications that are applied directly to the affected area as prescribed. Other forms of treatment include cryotherapy (freezing) using trichloroacetic acid (TCA) and bichloracetic acid (BCA), intralesional interferon injections, or laser surgery. These treatment modalities will remove the genital warts, but will not eliminate the HPV. There is always a chance that the genital warts will return and require repeat treatment. Ms. Dalton and her boyfriend should avoid intimate sexual contact until the genital wart lesions have healed (CDC, 2004; Linhart, 2007; Van Zandt, 2006).

Ms. Dalton should be educated about the importance of using a latex condom with every sexual encounter to help prevent the transmission of other STDs since oral contraceptives prevent pregnancy but offer no protection against the transmission of an STD or genital virus. The effect of condoms in preventing HPV infection is unknown. Genital areas not protected by a condom can become infected with HPV. However, condom use has been associated with a lower rate of cervical cancer (CDC, 2004).

10. Identify three priority nursing diagnoses appropriate for Ms. Dalton. Suggested priority nursing diagnoses to consider for Ms. Dalton include:

- Fear related to (r/t) outcome of biopsy, threat to well-being, and fear of incurable disease
- Acute pain r/t tissue damage (cervical biopsy procedure)
- Risk for fluid volume deficit r/t postprocedure complication (bleeding)
- Risk for infection r/t invasive procedure (biopsy)
- Ineffective health maintenance r/t deficient knowledge regarding HPV, transmission of STDs, and treatment
- Readiness for enhanced knowledge of testing and follow-up care
- Risk for ineffective coping r/t personal vulnerability in situational crisis

(Ackley & Ladwig, 2006).

11. A few weeks after her cone biopsy, Ms. Dalton calls her HCP and asks, "I saw on television that there is a new vaccine for HPV. Can I schedule an appointment to come in and get the vaccine?" What information should the HCP share with Ms. Dalton regarding the benefits of the HPV vaccine, its administration, cost, potential adverse effects, and if she is a candidate for the vaccine? The FDA approved the HPV vaccine (called Gardisil) in June 2006. There are approximately 30 types of genital-tract HPV. The vaccine targets four strains of HPV: HPV-16 and HPV-18, which account for 70% of all cases of cervical cancer, and HPV-6 and HPV-11, which are responsible for approximately 90% of genital wart cases. The vaccine is administered in three injections given over a one-year period at a cost of approximately $360 for all three doses. The second injection is given about two months after the initial injection, and the third dose is given four months after the second. Ms. Dalton should check to see if her health care insurance carrier will cover the cost or if she will need to pay out of pocket. The HPV vaccine has been approved for nonpregnant females aged 9 through 26 years. It is suggested that females receive the vaccine when they are 11 or 12 years old, and maximum benefit is offered when the vaccine is given prior to the female's first sexual experience. The vaccine only prevents infection with HPV. It does not prevent disease in the woman already infected with the virus. Ms. Dalton has been exposed to HPV-16. Receiving the vaccine will not have an effect on that type of HPV, but can still offer her protection against the three other types. The vaccine will not afford her protection against any other STDs and does not prevent pregnancy. Severe adverse reactions to the HPV vaccine are uncommon. The most common adverse effect is arm soreness at the site of the injection and a transient headache. She is currently within the age range approved for the vaccine and is not pregnant, but she would not be a candidate once she turned 27 years old or if she became pregnant. The HPV vaccine is not given to pregnant women since it imposes an increased risk of birth defects (ACS, 2006; Gupta, 2006).

References

Ackley, B., & Ladwig, G. (2006). *Nursing diagnosis handbook: A guide to planning care.* St. Louis, MO: Mosby.

American Cancer Society (ACS). (2005). *DES exposure: Questions and answers.* Retrieved August 25, 2006 from www.cancer.org.

American Cancer Society (ACS). (2006). *Detailed guide: Cervical cancer.* Retrieved August 25, 2006 from www.cancer.org.

Centers for Disease Control and Prevention (CDC). (2004). *Genital HPV infection: CDC fact sheet.* Retrieved August 25, 2006 from www.cdc.gov.

Chernecky, C. C., & Berger, B. J. (2004). *Laboratory tests and diagnostic procedures.* Philadelphia, PA: Elsevier.

Daniels, R. (2002). *Delmar's guide to laboratory and diagnostic tests.* Albany, NY: Delmar.

Erikson, J. M., & Field, R. B. (2007). Cancer. In F. Monahan, J. Sands, M. Neighbors, J. Marek, & C. Green (Eds.), *Phipps' Medical-surgical nursing: Health and illness perspectives* (p. 518). St. Louis, MO: Mosby Elsevier.

Gupta, N. E. (2006, July). What you should know about the HPV vaccine. *The Clinical Advisor,* 46–48.

Linhart, J. (2007). Female reproductive problems. In F. Monahan, J. Sands, M. Neighbors, J. Marek, & C. Green (Eds.), *Phipps' Medical-surgical nursing: Health and illness perspectives* (pp. 1697–1701). St. Louis, MO: Mosby Elsevier.

Lowdermilk, D. L. (2006). Assessment of the reproductive system. In D. Ignatavicius & L. Workman (Eds.), *Medical-surgical nursing: Critical thinking for collaborative care* (pp. 1781–1782, 1785–1786). St. Louis, MO: Elsevier Saunders.

Nissl, J. (2005). *Cone biopsy (conization) for abnormal cervical cell changes.* Retrieved August 25, 2006 from www.webmd.com.

Novak, K. (2006). Interventions for clients with gynecologic problems. In D. Ignatavicius & L. Workman (Eds.), *Medical-surgical nursing: Critical thinking for collaborative care* (pp.1846–1847). St. Louis, MO: Elsevier Saunders.

Smith, J. (2003). Cervical cancer and the use of hormonal contraceptives. *Lancet, 361* (9364), 1159–1167.

Van Zandt, S. (2006). Interventions for clients with sexually transmitted diseases. In D. Ignatavicius & L. Workman (Eds.), *Medical-surgical nursing: Critical thinking for collaborative care* (pp. 1891–1892). St. Louis, MO: Elsevier Saunders.

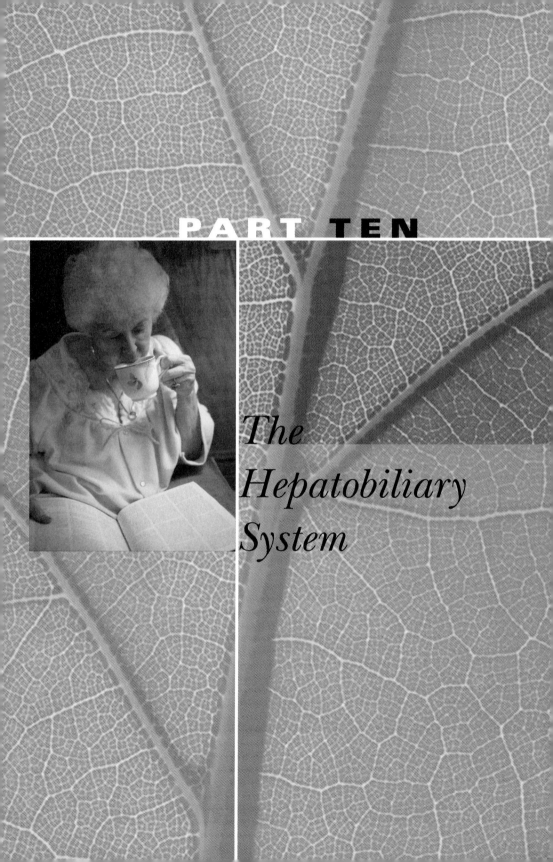

PART TEN

The
Hepatobiliary
System

Mr. Escobar

GENDER

Male

AGE

47

SETTING

- Hospital

ETHNICITY

- Black American

CULTURAL CONSIDERATIONS

PREEXISTING CONDITIONS

- Cirrhosis secondary to alcoholic hepatitis, hypertension (HTN), esophageal varices

COEXISTING CONDITIONS

- Esophageal varices, ascites

COMMUNICATION

DISABILITY

- Unemployed (on disability) for past four years

SOCIOECONOMIC

- Married, father of two boys (ages 19 and 17 years old), history of drinking one quart of hard liquor each day for three years prior to diagnosis of cirrhosis

SPIRITUAL/RELIGIOUS

PHARMACOLOGIC

- Lactulose (Cephulac); neomycin sulfate (Mycifradin Sulfate)

LEGAL

ETHICAL

ALTERNATIVE THERAPY

PRIORITIZATION

DELEGATION

THE HEPATOBILIARY SYSTEM

Level of Difficulty: Difficult

Overview: The client in this case presents with clinical manifestations of hepatic encephalopathy. The nurse must identify the abnormal laboratory findings and provide an explanation for their levels in this client's case. Priority nursing diagnoses for the client with hepatic encephalopathy are identified. Diagnostic testing reveals esophageal varices and a moderate amount of ascites. Ascites in the client with liver failure is discussed, and assessment of this condition reviewed. Rationales are offered for the prescribed medications and restricted diet that are part of the treatment plan. The nurse must convey an understanding of esophageal varices, what is accomplished in the banding procedure, and client instruction to prevent bleeding in the future.

DIFFICULT

Client Profile

Mr. Escobar is a 47-year-old male with a history of cirrhosis. He lives with his wife and teenage sons. His wife brought him to the emergency department today because she noticed that Mr. Escobar had increasing confusion and lethargy and was having difficulty walking. His wife states, "He is probably acting a little funny because he is sleep deprived. He hasn't slept very much in the past few days."

Case Study

Mr. Escobar is afebrile. His blood pressure is 136/68, pulse 88, and respiratory rate 18. His oxygen saturation is 98% on room air. He is awake, alert, and oriented to person only. His speech is slow and he appears tired. The nurse notices a foul odor to his breath. Upon physical examination, Mr. Escobar has a slightly distended abdomen. The health care provider (HCP) does not note any asterixis. The HCP requests an abdominal ultrasound, which reveals fatty infiltration of the liver, an enlarged spleen, a polyp in his gallbladder, and a moderate amount of ascites. Results of a complete blood count (CBC) reveal white blood cell count (WBC) 4.8 cells/mm^3, red blood cell count (RBC) 2.94 million/mm^3, hemoglobin (Hgb) 9.8 g/dL, hematocrit (Hct) 28.2%, and platelet count 89,000 mm^3. Results of a comprehensive metabolic panel (CMP) are sodium 145 mEq/L, potassium 3.6 mEq/L, chloride 112 mEq/L, and carbon dioxide 25 mEq/L. Mr. Escobar's glucose is 185. His blood urea nitrogen (BUN) is 42 mg/dL and creatinine is 1.6 mg/dL. Liver function tests (LFTs) reveal total protein 5.7 g/dL, albumin 3.1 g/dL, total bilirubin 1.8 mg/dL, aspartate aminotransferase (AST) 17 U/L, alanine aminotransferase (ALT) 14 U/L, and lactate dehydrogenase (LDH, LD) of 266 U/L. His prothrombin time is 13.1 seconds. His ammonia level is 124 μmol/L. Urinalysis results are within normal limits. The HCP schedules Mr. Escobar for a gastroscopy to rule out any gastrointestinal (GI) bleeding. Intravenous (IV) fluids of D 5½ NS are started at 100 mL per hour. Medications prescribed include lactulose and neomycin sulfate. The HCP admitting Mr. Escobar also prescribes daily weights, strict intake and output documentation, monitoring of stools for occult blood, neurological assessment every four hours, and a low protein, low sodium diet.

Questions

1. Mr. Escobar has cirrhosis. Briefly discuss the pathophysiology of this disease and its incidence in the United States.

2. Briefly explain how hepatic encephalopathy is related to cirrhosis.

3. Upon initial examination, the HCP did not note any asterixis. What is

Questions (continued)

asterixis, and how did the HCP assess Mr. Escobar for this condition?

4. Identify the characteristic clinical manifestations of hepatic encephalopathy consistent with Mr. Escobar's presentation.

5. Identify three priority nursing diagnoses for Mr. Escobar.

6. Identify which of the client's admitting laboratory results are abnormal and provide a rationale for why each is above or below the normal range.

7. Define ascites. Explain what causes ascites and how the nurse will assess for this condition.

8. Mr. Escobar has been prescribed 30 mL of lactulose every six hours and neomycin sulfate, 500 mg four times a day. Explain why each of these medications has been included in the client's medical management plan. What should the nurse teach Mr. Escobar regarding the potential adverse effects of each medication?

9. When should the nurse anticipate the onset of the effects of lactulose, and describe the therapeutic effects of lactulose on Mr. Escobar's bowel pattern. While evaluating the effectiveness of the lactulose, what finding would indicate a potential lactulose overdose?

10. Provide a brief rationale for the low-protein, low-sodium diet the HCP prescribed for Mr. Escobar.

11. A gastroscopy reveals that Mr. Escobar has esophageal varices, which are treated with banding. Briefly discuss what esophageal varies are and the banding procedure used to treat them.

12. Briefly explain how Mr. Escobar's hepatic encephalopathy is related to the esophageal varices.

13. Mr. Escobar is being discharged, and the nurse is educating the client about minimizing his risk of further injury. Provide a list of at least three precautions to decrease his risk of hemorrhage from future esophageal varices.

Questions and Suggested Answers

    1. Mr. Escobar has cirrhosis. Briefly discuss the pathophysiology of this disease and its incidence in the United States. Hepatic dysfunction is caused by damage to the liver either directly by a primary liver disease or indirectly from the obstruction of bile flow or impaired hepatic circulation. Liver dysfunction may be acute or chronic. Chronic dysfunction is more common than acute disease. Cirrhosis is a chronic, progressive liver disease that is characterized by fibrotic changes (scarring) in the liver and the formation of dense connective tissue and nodule formation that leads to degenerative changes and loss of function of hepatic cells. The disease processes that can lead to liver dysfunction include infectious agents (such as hepatitis), metabolic disorders, toxins and medications, and nutritional deficiencies. The most common cause of chronic liver disease is alcoholism (called Laënnec's cirrhosis). The parenchymal cells of the liver respond to noxious agents by replacing glycogen with lipids, creating hyperlipidemia, and producing fatty infiltration. There also may be necrosis of liver cells. In response, there is inflammatory cell infiltration and fibrous tissue forms. Eventually, chronic liver disease will cause a smaller, shrunken, fibrotic liver.

Liver disease and cirrhosis are the seventh leading cause of death in the United States among adults between the ages of 25 and 64 years old. Cirrhosis resulting from excessive alcohol ingestion has a poor prognosis, especially if the client continues to drink alcohol. More than 40% of the deaths related to cirrhosis are associated with alcohol abuse. Cirrhosis and alcoholic (Laënnec's) cirrhosis in particular occur twice as frequently in men than in women. Cirrhosis is more prevalent among black Americans than Caucasians (American Liver Foundation, 2005).

2. Briefly explain how hepatic encephalopathy is related to cirrhosis. Hepatic encephalopathy (also called portal-systemic encephalopathy) is a life-threatening complication of liver disease. Hepatic encephalopathy occurs in clients with liver failure and results from the accumulation of ammonia and other toxic metabolites in the bloodstream. In the client with liver failure, damaged liver cells are unable to metabolize ammonia and convert it to urea. Thus, the ammonia accumulates and enters the bloodstream. Ammonia is a central nervous system (CNS) depressant. An increased concentration of ammonia in the blood is toxic to the brain and causes dysfunction that manifests as hepatic encephalopathy. Central nervous system disturbances result, ranging from reduced mental alertness, confusion, and restlessness to loss of consciousness, seizures, and irreversible coma (Smeltzer & Bare, 2004; Smolen, 2005; Stalsbroten, 2007).

3. Upon initial examination, the HCP did not note any asterixis. What is asterixis, and how did the HCP assess Mr. Escobar for this condition? Asterixis refers to a flapping tremor of the hands. Some refer to this as "liver flap" or a "flapping tremor." To assess for asterixis, the HCP would ask Mr. Escobar to hold his arm out straight with his hand held upward in a dorsiflexed position. The HCP then looks for Mr. Escobar's hand to fall forward involuntarily and quickly return to the dorsiflexed position. The client with asterixis is unable to hold their hand steady. This condition makes handwriting and the ability to draw a line figure difficult. The inability to reproduce a simple figure, such as a star or a clock, is referred to as constructional apraxia. Daily assessment of the client's handwriting and ability to complete a line drawing exercise provides data regarding the progression of hepatic encephalopathy (Smeltzer & Bare, 2004).

4. Identify the characteristic clinical manifestations of hepatic encephalopathy consistent with Mr. Escobar's presentation. The characteristic clinical manifestations of hepatic encephalopathy that Mr. Escobar presented with include:

- Change in mental status (confusion)
- Motor disturbance (difficulty walking)
- Altered sleep pattern (His wife states, "He is probably acting a little funny because he is sleep-deprived. He hasn't slept very much in the past few days.")
  ○ Sleep pattern reversal is common in clients with hepatic encephalopathy. The client is often awake all night and sleeps throughout the day.

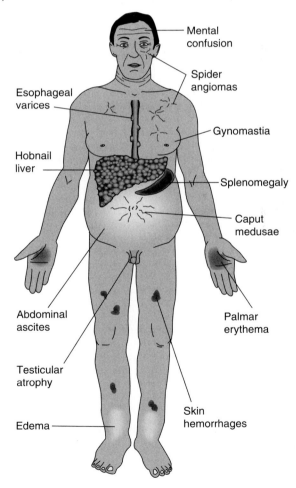

Clinical features of cirrhosis of the liver in the male

- Fetor hepaticus (foul odor to his breath)
  - ○ Some clients present with a sweet or slightly fecal odor to their breath. The odor has also been described as similar to freshly mowed grass or old wine. This pungent odor is thought to originate from the intestine.
- Serum ammonia level is elevated (124 μmol/L)
- Slightly distended abdomen with moderate amount of ascites noted on ultrasound
- Fatty infiltration of the liver noted on ultrasound

(Smeltzer & Bare, 2004).

5. Identify three priority nursing diagnoses for Mr. Escobar. Suggested priority nursing diagnoses include:

- Risk for injury (chemical, abnormal blood profile) related to (r/t) acute confusion, elevated ammonia levels, altered clotting factors, and decreased hemoglobin
- Risk for falls r/t difficulty with gait, sleeplessness, and confusion
- Disturbed thought processes r/t chronic organic disorder with increased ammonia levels (encephalopathy)
- Disturbed sleep pattern r/t physiological effects of illness (hepatic encephalopathy)
- Risk for deficient fluid volume: hemorrhage r/t active fluid volume loss secondary to bleeding from the GI tract (esophageal varices)
- Risk for excess fluid volume r/t compromised regulatory system (liver failure)
- Risk for infection (peritonitis) r/t inadequate primary defenses (stasis of body fluids and ascites)

(Ackley & Ladwig, 2006; Smolen, 2005).

6. Identify which of the client's admitting laboratory results are abnormal and provide a rationale for why each is above or below the normal range.

RBC 2.94 million/mm³: Below the normal range of 4.6 to 6.2 million/mm³

RBCs (erythrocytes) are the major carrier of hemoglobin, and thus oxygen, to cells and the carriers of carbon dioxide to the lungs for excretion. Blood loss can cause the normal levels of RBCs to decrease. Mr. Escobar has a history of esophageal varices and may have bleeding varices presently.

Hgb 9.8 g/dL: Below the normal range of 14 to 18 g/dL

Hgb is the main intracellular protein of erythrocytes. The amount of hemoglobin per 100 mL of blood is an indicator of the oxygen-carrying capacity of the blood. Decreased levels in Mr. Escobar's case most likely indicate blood loss, perhaps secondary to esophageal varices. The client with low levels of Hgb will often feel fatigue, lethargy, and have pallor of the skin.

Hct 28.2%: Below the normal range for males of 40 to 54%

Hct is the percentage of RBC mass to the original blood volume. The Hct depends on the number of RBCs (which in Mr. Escobar's case are decreased) and the average size of the RBCs. Clients who are losing blood, such as from bleeding esophageal varices, will have lower than normal levels of Hct.

Platelet count 89,000 mm³: Below the normal range of 150,000 to 450,000 mm³

When pressure increases in the portal venous system, damage to the spleen occurs, and the spleen can become enlarged (splenomegaly is noted on Mr. Escobar's ultrasound). Enlargement of the spleen destroys blood cells, especially platelets. Low platelet levels in the blood (thrombocytopenia) increase the client's risk of hemorrhage and anemia.

Chloride 112 mEq/L: Above the normal range of 98 to 106 mEq/L

Chloride is a major extracellular anion that, in combination with sodium, maintains osmolality and water balance. Serum chloride is elevated in clients with alcoholism.

Glucose 185 mg/dL: Above the normal range of 70 to 115 mg/dL

The liver plays a major role in the metabolism of glucose and in the regulation of blood glucose concentration. In the healthy client, the glucose from a meal is taken from the GI tract to the liver by the portal vein and converted into glycogen. Glycogen is stored in liver cells (hepatocytes) and is converted back into glucose and released into the bloodstream as needed to maintain a normal level of glucose within the body. This process is altered in the client with liver dysfunction and results in increased levels of glucose in the bloodstream.

BUN 42 mg/dL: Above the normal range of 5 to 20 mg/dL and *Creatinine 1.6 mg/dL:* Above the normal range for males age 40–50 years of 0.75 to 1.33 mg/dL

The BUN measures the nitrogen fraction of urea, which is the end product of protein metabolism. Urea is formed from ammonia by the liver and excreted by the kidneys. BUN exists in a normal ratio with creatinine. These two values often rise together in pathological conditions, such as compromised renal function, which can occur with ascites when there is a decrease in extracellular fluid volume.

Total protein 5.7 g/dL: Below the normal range of 6 to 8 g/dL and *Albumin 3.1 g/dL:* Below the normal range of 3.4 to 4.8 g/dL

A serum protein test measures the total protein level in the blood. The value includes the measurement of albumin, globulin, and the albumin/globulin ratio. Since the liver plays a role in protein metabolism, the level of albumin is decreased in clients with liver failure.

Total bilirubin 1.8 mg/dL: Above the normal range of 0 to 1.3 mg/dL

Bilirubin is a pigment that is derived from the breakdown of hemoglobin. Liver cells (hepatocytes) remove bilirubin from the blood and modify it through conjugation to glucuronic acid rendering it more soluble in aqueous solutions. The conjugated bilirubin is then secreted by the hepatocytes into adjacent bile canaliculi (narrow tubular channels) and carried in the bile to the duodenum. Elimination of bilirubin in the bile is the major route of excretion. In the client with liver disease, the concentration of bilirubin in the blood is often increased because of impaired bile flow (i.e., gallstones in bile ducts), or because of the destruction of RBCs. Some clients develop jaundice from an increased concentration of bilirubin in the blood.

LDH 266 U/L: Above the normal range of 48 to 115 U/L

LDH is an intracellular enzyme found in almost all body tissues. It is released as a result of tissue damage. The highest concentrations are found in organs such as the heart, liver, kidneys, and skeletal muscles. When an organ is damaged from ischemia, such as in cirrhosis, LDH levels are elevated. This test is used as a marker for biliary cholestasis (suppression of bile flow). This value is often elevated in clients with a history of alcohol abuse.

Ammonia 124 μmol/L: Above the normal range of 11 to 32 μmol/L

The healthy liver converts metabolically generated ammonia and ammonia produced by bacteria in the intestine into urea. This process facilitates the excretion of ammonia, a potential toxin, through the urine. A diseased liver has impaired protein metabolism and is unable to convert the ammonia for excretion and a toxic level of ammonia builds up in the bloodstream.

(Chernecky & Berger, 2004; Daniels, 2002; Murphy, 2006; Smeltzer & Bare, 2004; Smolen, 2005)

7. **Define ascites. Explain what causes ascites and how the nurse will assess for this condition.** Ascites is the accumulation of free fluid in the peritoneal cavity of the abdomen. The obstructed blood flow through a diseased liver results in increased blood pressure throughout the portal venous system, called portal hypertension. Two major consequences of portal hypertension are ascites and varices. Ascites can occur in clients with cancer, kidney disease, heart failure, and from circulatory changes within a diseased liver. Portal hypertension, an increase in capillary pressure, and the obstruction of blood flow through the liver contribute to

the accumulation of fluid. In addition, the diseased liver cannot properly metabolize aldosterone, which increases sodium and water retention by the kidneys. This sodium and water retention, the increased intravascular fluid volume, and decreased ability of the liver to synthesize albumin result in the shift of fluid from the vascular system into the peritoneal space. When this shift occurs, the kidneys respond by retaining more sodium and fluid in an effort to maintain vascular fluid volume, and the process becomes self-perpetuating. Mr. Escobar has a moderate amount of ascites as noted on his physical examination and ultrasound. However, the client with liver failure may accumulate large amounts (15 mL or more) of albumin-rich fluid in their peritoneal cavity (ascites). The client with ascites will have an increased abdominal girth and rapid weight gain. Percussion of the abdomen will reveal a dullness over the area of fluid accumulation and a fluid wave may be detected. To assess for a fluid wave, the nurse places their hands along either side of the client's flank. Striking one flank sharply with the fingertips, the nurse feels for the impulse of a fluid wave transmitted to the opposite hand. A second nurse should apply pressure by placing their hand along the midline of the client's abdomen (with the ulnar side against the client's abdomen) during this assessment to prevent the fluid shift from being transmitted through the tissues of the abdominal wall, resulting in a false-negative assessment. A fluid wave is likely to be detected only in clients with a large volume of ascites. The distended abdomen may cause discomfort and make breathing difficult. Striae (streaks or lines) and distended veins may be observed over the abdominal wall, and fluid and electrolyte imbalances will occur (Smeltzer & Bare, 2004).

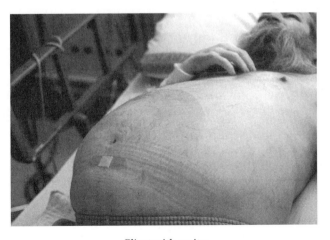

Client with ascites

8. Mr. Escobar has been prescribed 30 mL of lactulose every six hours and neomycin sulfate, 500 mg four times a day. Explain why each of these medications has been included in the client's medical management plan. What should the nurse teach Mr. Escobar regarding the potential adverse effects of each medication? *Lactulose* is a synthetic sugar used as a laxative. This laxative is administered to reduce serum ammonia levels and thus hepatic encephalopathy. Lactulose acts to help promote the excretion of ammonia through the stool, and is effective in reducing ammonia levels by 50%. Lactulose is effective because it acts to reverse the normal passage of ammonia from the GI tract into the bloodstream and promotes evacuation of the bowel by increasing peristalsis, which decreases the amount of ammonia absorbed by the bowel. Lactulose also changes the fecal flora to organisms that do not convert urea to ammonia. Potential adverse effects Mr. Escobar should be aware of include diarrhea, intestinal bloating, and cramps, which usually disappear in a few days to one week. Some find the sweet taste of lactulose objectionable. The taste can be masked by diluting lactulose with a full glass of water or fruit juice. Low potassium levels (hypokalemia) in the blood and dehydration can result from frequent bowel movements. These potential adverse effects will be monitored through nursing assessment, intake and output analysis, and by serum laboratory testing (Skidmore-Roth, 2005; Smeltzer & Bare, 2004; Stalsbroten, 2007).

Neomycin sulfate is an antibiotic (aminoglycoside) that interferes with bacterial protein synthesis. This antibiotic reduces the number of intestinal bacteria responsible for ammonia production and thus reduces the absorption of ammonia into the bloodstream. Reducing the intestinal flora, however, can result in the adverse effects of diarrhea and a deficiency of vitamin K. Some clients report changes in hearing, ringing in their ears (tinnitus), or dizziness while taking neomycin sulfate and should be assessed for such changes during treatment. There exists a potential interaction between neomycin sulfate and lactulose. This interaction can decrease the therapeutic effectiveness of lactulose. Therefore, a longer length of treatment with lactulose may be necessary to reduce the serum ammonia levels (Skidmore-Roth, 2005; Smolen, 2005; Spratto & Woods, 2006).

9. When should the nurse anticipate the onset of the effects of lactulose, and describe the therapeutic effects of lactulose on Mr. Escobar's bowel pattern. While evaluating the effectiveness of the lactulose, what finding would indicate a potential lactulose overdose? The exact onset of lactulose's therapeutic effect is unknown. Lactulose is administered until the client's stools are soft. While taking lactulose, Mr. Escobar should have two to four soft stools each day. If the nurse should note an increase in the frequency of stools or watery diarrhea, the HCP should be notified since this can be an indication of lactulose overdose. The nurse also should monitor Mr. Escobar's serum potassium level for hypokalemia and for any clinical manifestations of dehydration, which should be reported to the HCP promptly (Smeltzer & Bare, 2004; Stalsbroten, 2007).

10. Provide a brief rationale for the low-protein, low-sodium diet the HCP prescribed for Mr. Escobar. A low protein diet is recommended for the client with hepatic encephalopathy to minimize the breakdown of dietary protein and subsequent conversion into ammonia, which is then absorbed by the GI tract into the bloodstream. Low protein diets help to prevent further elevation of serum ammonia and severity of the hepatic encephalopathy. Daily protein intake should be between 1 and 1.5 g per kilogram (40 to 60 g per day). A low sodium diet has been prescribed for Mr. Escobar to help manage his hypertension, as well as decrease sodium retention and further fluid accumulation (ascites).

11. A gastroscopy reveals that Mr. Escobar has esophageal varices, which are treated with banding. Briefly discuss what esophageal varices are and the banding procedure used to treat them. Esophageal varices are swollen, dilated, tortuous veins most often occurring in the submucosa of the lower esophagus. They can develop higher up in the esophagus as well as in the stomach. The primary cause of esophageal varices in the client with liver failure is an obstruction of the portal venous circulation through the liver, resulting in portal hypertension. Because the portal vein is obstructed, blood from the GI tract and spleen look for pathways through collateral circulation forming new routes back to the right atrium. This collateral circulation creates increased pressure in the vessels within the submucosa of the lower esophagus and upper part of the client's stomach. Because collateral vessels are tortuous and fragile, they bleed easily. Bleeding esophageal varices can be a life-threatening emergency since significant blood loss can lead to hypovolemic shock.

In the banding procedure, an endoscope is loaded with an elastic rubber band and passed directly over each bleeding varix. After suctioning the varix into the tip of the endoscope, the rubber band–like ligature is slipped over the varix. Necrosis of the strangulated varices eventually results, and the varices slough off. Banding controls the bleeding and is effective in reducing the rate of rebleeding, thus reducing mortality (Smeltzer & Bare, 2004).

12. Briefly explain how Mr. Escobar's hepatic encephalopathy is related to the esophageal varices. Varices are "varicosities that develop from elevated pressures transmitted to all of the veins that drain into the portal system. They are prone to rupture and often are the source of massive hemorrhages from the upper gastrointestinal tract and the rectum" (Smeltzer

& Bare, 2004, p. 1082). Clients with liver disease also have blood clotting abnormalities that increase the likelihood of bleeding. The enzymatic and bacterial digestion of blood proteins in the GI tract provides the greatest source of ammonia. GI bleeding, such as the bleeding from esophageal varices, increases the digestion of blood in the intestines and leads to increased ammonia levels in the blood. Excessive ammonia levels result in disturbed brain function manifested as hepatic encephalopathy.

13. Mr. Escobar is being discharged, and the nurse is educating the client about minimizing his risk of further injury. Provide a list of at least three precautions to decrease his risk of hemorrhage from future esophageal varices. Mr. Escobar should be instructed to take the following precautions to help decrease his risk of bleeding from future esophageal varices. The client, his wife, and sons should be taught how to assess a pulse and how to use an automatic blood pressure cuff, which they can purchase for use at home.

- Monitor for signs of bleeding such as:
  - blood pressure below 90/60 mmHg
  - bloody or black, tarry stools (melena)
  - cool, clammy skin
  - decreased level of consciousness
  - diminished orientation to person, place and/or time
  - heart rate above 100 beats per minute
  - restlessness
  - vomiting blood (hematemesis)
- Avoid irritating fluids such as colas and alcohol.
- Avoid lifting heavy objects to prevent muscular exertion.
- Avoid vigorous physical exercise.
- Chew food carefully and into small pieces to avoid irritation of varices by bulky, poorly chewed foods.
- Consult his HCP if he has gastroesophageal reflux since the reflux of acidic gastric juices can cause esophageal erosion and irritation of varices.
- Consult his HCP before taking salicylates, which can erode the esophageal mucosa.
- Do not strain to have a bowel movement.
- Sneezing, coughing, and vomiting increase the risk of rupturing esophageal varices. Monitor for signs of bleeding if he has episodes of vomiting or frequent and forceful sneezing and/or coughing.

(Smeltzer & Bare, 2004; Smolen, 2005)

References

Ackley, B., & Ladwig, G. (2006). *Nursing diagnosis handbook: A guide to planning care.* St. Louis, MO: Mosby.

American Liver Foundation. (2005). *Hepatitis and liver disease in the United States.* Retrieved October 16, 2006 from www.liverfoundation.org.

Chernecky, C. C., & Berger, B. J. (2004). *Laboratory tests and diagnostic procedures.* Philadelphia, PA: Saunders.

Daniels, R. (2002). *Delmar's guide to laboratory and diagnostic tests.* Albany, NY: Delmar.

Murphy, M. B. (2006). Interventions for clients with liver problems. In D. D. Ignatavicius & M. L. Workman (Eds.) *Medical-surgical nursing: Critical thinking for collaborative care* (pp. 1368–1374). St. Louis, MO: Elsevier Saunders.

Skidmore-Roth, L. (2005). *Mosby's drug guide for nurses.* St. Louis, MO: Elsevier Mosby.

Smeltzer, S., & Bare, B. (2004). Assessment and management of patients with hepatic disorders. In L. Brunner & D. Suddarth (Eds.) *Textbook of medical-surgical nursing* (pp. 1074–1093). Philadelphia, PA: Lippincott Williams & Wilkins.

Smolen, D. M. (2005). Management of clients with hepatic disorders. In J. M. Black & J. H. Hawks (Eds.) *Medical-surgical nursing: Clinical management for positive outcomes* (pp. 1335–1359). St. Louis, MO: Elsevier.

Spratto, G. R., & Woods, A. L. (2006). *PDR nurse's drug handbook.* Clifton Park, NY: Thomson Delmar Learning.

Stalsbroten, V. L. (2007). Hepatic, biliary tract, and pancreatic dysfunction: Nursing management. In R. Daniels, L. J. Nosek, & L. H. Nicoll (Eds.), *Contemporary medical-surgical nursing* (p. 1717). Clifton Park, NY: Thomson Delmar Learning.

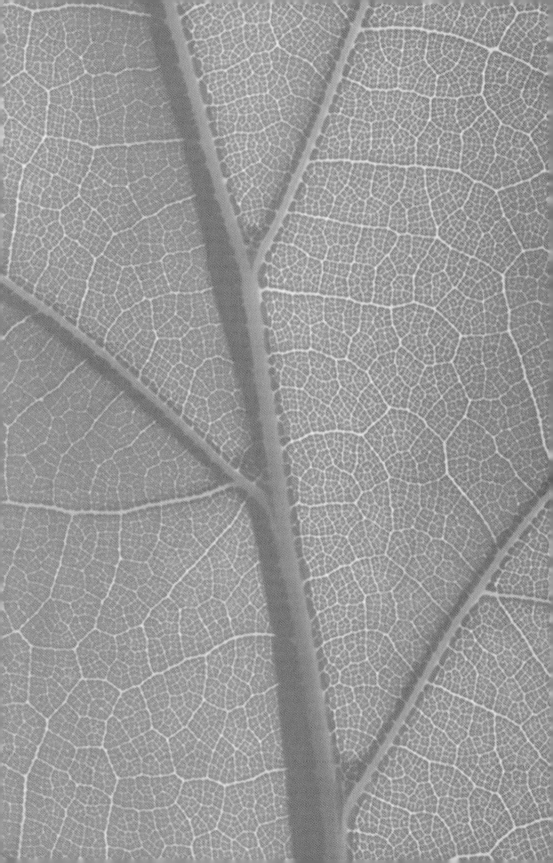

Index

Page numbers in *italics* indicate figures/tables.

A

Abdominal pain, in acute pyelonephritis, 19
ABG results, bronchitis and pneumonia, 63–64
Acetaminophen
    treatment of CAP, 64–65
    use in bacterial meningitis, 174
Achalasia, 3–12
Activities of daily living, RA, 111, *111*
Advance directive, 189–190
Age, risk factor for hypertension, 78
Albuterol, treatment of CAP, 64–65
Alcohol use
    diabetes and, 212–213
    risk factor for hypertension, 78, 81
Allograft, in burn patients, 160
Alpha blockers, selective and nonselective, treatment
    of BPH, 243
American Chronic Pain Association, 114
American Urological Association BPH Symptom Index
    Questionnaire, 241–242
Amlodipine, actions, 146–147
Anemia, renal failure and, 34
Aquathermia pad, use in diabetic patient, 147–149
Arthritis Foundation, 114
Ascites, 268–269, *269*
Ascorbic acid (Vitamin C), prevention of UTI, 21
Asterixis, in liver disease, 264
Atenolol, indications for, 109
Autograft, in burn patients, 160

B

Bacterial meningitis, 167–177
    age and gender, 171
    medications, 174–175
    precautions required, 175–176
Banding procedure, for esophageal varices, 271–272
Barium swallow, in achalasia, 2
Benign prostatic hypertrophy (BPH), 235–247
    clinical manifestations, 237–238, *239*
    potential complications, 242
    TURP for, 244–247
Bipolar disorder, 209–217
Blood pressure
    classifications in adults, *77*
    systolic and diastolic readings, 75–76
Body weight
    achalasia and, 8
    reduction for hypertension, 81–82
Borrelia burgdorferi, 119–120, 122
Breathing pattern, with hemothorax, 45
Broca's area, stroke and, 185–186
Bronchitis, 51–69
    causes, pathophysiology, and symptoms, 55
    other symptoms, 54–55

Bruit, over thyroid gland, 203
B-type natriuretic peptide assay (BNP), bronchitis and
    pneumonia, 52
Burdzinski's sign, in meningitis, 170–171
Burn injury, 151–163. *see also* specific type
    contracture with, 160
    decrease of scarring, 162
    description of each degree of injury, 156–157, *158*
    edema in, 157
    EMT first aid interventions, 154–155
    environmental temperature control for client, 161
    fluid replacement, 159
    psychological reactions, 161
    Rule of Nines, 155, *155*
    skin grafts, 160
    splint use, 161–162

C

Caffeine, risk factor for hypertension, 78, 81
Caregiver issues
    bipolar disorder, 216
    spinal cord injury, 135–136
Ceftriaxone sodium
    treatment of CAP, 64–65
    use in bacterial meningitis, 174
Cellulitis, 141–149
    definition and clinical manifestations, 143
Centers for Disease Control and Prevention (CDC), HSV
    infection report, 227, 233
Cerebral cortex, *186*
Cervical cancer, HPV infection and, 251–254
Cervical dysplasia, 249–258
Cervical epithelial neoplasia I (CIN I), 254
Chemical burns, 154
Chest drainage system, hemothorax, 46, *46–47*
Chest pain, symptom of achalasia, 8
Chest tube, for hemothorax, 45, 47
Chlamydia, swab culture for testing, 228
Chlamydia trachomatis, 228
Cholecystitis, 85–99
    clinical manifestations, 88
    pathology of, 87–88
Cholesterol, 79
Chronic lymphocytic leukemia (CLL), 85–99
    clinical manifestations, 91
    etiology and prognosis, 92
    incidence and greatest risks, 91
    pathophysiology of, 90
    stages, 91–92
    treatment options, 92–93
    ways to reduce risk of infection, 93–94
Chronic obstructive pulmonary disease (COPD),
    57, 66
Chronic renal failure, 25–36
Cirrhosis, pathophysiology, clinical manifestations, *266*

Clopidogrel bisulfate, actions, 146–147
Colposcopy, use in HPV, 250, 252–253
Communication, client and nurse, 42–49
Community-acquired pneumonia (CAP), 56–57
Comprehensive metabolic panel (CMP)
    for acute pyelonephritis, 16
    bronchitis and pneumonia, 52
Computed tomography (CT)
    meningitis, 168, 172
    stroke, 180
Cone biopsy, for CIN I, 254
Continuous ambulatory peritoneal dialysis (CAPD),
    25–36, 30
Continuous bladder irrigation, purpose in BPH, 245–246
Contracture, in burn injury patient, 160
Cranberry juice, prevention of UTI, 21, 22
Cystography, diagnosis of BPH, 236, 240
Cystoscope, 241

D

Deer tick, 120
Depression, risk with life-threatening illness, 94–97
Dexamethasone, use in bacterial meningitis, 174
Dextromethorphan, cough medicine, 66
Dextrose (D50), intravenous, for hypoglycemia, 213–214
Diabetes, 27–28, 209–217
    proper foot care, 145–146
    type 1 and 2, 144–145
    use of aquathermia pad, 147–149
Diet. see Nutrition
Dietary Approaches to Stop Hypertension (DASH), 73–84
Disease-modifying antirheumatic drugs (DMARD), 110
Do-not-resuscitate (DNR) order, 189–190
Doxazosin mesylate, treatment of BPH, 243
Doxycycline, for Lyme disease, 122–123
Drug abuse, diabetes and, 212–213
Durable power of attorney, 189–190
Dysphagia, symptom of achalasia, 8

E

Edema, burn injury patient, 157
Electrical burns, 154
Electrocardiography (ECG, EKG)
    bronchitis and pneumonia, 52
    meningitis, 168
Endocrine system, 200
Endoscopy, in achalasia, 2
End-stage renal failure, 25–36
Enoxaparin, use in stroke patient, 191
Enterobacter, HAP infection, 57
Erectile dysfunction, after TURP, 247
Erythema migrans, Lyme disease, 121
Erythromycin, treatment of CAP, 64
Escherichia coli (E.coli), acute pyelonephritis, 16–18
Esophageal dilation procedure, for achalasia, 9–10
Esophageal manometry, in achalasia, 2
Esophageal varices
    future hemorrhage risk, 272
    with hepatic encephalopathy, 271–272
Esophagomyotomy, for achalasia, 9–11
Essential hypertension, 76
Ethnicity, risk factor for hypertension, 78
Exercise
    diabetes and, 212–213
    reduction for hypertension, 82
Exophthalmos, Graves' disease, 200–201, 201
Expressive aphasia, stroke patient, 183

F

Fall injuries, renal failure patients, 33
Family dynamic
    bipolar disorder and, 216
    in life-threatening illness, 96–97
Family history, risk factor for hypertension, 78
Fear, in life-threatening illness, 94–95
Fever, symptom of acute pyelonephritis, 17–18
Finasteride, treatment of BPH, 242–243
Fish oil, for RA, 112
Flaxseed oil, for RA, 112
Foley catheter, 245
Folic acid, for RA, 104, 110–111
Foot care, diabetic patients, 145–146
Free tetraiodothyronine. see Thyroxine (T₄)
Full code, definition, 186–187
Furosemide, indications for, 109

G

Gallbladder. see Cholecystitis
Gastroesophageal reflux disease (GERD), 6, 10
Gender, risk factor for hypertension, 78
Genital herpes virus (HSV)
    clinical manifestations, 227–228
    development of vaccine, 233
    future outbreaks, 232–233
    HIV testing and, 230–231
    hygiene during treatment, 229
    medication mechanism of action, 229
    psychological consequences, 230
    sexual activity with, 229
    visual examination, 227
Glipizide, client education, 146
Glomerular filtration rate, 27–29
Goiter, Graves' disease, 205
Gonorrhea, swab culture for testing, 228
Graves' disease
    exophthalmos, 200–201, 201
    goiter, 205

H

Halitosis, achalasia and, 8
Health care proxy, 189–190
Health Insurance Portability and Accountability Act of 1996
    (HIPAA), 43
Hemiplegia, after stroke, 184–185
Hemodialysis, versus peritoneal dialysis, 31
Hemorrhagic infarction, 182–183
Hemothorax, 39–50
Hepatic encephalopathy, 261–273
    cirrhosis relations, 264
    clinical manifestations, 265–266, 266
Herpevac Trial for Women, 233
Heterograft (xenograft), in burn patients, 160
Hill-Burton Act (Title VI), 43
Hospital-acquired pneumonia (HAP), 56–57
Human immunodeficiency virus (HIV), testing, 230–231
Human papillomavirus-16 (HPV-16), 249–258
    clinical manifestations and cancer relationship, 251
    partner notification, 255–256
    vaccine (Gardasil), 256–257
Hydrochlorothiazide
    adverse effects, 79–80
    for hypertension, 79
Hydrocodone/acetaminophen, for Lyme disease,
    122–123

Hypercholesterolemia/dyslipidemia, risk factor for hypertension, 78
Hyperkalemia, in chronic renal failure, 28
Hyperphosphatemia, renal failure and, 32
Hypertension, 73–84
    follow-up, 83
    primary and secondary, 76–77
    risk factors, 78–79
    symptoms, 77
Hyperthyroidism
    clinical manifestations, 200–201
    lump or goiter, 204–205, *205*
Hypoglycemia
    clinical manifestations, 212
    definition, 211–212
    hypothermia and, 213
Hypothermia, hypoglycemia and, 213
Hypothyroidism
    after RAI therapy, 206–207
    clinical manifestations, 200–201
Hypoxemia, 64

I
Idiopathic hypertension, 76
Incentive spirometer (IS), 52, *61*, 61–62, 65
    use in spinal cord injury, 134
Infection
    with CLL, 93
    with hemothorax, 45
Influenza vaccine, 149
Inhalation burns, 154
    assessment, 156
Intravenous pyelography (IVP)
    acute pyelonephritis, 16, 19
    diagnosis of BPH, 241
Ischemic infarction, 182–183

J
Joints of the hand, *106*

K
Kernig's sign, in meningitis, 170–171
Ketorolac tromethamine, use for acute pyelonephritis, 19–20
Klebsiella pneumonia, 57

L
Laboratory tests
    achalasia, antinuclear antibody (ANA) test, 2–3
    acute pyelonephritis
        CBC with diff, 16
        urinalysis (U/A C&S). 16
    benign prostatic hyperplasia (BPH)
        CBC, 236, 240
        creatinine, 236, 240
        prostate-specific antigen (PSA), 236, 240
        serum blood urea nitrogen (BUN), 236, 240
        urinalysis (U/A C&S), 236, 240
    bronchitis and pneumonia
        CBC, 52
        significance, 62–63
    cholecystitis, CBC and CMP, 86
    chronic renal failure
        blood urea nitrogen, 28
    hepatic encephalopathy
        blood urea nitrogen (BUN), 262

        CBC, 262, 266268
        comprehensive metabolic panel (CMP), 262
        liver function tests, 262
    Lyme disease
        ELISA, 118, 122
        immunoglobulin M and G Western blot test, 118
    meningitis
        basic metabolic panel (BMP), 168
        CBC, 168
        urinalysis, 168
        urine culture and sensitivity, 168
    rheumatoid arthritis
        antinuclear antibody (ANA) test, 104, 108
        C-reactive protein test, 104, 108
        erythrocyte sedimentation rate (ESR), 104, 108
        rheumatoid, 104, 108
    STDs
        dipstick urine, 225–226, *226*
        urinalysis, (U/A C&S), 225–226
    thyroid disease
        thyroid stimulating hormone (TSH) 198, 203–204
        thyroxine or T_4, 198, 203–204
Lactulose, for hepatic encephalopathy, 270
Language barrier, client and nurse, 42–49
Laparoscopic cholecystectomy, 89
Leukemia, 85–99
    types, 90
Leukocytosis, 89
Levofloxacin
    for cellulitis, 142
    use for acute pyelonephritis, 19–20
Levothyroxine sodium, for hypothyroidism, 206–207
Lifestyle changes
    after CAP, 67
    genital herpes, 231
    peritoneal dialysis, 35
    reduction of hypertension, 80–81
Lithium, toxicity, 213
Lumbar puncture, meningitis, 168, 172–174
Lycopene, treatment of BPH, 243
Lyme disease, 117–126
    client and family education, 124–125
    deer tick, *120*
    definition, 119
    Erythema migrans, *121*
    transmission and incubation period, 119–121

M
Malaise, in acute pyelonephritis, 19
Mantoux test, 58–61, *60*
Marijuana use, diabetes and, 212–213
Medical interpreter, 42–43
Meningitis, 167–177
    causes and pathophysiologic changes in brain, 169–170
    hearing loss, 174
    isolation, 171
    precautions, 171–172
    serum drug screening in, 174
Methotrexate, for RA, 104, 110
Metoclopramide, after esophagomyotomy, 10–11
Monoamine oxidase (MAO) inhibitors, hypoglycemia and, 213
Morphine sulfate, use in bacterial meningitis, 175
Mycobacterium tuberculosis, 58–61

N

Nasogastric tube, use in burn injury patients, 156
National Kidney Foundation, five-stage classification system
    for CKD, 28–29, 29
Nausea/vomiting, in acute pyelonephritis, 19
Neisseria gonorrhoeae, 228
Neisseria meningitidis, 174
Neomycin sulfate, for hepatic encephalopathy, 270
Nonsteroidal anti-inflammatory drugs (NSAIDS),
    for RA, 104
NovoLog insulin, sliding scale, 146
Nutrition
    achalasia and, 8
    healing of pressure ulcer, 132
    hyperthyroidism, 202
    low protein diet for hepatic encephalopathy, 271
    renal failure diet, 32–33
    risk factor for hypertension, 79

O

Obesity, risk factor for hypertension, 78
Occupational therapy, for RA, 111, *111*
Ondansetron hydrochloride, use for acute pyelonephritis,
    19–20
Oxygen, treatment of CAP, 64

P

Pap smear, 250, 255
Paraplegia, 129–130
Parkland Formula, fluid replacement in burn
    patients, 159
Percutaneous endoscopic gastrostomy (PEG), use in stroke
    patient, 190–191
Periorbital edema, with hyperthyroidism, 203
Peritonitis, complication of peritoneal dialysis, 34–35
Phlebitis, IV access site, 216
Physical therapy (PT), for RA, 111
Pneumococcal vaccine, 149
Pneumonia, 51–69
    other symptoms, 54–55
    pathophysiology and causes, 56
    risk factors, 57–58
Prazosin hydrochloride, treatment of BPH, 243
Prehypertension, 76–77
Pressure ulcer, with spinal cord injury, 130–133
Progressive systemic sclerosis (PSS), 5–6
Prostate, function, 237, *239*
Pseudomonas aeruginosa, HAP infection, 57
Pyelonephritis, acute, 15–23

Q

Quality of life
    in life-threatening illness, 95–96
    Lyme disease, 123–124

R

Radiation burns, 154
RAI therapy
    for hyperthyroidism, 205–206
    laboratory tests before treatment, 206
    potential adverse effects, 206
RAI uptake test, in suspected hyperthyroidism, 204
Regurgitation, symptom of achalasia, 8
Respiratory symptoms, achalasia and, 8
Respiratory syncytial virus (RSV), 57
Rheumatoid arthritis (RA), 103–115
    client education, 113–114

    clinical manifestations, 105–106
    incidence and predisposing factors, 106–107
    laboratory tests, 104–108–109
    pathophysiology, 107–108
    symptoms and course of disease, 113
Rib fractures, 39–50
Rule of Nines, 155, *155*

S

Salicylates, hypoglycemia and, 213
Saw palmetto, treatment of BPH, 243
Scleroderma, 5–6
Sequential compression devices (SCDs), for BPH, 246
Serum drug screen, in meningitis patient, 174
Seventh Report of the Joint National Committee
    on Prevention, Detection, Evaluation, and
    Treatment of High Blood Pressure (JNV VII),
    73–84
Sexually transmitted disease (STD), 221–234, 249–258
Skin grafts, burn patients, 160
Sodium intake, reduction of hypertension, 81
Spinal column, lateral and posterior views, *131*
Spinal cord injury, 127–137
    caregiver issues, 135–136
    incidence and risk, 129
    physiological issues, 133
    resource organizations, 136–137
    sexuality concerns, 134–135
    spasticity, 133–134
Splint, in burn patients, 161–162
Staphylococcus aureus, HAP infection, 57
Streptococcus pneumoniae, 174–175
Stroke, 180–193
    clinical manifestations, 183–184
    culture and religion role in, 191–193
    deficits after, 184
    expressive aphasia, 183
    hemiplegia after, 184–185
    hemisphere affected, 186
    pathophysiology, 182–183
    risk factors, 183
Sulfonamides, hypoglycemia and, 213
Swallowing difficulty, symptom of achalasia, 8
Synthetic skin graft, in burn patients, 160

T

Tamsulosin hydrochloride, treatment of BPH, 243
Terazosin, treatment of BPH, 243
Tetanus toxoid, use in burn injury patients, 156
Tetraplegia (quadriplegia), 129–130
Thermal burns, 153–154
Thyroid disease, 197–207
Thyroid gland
    anatomy, hormone production, and function,
    199–200
    bruit, 203
Thyrotropin releasing hormone (TRH), 199
Thyroxine (T_4), 198, 199, 204
Tissue plasminogen activator (tPA), 187
    clinical indications and contraindications,
    188–189
Tramadol hydrochloride, for cellulitis, 142
Transient ischemic attack (TIA), 182–183
Transurethral resection of the prostate (TURP)
    sexual dysfunction after, 247
    for symptomatic BPH, 244–247
Triiodothyronine (T_3), 199, 204
Tuberculosis, 58–59

U

Ultrasonography
    abdominal, hepatic encephalopathy, 262
    bladder, diagnosis of BPH, 236, 240
    gallbladder, 86
Uncertainty, in life-threatening illness, 95
Urinary catheter
    diagnosis of BPH, 241
    use in burn injury patients, 156
Urinary tract infection (UTI)
    health promotion behaviors for prevention,
        21–22
    relation to acute pyelonephritis, 16–19
Urine specimen, clean-catch, 222–223,
    225
Urodynamics, diagnosis of BPH, 241

V

Valacyclovir hydrochloride, for genital herpes, 229
Valsartan, indications for, 109
Viral meningitis, 167–177
Viral pneumonia, 56–57
Voiding changes, symptom of acute pyelonephritis, 17–18

W

Water seal, chest drainage system, 46, *46–47*
Wernicke's area, stroke and, 185–186

X

X-ray
    chest, bronchitis and pneumonia, 52, 58
    kidney, ureter, bladder, for acute pyelonephritis, 16, 19

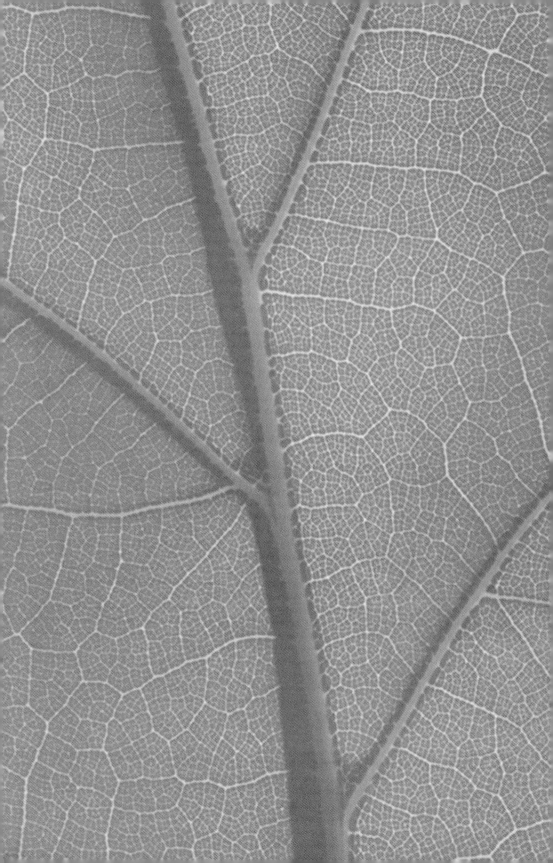